Herbs and Spices - New Advances

Edited by Eva Ivanišová

Published in London, United Kingdom

Herbs and Spices - New Advances
http://dx.doi.org/10.5772/intechopen.104270
Edited by Eva Ivanišová

Contributors
Archana A. Yelmate, Sanjay S. Thonte, Kranti L. Satpute, Pakiso Moses Makhoahle, Seema Bisht, Acharya Balkrishna, Bhaskar Joshi, Anupam Srivastava, Vijaya Sadashiv Rabade, Ashwini Ingole, Purushottam Gangane, Vidya Sabale, Ujwala Mahajan, Yash Narendra Kale, Madonna Ngwatshipane Mashabela, Peter Tshepiso Ndhlovu, Wilfred Otang Mbeng, Mojtaba Afshari Babazad, Hamed Zandavar, Dharini Chittaragi, Jalaja S. Menon, Jacqueline Naalamle Amissah, Frank Opoku-Agyemang, Jessica Naa Offeibea Dodoo, Kathleen Gilday, Theophilus Elorm Hlomador, Anka Trajkovska Petkoska, Anita Trajkovska-Broach, Nguyen Trung Thanh, Le Thi Thanh Huong, Nguyen Phu Hung, Do Van Hai, Hosakatte Niranjana Murthy, Boris Nemzer, Diganta Kalita, Marizvikuru Mwale, Wiseman Ndlovu, Nyambeni Ronald Mudimeli, Ola Segun Obadire, Joseph Francis, Tshianeo Mellda Ndou, Eva Ivanišová, Judita Lidiková, Natália Čeryová, Tomáš Tóth, Janette Musilová, Alena Vollmannová, Kushvara Mammadova

First published in London, United Kingdom, 2023 by IntechOpen
IntechOpen is the global imprint of INTECHOPEN LIMITED, registered in England and Wales, registration number: 11086078, 5 Princes Gate Court, London, SW7 2QJ, United Kingdom

British Library Cataloguing-in-Publication Data
A catalogue record for this book is available from the British Library

Additional hard and PDF copies can be obtained from orders@intechopen.com

Herbs and Spices - New Advances
Edited by Eva Ivanišová
p. cm.
Print ISBN 978-1-83768-474-8
Online ISBN 978-1-83768-475-5
eBook (PDF) ISBN 978-1-83768-476-2

For EU product safety concerns:
IN TECH d.o.o., Prolaz Marije Krucifikse Kozulić 3, 51000 Rijeka, Croatia,
info@intechopen.com or visit our website at intechopen.com.

Meet the editor

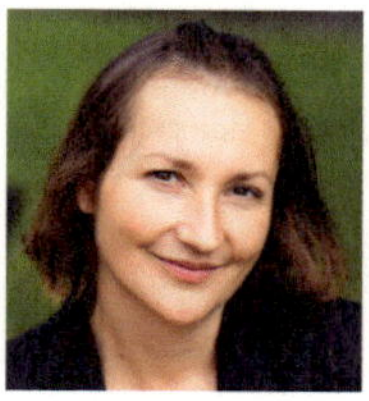

Ing. Eva Ivanišová, Ph.D., is an assistant professor at the Institute of Food Sciences, Faculty of Biotechnology and Food Sciences, Slovak University of Agriculture, and head of the Laboratory of Fats and Oils of the AgroBioTech Research Centre. Her field of study is food technology, particularly plant raw materials and foodstuffs, foods enriched with medicinal plants, lesser-known types of fruits and vegetables, and alternative food sources such as edible insects and flowers. She has published more than 480 scientific works in international and domestic journals, for which she has received more than 635 citations in indexed databases.

Contents

Preface

"The doctor cures, nature heals"

-Hippocrates.

Nowadays, most people want to be healthy and strong, but modern hectic lifestyles can lead to diseases and health problems. For many, synthetic drugs are the most common treatment for illnesses, but their side effects can sometimes be dangerous. Alternative methods of treatment can be much safer, and more and more people are looking for effective and time-proven natural remedies.

Medicinal plants have an incredible history of serving humanity on almost every continent of the world. They are one of the basic sources of nutrition in terms of their content, and their use in medicine has been known since the beginning of civilization. Industrialization and busy lifestyles produce free radicals, which can cause disease and other adverse health effects. Plants used in traditional medicine contain a large number of antioxidants, such as polyphenols, carotenoids, tocopherols, glutathione, ascorbic acid, and enzymes with antioxidant activity, which help the body fight against dangerous oxidative damage. There are around 4,000 medicinal species known in Europe, 500 of which are medicinal plants. Currently, there is a trend of using medicinal plants not only in traditional medicine but also in the food, pharmaceutical, and cosmetic industries as well as in modern gastronomy to increase the sensory and biological value of food via plant polyphenols. The most widespread form of administration is in the form of tea.

In medicine, plants find unlimited use for treating numerous diseases, such as diseases of the digestive, respiratory, and urinary systems, skin problems, and more. They also have a positive effect on substance metabolism and are characterized by excellent detoxification, anti-inflammatory and antibacterial properties, and several other therapeutic effects. Due to their antioxidant and antimicrobial effects, medicinal plants can also be used in preserving food and increasing food's biological value.

Spices are all the aromatic parts of plants used to flavor food. These parts can be fresh, dried, or otherwise prepared. Spices are included in the group of snacks that have a negligible caloric value but have stimulating effects either directly on the digestive system or indirectly on the nervous system. They serve to aromatize and enhance the taste and smell of food. Spices are valued not only because they add taste and aroma to food but also because they have antioxidant effects. They are antioxidant substances that extend the shelf life of food by protecting it from oxidation, which causes undesirable sensory changes in food. In recent years, several beneficial physiological effects of spices on the human body have been experimentally documented. These are mainly beneficial antioxidant and hypolipidemic effects on the human body.

This book gives an overview of medicinal plants and spices used in different parts of the world in folk medicine, pharmacy, food industry, gastronomy, and agriculture. It provides interesting information on the nutritional, therapeutic, antioxidant, and antimicrobial effects of medicinal herbs and spices, discusses their bioaccessibility and bioavailability as well as their risks and benefits, and presents research on the use of spices as nutraceuticals and in ethnoveterinary practices.

This book is a useful resource for researchers, students, and readers interested in nature and who believe that plants can be used to improve health as well as agriculture, foods, medicines, cosmetics, and veterinary practice.

Eva Ivanišová
Institute of Food Sciences,
Slovak University of Agriculture in Nitra,
Nitra, Slovak Republic

Section 1

Spices

Chapter 1

Bio-Colours From Spices

Dharini Chittaragi and Jalaja S. Menon

Abstract

Colour is an important aspect influencing every moment of our life. It may be the clothes we wear, furnishings of our home, religious ceremonies and even the food we relish. Colour is a molecule that absorbs certain wavelengths of visible light and transmits or reflects others. There are four different types of colours viz., natural colours, nature identical colours, synthetic colours and inorganic colours. Bio-colour is a dye or pigment of biological origin (plants, insects, animals or microbes) that imparts colour when applied to food, drug, textiles or cosmetics. Bio-colours are classified into five groups viz., anthocyanin, betalain, carotenoid, chlorophyll and caramel. Spices are generally used for seasoning and flavouring. Some spices can also be used as bio-colourants. The common spices used as colourants are turmeric (curcumin), paprika (capsanthin), saffron (crocin), tamarind (leucoanthocyanidine) and kokum (anthocyanin). Use of colour is regulated by laws, such as U.S. Food and Drug Act (1960) and Food Drug and Cosmetic Act (1938). Although bio-colourants have potential benefits, the tedious extraction procedures, low colour value and instability during processing hinder their popularity. More detailed studies on the production and stability of bio-colours are necessary for their promotion in various sectors.

Keywords: natural colours, spice extracts, permissible limit, FDA, health concern

1. Introduction

Colouring is an important aspect of our lives for many decades. It may be the clothes we wear, furnishings of our home, religious ceremonies and even the food we relish. The various evidence related to synthetic colours usage showed harmful effects over the years, now a day's need of consumers is shifting towards bio-colours. There is an emerging trend for the use of bio-colours as they are available naturally and are non-renewable [1].

A recent survey conducted in northern Kerala revealed excessive use of synthetic colours in sugar-based confections, posing a serious health risk, especially for children. Out of the 14 samples collected from different locations showed 97 per cent of non-permitted colours. On analysis about 82 per cent showed the higher level of permitted colours than the required limit (more than 100 ppm) [2].

Colour is a molecule that absorbs certain wavelengths of visible light and transmits or reflects others [3]. It will correct the natural variations in colour and enhance the colours that occur naturally. It is added mainly to maintain or improve the safety and freshness of the food material. It will also improve taste, texture, appearance and thereby its nutritional value [4].

Colours are mainly classified into four different types *viz.*, **Natural colours** are pigments obtained from living organisms such as caramel, anthocyanin, betaline. **Nature - identical colours** are man-made pigments which are also found in nature - *e.g.* Carotene. **Synthetic colours** are man-made colours that are not found in nature, these are often azo-dyes and Allura red and **Inorganic colours** are non-edible which are used in paints and plastics [5].

2. Bio colours

Any dye or pigment, of biological origin (plants, insects, animals or microbes) impart colour when applied to food, drug, textiles or cosmetics. Bio means natural and colouring means anything used for colouring purposes [6].

2.1 History

From time immemorial, colour has been an important criterion for the acceptability of products like textiles, cosmetics, food and other items.

- The earliest written record of the use of natural dyes was found in China dated 2600 BC.
- According to the reports, the product appearance was enhanced by the addition of natural extracts and wine by Egyptian candy makers during 1500 BC.
- During the Indus Vedic period (2500 BC) the dyeing was known in the Indian subcontinent and later it has been replaced with the new coloured cloth garments including the Mohenjo-Daro and Harappa civilization (3500 BC) madder dye.
- The cochineal dye was used by the people of Aztec and Maya culture periods of Central and North America.
- Saffron is mentioned in the Bible.
- Use of natural bio-colourants in food is known from Japan in the Shosoin text of the Nara period (Eighth century), which contains references regarding colouring soybean and adzuki-bean cakes.

2.2 The need for bio-colourants

- They are stable in their nature during different process.
- They maintain their character during uneven climatic conditions.
- They will enhance the product colour and retains its quality.
- They reduce the vitamin loss and maintains the original flavour.
- Their addition will meet the people demand and is considered as a consumable food.

Bio-colours can be classified into three main classes [7].

1. Anthocyanin

2. Betalain

3. Carotenoids

4. Chlorophyll

5. Caramel

Anthocyanins, a group of water-soluble pigments, impart red to blue colours (250–650 nm). Betalains yield betacyanin (red) and betaxanthin (yellow) pigments. Carotenoid groups are responsible for the yellow and orange pigments (250–650 nm). Chlorophylls are found in two forms: chlorophyll a (blue-green) and b (yellow-green). Caramel is obtained by heating carbohydrates, which imparts a brown colour.

2.3 Insects

The bodies of some scale insects produce carminic acid- a red/purple colour called Cochineal (*Dactylopius coccus*). They consume cactus leaves as their food and their bodies are allowed to dry and crushed to get the red colour. These are mainly used in Africa, Spain and Central America.

2.4 Microbes

Microbes like *Monococous* sp. (Carotenoids) *Dunaliella salina* and *Blakeslea trispora* (β-carotene) *Arthrospira platensis* (*spirulina* bacteria) produce certain bio-colours. Phycobiliproteins, algae belonging to Rhodophyta and Chlorophyta produces red and blue colours.

2.5 Animals

Sea fishes (*Hexaplex trunculus*) produces purple colour from its shell due to the presence of bromine. It is mainly used in the fabrics and textile industries.

2.6 Advantages of bio-colours

Bio-colourants are gaining importance because of health, hygiene, nutrition, pharmaceutical activities, fashion and environmental consciousness. Some of the advantages of using bio-colours are:

- They are protective in their action thereby prevents from cell degradation.

- They are having anti-microbial properties and thereby increase the shelf life.

- They will enhance the nutritional quality of the food as they are rich sources of carbohydrates, minerals and vitamins.

- They will strengthen the human immune system as they have free radical scavenging properties.
- They are non - carcinogenic and safe.

3. Spices as colourants

The spices are the food additives that are mainly added to impart flavour. Besides, they can also be used as a colouring agent due to the presence of several chemical compounds, the principal compound responsible for the colour are the carotenoids, such as beta carotene, lutein, and neoxanthin [8].

The most common spices used for colouring are turmeric, red pepper, saffron, kokum and tamarind. Other compounds that provide these colouring properties to spices are flavonoids with yellow colours – curcumin and chlorophyll with green (**Table 1**). Spices provide strong colour pigments commonly between orange, yellow, and red, this can be advantageous since spices can be used as natural colourants especially for food. Using spices as colourants in food is a natural alternative that avoids the use of conventional synthetic colourants.

3.1 Turmeric

Curcuma longa L. belongs to the family Zingiberaceae. It is mainly used as a food additive, preservative and colouring agent. The economic part is a rhizome that yields a phenolic compound Curcumin (3–4%). Some of the varieties rich in Curcumin are CIM-Pitamber (12.1%), Suroma (9.3%), Rajendra Sonia (8.1%), Varna (7.8%) and cultivars such as Wayanad Local (9.5%) and Duggirala (7.5%) [15].

3.2 Properties of curcumin

- Orange-yellow crystalline powder
- Stable at high temperatures and in acids, but unstable in alkaline conditions

Crop	Part used	Pigment	Colour shade	Applications	Reference
Turmeric	Rhizome	Curcumin	Yellow	Food colourant	[9]
Chilli	Pericarp	Capsanthin	Red	Culinary preparation	[10]
Saffron	Stigma	Crocin	Yellow-Orange	Colourant in sweet preparations	[11]
Tamarind	Pulp Seed	Leucoanthocynidine Tannin	Red Brown	Textiles Dye	[12]
Kokum	Rind	Anthocyanin	Red	Beverages, textiles	[13]
Fenugreek	Seed	Carotenoid	Yellow	Dye	[9]
Sea fennel	Leaves	Phycocyanin	Green	Colourant in food	[14]

Table 1.
Spice bio-colours and their applications.

- Light-sensitive in nature
- First isolated by Roughley and Whiting [16]
- Structure of curcumin ($C_{21}H_{20}O_6$)
- Melting point: 176–177°C
- Hydrophobic in nature- Soluble in ethanol, alkali, ketone and chloroform
- Absorption maxima: 420 nm

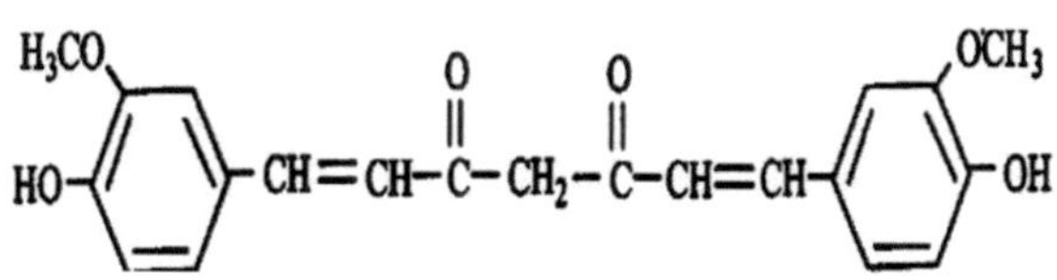

3.3 Extraction of curcumin

Curcumin is extracted from the dried root of the rhizome *C. longa*. For extraction, the raw materials are crushed to make into powder form and are treated with a specific solvent to obtain the required coloured compound. After distillation, the obtained product called as oleoresin is a mixture of volatile oils along with other extracts produces about 25–35 per cent coloured compound. The oleoresins are then subjected to further washes using selective solvents that can extract the curcumin pigment from it. This process yields a purified food colour which is known as Curcumin. It contains 90 per cent colouring matter and very little volatile oil and other dry matter. The extractability and regulatory criteria depend on the selection of solvent [17].

3.4 Chilli

Capsicum annuum is one of the major spices used as a natural flavouring and colouring agent. Its extract contains carotenoid pigment Capsanthin which has a major role in the food industry. Paprika oleoresin is manufactured by solvent extraction of the dried capsicum pods. One kg of pods yields 90 to 120 g of extract. Varieties and cultivars rich in capsanthin: KTPL - 19 (233.70 ASTA), Bydagi chilli (159.9 ASTA), Kashmiri chilli (54.1 ASTA), Sanam S-4 (70.4 ASTA) [18].

3.5 Properties of Capsanthin

- Capsanthin is fat and lipid-soluble
- Capsanthin increases proportionally with advanced stages of ripeness
- It is more stable at neutral pH
- Colour saturation level: 100 mg/kg (ppm) colouring matter
- It is sensitive to heat.

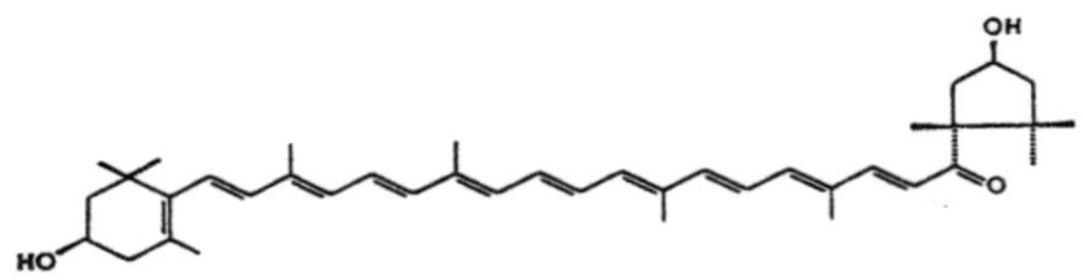

Saffron

Crocus sativus L., a perennial flowering plant and most expensive spice in the world. The economic part is the dried stigmas which are the source of a natural dye. It is mainly used as a colouring agent, for dyeing silk and fabric rugs, painting, cooking and as medicine. The Colouring principle: Crocin (4–6%) isolated in the crystalline state by Karrer et al. [19].

Properties of Crocin

- Crocin: Soluble in hot water, giving an orange-coloured solution
- Sparingly soluble in absolute alcohol, ether and other organic solvents
- Golden yellow pigment
- Absorption spectrum: 435 nm [20]

Cultivars of saffron

- Kashmiri saffron: Famous for its thin and longer stigma throughout the world.
- Spanish saffron: Highest Crocin content with thicker stigma.

Extraction technique

- Saffron Stigma (10 g) were suspended in 80% ethanol at 0°C and extracted for 2 minutes
- Centrifugation at 4000 rpm for 10 min and the supernatant was separated
- 25 ml of 80% ethanol to the sediment and the extraction is repeated
- Crystal storage: thick-walled glass container at –5°C for 24 days in darkness
- Obtained crystals were separated from solution washed with acetone
- Dissolved in 120 mL ethanol 80% at –5°C in darkness for 20 extra days for re-crystallisation which yields 1.2 g of crystals [21].

Kokum

Garcinia indica well-known tropical fruit, widely used in South Indian and Konkan delicacies for imparting colour and flavour. The economic part is the dried outer cover of fruit which contain a very high concentration of anthocyanins (2.4/100 g of kokum fruit).

Properties

- The red colour in Kokum is due to the presence of anthocyanin
- The colouring compound is cyanidin 3-glucoside ($C_{21}H_{21}O_{11}$; MW: 449.38 g)
- Bright red colour at a pH of 2 to 3
- Stable at high temperature and water-soluble

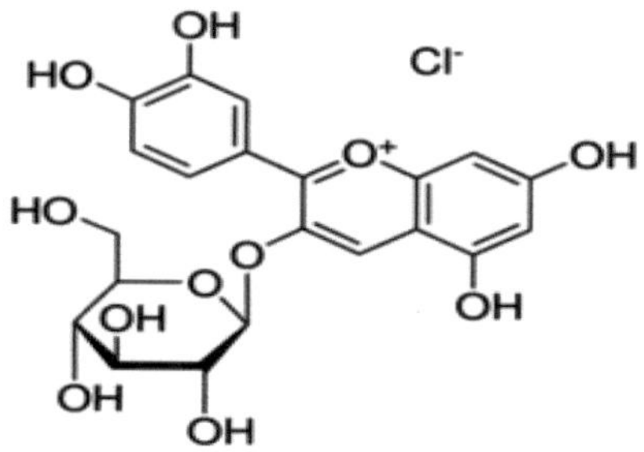

Extraction of anthocyanin

- The fruit pulp is extracted by manual method.
- It is mixed in a 1:2 ratio with acidified water (0.1% hydrochloric acid).
- Then the mixture was subjected to a hydraulic press.
- The extract was filtered using a muslin cloth and stored in a cold room at 4–5°C.

Tamarind

Tamarind is one of the most important multipurpose trees which is grown in farmland and also occurs naturally in the forests. The red tamarind is a rare mutant and its availability is not well known. The red tamarind fruit contains rosy red pigments. The red colour is due to the presence of water soluble red-rose anthocyanin pigment.

Extraction of Leucoanthocyanidine

- It involves maceration and refrigerated storge of the prematured fruit whole night in a solution of acidified methanol (0.01% HCl in methanol) [22–24].
- The process is continued to obtain the end point with least colour and the filtrates were added together.
- The product was subjected to rotary evaporator to remove the solvent at 40°C under vacuum.
- Finally purify the product to obtain the pigment [12].

4. Sea fennel as a new spice-colourant

The sea fennel (*Crithmum maritimum* L.) belongs to the family Apiaceae of grows wild on maritime rocks, piers, sandy beaches along the Mediterranean sea. This is consumed as a traditional vegetable due its sensory traits like salty and similar tastes to celery, common fennel and peel of green citrus along with some pungency in many countries.

Bio-colours as health enhancers

Bio-colourants are prepared from renewable sources and the majority are of plant origin. In addition to food colouring, bio-colourants also act as anti-oxidant (chilli), anti-obesity (kokum), anti-carcinogenic (turmeric), anti-asthmatic (tamarind) and anti-depressant (saffron) and thereby prevent several diseases and disorders in human beings [25].

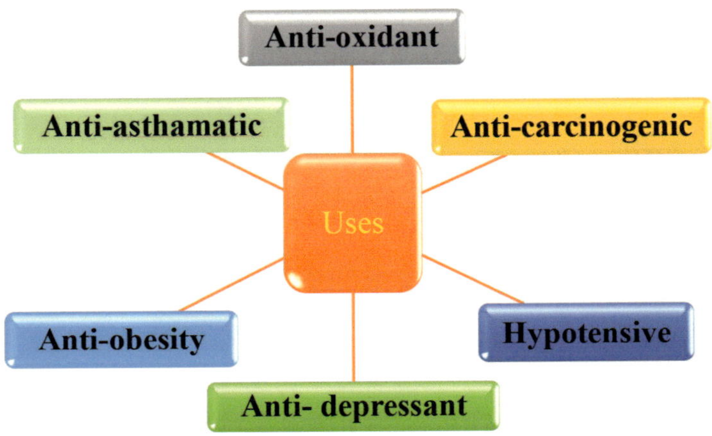

5. Food colour laws and regulations

The use of colour is regulated by some laws and regulations and will also provide information about its components. Some of them are:

- 1906 - US Food and Drug Act (FDA) - Prevents the use of misbranded colours.
- 1938 - Federal Food, Drug and Cosmetics Act - Inspection on the usage of colours in cosmetics and drugs.
- 1960 - FDA approved list of colours to be used in the food industry.
- 1990 - Nutrition Labelling and Education Act - This mainly regulates the labelling of food products and also their nutrient contents.
- 2006 - Regulation of colouring additive to food is mainly regulated by FSSAI in the case of exports.

5.1 Bio-colours approved by FDA

Natural biocolourants are exempt from the certification category of FDA, and European Union for food use and are annatto extract, beet, canthaxanthin, carotene, *Dactylopuis coccus* extract etc. (**Table 2**).

5.2 Market trend for bio-colours

The growth rate is going to be large for naturally derived colours with a predicted annual growth rate of 5–10%. The natural food colour reached the US 1 billion dollar in the market throughout the world. This trend is increasing day by day as natural colours are preferred by the consumers in the food related industries over the harmful synthetic colours (**Table 3**).

5.3 Applications of bio-colours

Drawbacks

Even though biocolours have several applications, but they also got certain limitations like sensitivity to low pH and heat sensitive, etc.

Lack of eyesight:

Food gives a great palatability only if it is consumed natural. But the natural colours are not that much attractive as compared to synthetic colours.

Lack of wide applications:

These are product specific in nature. Beet colour is only used in soda as it turns blue in milk. This also not suitable in the baking industry.

Lack of colour stability and fading:

These colours change its nature sometimes and are failed to maintain their originality.

Colour	EEC	Source	Year (approved)
Bixin, nor-Bixin	E160b	Annatto	1963
Capsanthin	E160c	Chilli	1966
Crocin	E164	Saffron	1966
Curcumin	E100	Turmeric	1966
Lutein	E161b	Marigold	1968
Lycopene	E160	Tomato	2006
Carmine	E120	Cochineal	2009

Table 2.
List of Bio-colours approved by FDA.

Name of the organisation	Product
Roche products Pvt. Ltd., Australia	Carotenoids
Synthetic industrial chemicals Ltd., India	Xanthophylls
Bush boake allen company, USA	Natural colours
Aarkay food products Ltd., Gujarat	Fruit and vegetable powders
Vinayak ingredients Pvt. Ltd., Mumbai	Natural colours
Synthite industries Ltd., kolenchery, Kerala	Lutein

Table 3.
Companies dealing with bio-colours.

Heat Sensitivity:

They are susceptible to heat and losses its main trait.

Higher price and lesser availability:

These are highly priced and are not easily available in the commercial market as that of other products.

6. Conclusion

The demand for natural colourants is high now a days. Spices are the one of the main ingredients in Indian food diet on daily basis. Pigments obtained from these spices are natural with health benefits and are seeking the attention of the consumers.

Although bio-colourants have potential benefits, the tedious extraction procedures, low colour value and instability during processing hinder their popularity. Encapsulation is one of the new technique to reserve the available natural pigments. Microencapsulation and nanoencapsulation are the methods to overcome the environmental drawbacks and increase its bioavailability. More detailed studies on the production and stability of bio-colours are necessary for their promotion in various sectors.

Author details

Dharini Chittaragi[1*] and Jalaja S. Menon[2]

1 Department of Spices and Plantation Crops, Tamil Nadu Agricultural University, Coimbatore, India

2 Department of Plantation Crops and Spices, Kerala Agricultural University, Thrissur, India

*Address all correspondence to: chitti.smile3@gmail.com

References

[1] Aberoumand A. A review article on edible pigments properties and sources as natural biocolorants in foodstuff and food industry. World Journal of Dairy & Food Sciences. 2011;**6**(1):71-78

[2] Nandakumar T. Synthetic food colours pose health risk - The Hindu, 31 Oct. 2015. 2015. p. 9

[3] FDA [Food and Drug Administration]. 1960. Colour additive ammendment. [on-line]. Available from: https://www.fda.gov/default.htm. [16 Dec. 2017]

[4] Naidu MM, Sowbhagya HB. Technological advances in food colours. Chemical Industry Digest. 2012:79-88

[5] Downham A, Collins P. Colouring our foods in the last and next millennium. International Journal of Food Science and Technology. 2000;**35**:5-22

[6] Pattnaik P, Roy U, Jain P. Biocolours: New generation additives for food. Indian Food Industry. 1997;**16**(5):21-32

[7] Sharma D. Understanding biocolour-A review. International Journal of Scientific and Technology Research. 2014;**3**(1):294-299

[8] Kadu P, Waghmare P, Patingrao D. Extraction, isolation, purification and identification of curcumin. European Journal of Biomedical and Pharmaceutical Sciences. 2015;**2**(3):108-123

[9] Selvam MR, Athinarayanana G, Nanthinib RUA, Singh AJA, Kalirajana KP, Selvakumard M. Extraction of natural dyes from *Curcuma longa, Trigonella foenum graecum* and *Nerium oleander* plants and their application in antimicrobial fabric. Industrial Crops and Products. 2015;**70**:84-90

[10] Arimboor R, Babu R, Menon NKR, Lekshmi P, Chandrasekhar, Moorkoth V. Red pepper (*Capsicum annuum*) carotenoids as a source of natural food colors: Analysis and stability - A review. Journal of Food Science and Technology. 2015;**52**(3):1258-1271

[11] Raja SM, Pareek PK, Shakyawar DB, Sarfaraz AW, Nehvi FA, Asif H. Extraction of natural dye from saffron flower waste and its application on pashmina fabric. Advances in Applied Science Research. 2012;**3**(1):156-161

[12] Mayavel A, Singh GB, Durai A, Murugeasan S. Evaluation of colour and stability of anthocyanin in red tamarind (*Tamarindus indica* L.). International Journal of Advanced Life Sciences. 2012;**5**(2):137-144

[13] Vasundhara M, Radhika B, Thara BS, Priyanka R, Jayaram A. Organic colours for ayurvastra from kokum fruits and rinds. Journal of Medicinal Plants Studies. 2016;**4**(6):104-107

[14] Rennan M, Gonnella M. The use of the sea fennel as a new spice-colorant in culinary preparations. International Journal of Gastronomy and Food Science. 2012;**1**:111-115

[15] Geethanjali A, Lalitha P, Firdhouse MJ. Analysis of curcumin content of turmeric samples from various states of India. International Journal of Pharma and Chemical Research. 2016;**2**(1):55-58

[16] Roughley PJ, Whiting DA. Whiting. Experiments in the biosynthesis of curcumin. Journal of the Chemical Society, Perkin Transactions. 1973;**1**:2379-2388

[17] Bagchi A. Extraction of curcumin. Journal of Environmental Science,

Toxicology and Food Technology. 2012;**1**(3):1-16

[18] Basavaraj M, Kumar PGP, Sathyanarayanareddy B, Jagadeesha RC. Effect of drying on colour degradation and rheology in red chilli cv BYADAGI. The Asian Journal of Horticulture. 2008;**3**(2):253-255

[19] Karrer P, Helfenstein A, Wehrli H, Wettstein A. Plant pigments. XXV. On the constitution of lycopene and carotene. Helvetica Chimica Acta, German. 1930;**13**:1084-1099

[20] Bolhassani A, Khavari A, Bathaie ZS. Saffron and natural carotenoids: Biochemical activities and anti-tumor effects. Biochimica et Biophysica Acta. 2014;**1845**:20-30

[21] Hadizadeh F, Mohajeri SA, Seifi M. Extraction and purification of crocin from saffron stigmas employing a simple and efficient crystallization method. Pakistan Journal of Biological Sciences. 2010;**13**(14):691-698

[22] Lenora LM, Sureshbabu D, Sumathi R, Mayavel A, Murugesan S, Senthilkumar N. Anthocyanin from red tamarind, vs rhodocarpa as a potential natural pigment for use in textile industry. International Journal of Recent Trends in Science and Technology. 2017;**23**(1):15-17

[23] Muringatheri M. Kerala Agricultural University identifies plants to make natural dyes - The Hindu, 12 May 2015. 2015. p. 8

[24] Parmar M, Phutela UG. Biocolours: The new generation additives. International Journal of Current Microbiology and Applied Sciences. 2015;**4**(7):688-694

[25] Vikram N, Kewat NR, Singh RP, Singh PR, Singh P. Natural edible colour and flavours used as human health (review article). International Journal of Pharmaceutical Sciences and Research. 2015;**6**(11):4622-4628

Chapter 2

An Insight on Nutraceutical Influences of Spice and Condiments: Serve as a Flavor and Immunity Enhancer from Ages

Acharya Balkrishna, Bhasker Joshi, Anupam Srivastava and Seema Bisht

Abstract

Spice is a dried aromatic or pungent plant substance such as root, stem, bark, leaves, bud, flower, fruit, seeds, etc., used as a flavor modifier in many culinary practices. A historical wisdom supports their use as an ingredient for flavoring the food and medicinal uses in various kind of healing systems. Spice and condiments not only enhance the sensory quality of food whereas they boost the immune system and give healthy nutrition which prevents the risk of chronic diseases. The ancient study also reveals that an adequate amount of daily intake of spices balances the three doshas (tridoshas) of the human body such as Vata, Pitta and Kapha. The imbalance of these doshas effect directly immune health and makes the body susceptible to disease. These plants have special chemical compounds which are responsible for their aromatic or pungent flavor and therapeutic actions. Due to the richness of phytochemicals, spice & condiments supports pharmaceutical, cosmetics, perfumery and several other industries world-widely.

Keywords: medicinal plants, nutraceutical, phyto-chemistry, traditional uses

1. Introduction

Since the ancient era humans and plants had a complex relationship in which humans always depended on forests for many reasons like clean air, food, water, nutrition, energy, fuel, clothing, and shelter. They have the biggest role in the survival and growth of all living organisms that exist on the planet. Our forests have been playing an important role in the economic development and medicinal health of humans. The world's vegetation is rich in many special plants with those dried parts such as roots, stems, bark, leaves, bud, flowers, fruit, seeds, etc., known for their special aroma and pungent flavors, which are called spices. Over the centuries, these dried parts come to use in many culinary practices for enhancing taste and flavor as well as preservative and coloring agents. Special chemical constituents are responsible for the aromatic and pungent properties of plants which not only enhance the taste of our food but also keep us away from many diseases. So, these parts have been used in many traditional healing systems for ages.

The history of spices is very long with their use in various ways during ancient times. Indian food is famous for its special taste, color, and aroma in the world which explains the diversity of spices and condiments in their land. Since the beginning of human history, all of India's spices have been strongly associated with its culture, traditions, preservation, and healing system. The maritime route called as spice route was developed in 3000 BCE before the silk route (land route), it was the biggest network that linked the east with the west. This route stretches from Japan's west coast through Indonesia's island, India to Middle Eastern lands to Europe through the Mediterranean. This spice route served as a bridge for religious and cultural contacts among many parts of the world. During ancient times spices were largely used for medicinal purposes than use in food preparation. At that time, India had become the center of the world's spice trade due to its top position in spice production. At present, India contributes 70% to the global production of spices and ranks first in the world among major spice-producing countries [1–3].

2. Ancient uses of spices & condiments

Since ancient spices were closely related to culture, and traditional activities for good health worldwide. The prestigious Hindus holy book 'Ramayana' and literature from the 1st century AD of the Roman Empire both make reference to the clove. In Ayurveda, small cardamom was known for its medicinal values which also mentions as '*ela*' in various Ayurvedic Sanskrit texts on medicine '*Charaka Samhita*', '*Sushruta Samhita*' and *Ashtanga Hridaya*. In 1555 BCE Ancient Egyptians recorded the use of coriander, fennel, juniper, cumin, garlic, and thyme. Garlic was also used for worship by ancient Egyptian and also have been found in the tomb of king Tutankhamen who ruled Egypt until 1338 BC. As early as 3000 BCE, the farmers of Mesopotamia cultivated garlic and it is also found that garlic was used in the treatment of intestinal disorders and for lowering blood cholesterol levels due to having fibrinolytic activity. Cardamom and cinnamon were used as spices in ancient Egypt. In the first century Greek physician, Pedanius Dioscorides published a plant monograph of 600 herbs which has a description of all the use of herbs for health benefits [1, 2, 4–7].

2.1 An insight on ayurvedic uses

Ayurveda is the ancient natural medical system that evolved more than 5000 years ago in the Himalayas. The ayurvedic healing system directly depends on three forces of energies known as *Doshas* such as *Vata* (air) -*Pitta* (fire) -*Kapha* (water). These three doshas are primary functional energies of the human body which are strongly related to five elements of nature such as Earth (Prithvi), Air (Vayu), Water (Jala), Fire (Teja), and Space (Aakash). The relationship between elements of nature with three doshas is *Vata Dosha*- a catabolic dosha formed by a combination of air and space (air is an active element in vatta and space acts as a regulatory element), *Pitta Dosha*- a metabolic dosha formed by a combination of fire and water (fire is an active element, and water helps to regulate or control fire), and Kapha- an anabolic dosha formed by a combination of earth and water (earth is an active element, and water acts as the regulatory element). Elements of nature energized the human body in the form of three doshas which balance the energy for good health. The balance of

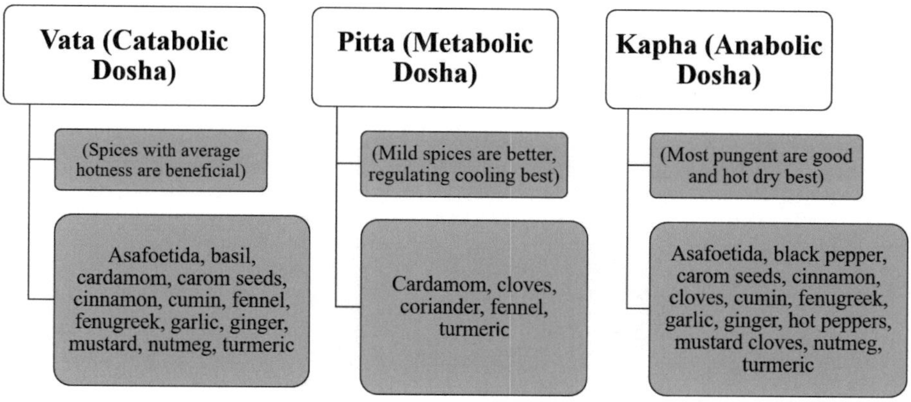

Figure 1.
Spice & condiments use to pacify three doshas. Source: [14].

tridoshas is unique to each person and different from one individual to another, which represents the body's natural state of equilibrium. The balance of these doshas produces good or bad consequences in the entire body [8–11].

"*Vaata pitta sleshmaana eva deha sambhava hetavah Taireva avyaapannaih adho madhyordhwa sannivishtaih Sariramidan dharyute aagaaramiya stoonaabhistisnubhih*".

Ayurvedic texts have a great description of the uses of spices and condiments in the prevention of diseases caused by these three doshas. For instance, the use of clove as a painkiller in dental emergencies, turmeric for microbial infection, skin disease and jaundice, basil for heart diseases, cinnamon to stimulate circulation, cardamom for headache, and mouth infections [2, 12]. An adequate amount of spice intake plays a vital role to pacify tridoshas [9, 13]. Some spices & condiments used to pacify three doshas are as follows (**Figure 1**).

3. Spice & condiments

Spice is an aromatic and pungent dried part of the plants such as roots, stems, bark, leaves, bud, flowers, fruit, seeds, etc., which are used as food adjuncts for aroma and

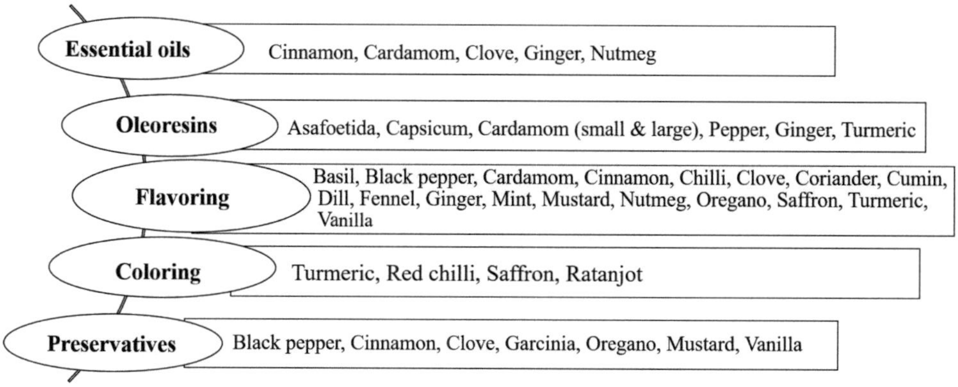

Figure 2.
Spice & condiments for value-added products.

S.N.	Common name (Botanical name)	Native range	Production rank in the world	Parts use	Principle phytochemical compound	Pharmacological activity
1.	**Asafoetida** [20–22] (*Ferula assa-foetida* L.)	Iran	Afghanistan, Iran	Latex from rhizome	Asaresinotannols, ferulic acid, umbelliferone	Antioxidant, Antispasmodic, Hypotensive, Hepatoprotective, Antimicrobial, Anticancer, Anthelmintic
2.	**Aniseed** [20, 21, 23] (*Pimpinella anisum* L.)	SE. Turkey to Central Israel	Mexico, The Netherlands, Spain	Fruit	Anethole, anisaldehyde	Antibacterial, Antifungal, Anti-inflammatory, Antispasmodic, Anti-ulcer,
3.	**Basil/sweet basil** [20, 21, 24] (*Ocimum basilicum* L.)	India	India	Leaves, Seeds	Linalool, 1,8, cineol, eugenol, methyl eugenol, methyl chavicol	Antibacterial, Anticonvulsant, Anti-inflammatory, Antioxidant, Insecticidal, Larvicidal
4.	**Basil/ holy basil** [20, 21] (*Ocimum tenuiflorum* L.)	Indian subcontinent	India	Leaves, Seeds	Methylchavicol, linalool, methyl eugenol	Antiasthmatic, Anti-carcinogenic, Anti-inflammatory, Antimicrobial, Antioxidant, Antistress
5.	**Indian bay leaf** [20, 21] (*Cinnamomum tamala* (Buch.-Ham.) T.Nees & C.H.Eberm.)	Himalaya to China and Indo-China	India	Leaves	Eugenol, β-pinene, caryophyllene, spathulenol, acetyl eugenol	Antibacterial, Antidepressant, Anti-diabetic, Antifungal, Carminative, hypolipidemic, Sedative
6.	**Black pepper** [20, 21, 23] (*Piper nigrum* L.)	India	Vietnam, Indonesia, and India	Fruit	Piperine, β-caryophyllene, chavicine	Analgesic, Antiseptic, Antispasmodic, Antitoxic, Diaphoretic, Digestive, Diuretic, Febrifuge, Laxative, Phrodisiac, Rubefacient
7.	**Cardamom** (small) [20, 21, 23] (*Elettaria cardamomum* (L.) Maton)	India	India, Guatemala	Fruit	1,8-cineole, α-terpinyl acetate	Anti-inflammatory, Antimicrobial, Antiseptic, Antispasmodic, Carminative, Digestive, Diuretic, Stimulant, Stomachic, Tonic
8.	**Cardamom** (large) [20, 21, 23] (*Amomum subulatum* Roxb.)	Eastern Nepal, India, Bhutan	Nepal, India Bhutan	Fruit	1,8-cineol, terpinyl acetate, limonene	Anthelminthic, Antibacterial, Anti-inflammatory, Aphrodisiac, Antiseptic, Antispasmodic (neuromuscular), Anti-ulcerogenic

S.N.	Common name (Botanical name)	Native range	Production rank in the world	Parts use	Principle phytochemical compound	Pharmacological activity
9.	**Carom seeds /Ajowan** (*Trachyspermum ammi* (L.) Sprague) [2, 20, 21, 23]	Egypt	India	Seeds	Thymol, γ-terpenene	Antibacterial, Antihypertensive, Anti-inflammatory, Antimicrobial, Antinociceptive, Antioxidant, Antispasmodic, Broncho-dilating Cytotoxic, Diuretic Hypolipidemic,
10.	**Chili** [20, 21, 23] (*Capsicum frutescens* L.)	Bolivia to Brazil	India, China, Thailand	Fruit	Capsaicin	Aflatoxigenic, Anthelmintic, Anticancerous, Anti-inflammation, Antioxidant, Insecticidal
11.	**Cinnamon** [20, 21, 23] (*Cinnamomum verum* J.Presl)	Sri Lanka	Sri Lanka, India	Stem, bark	Eugenol, benzyl benzoate, cinnamaldehyde	Antibacterial, Antidiabetic, Anti-inflammatory, Antioxidant, Antipyretic, Immunological effects, Insecticidal,
12.	**Clove** [2, 20, 21, 23] (*Syzygium aromaticum* (L.) Merr. & L.M.Perry)	Indonesia	Indonesia, Malaysia, Tanzania	Buds	Eugenol, eugenyl acetate	Anesthetic, Antibacterial, Anticancerous, Anti-inflammatory, Antioxidant, Antipyretic, Antithrombotic, Antiviral, Insecticidal,
13.	**Coriander** [2, 20, 21, 23] (*Coriandrum sativum* L.)	E. Medit. to Pakistan	India, Morocco, Russia	Fruit	Linalool	Aflatoxin, Antimicrobial, Antioxidant, Insecticidal,
14.	**Cumin** [20, 21, 23] (*Cuminum cyminum* L.)	The Mediterranean to India	India, Syria, Iran, Turkey	Fruit	Cuminaldehyde, b-pinene, cis-β-farnesene	Antimicrobial, antioxidant, antispasmodic, carminative, chemoprotective, stimulant
15.	**Curry leaf** [20, 21, 23] (*Murraya koenigii* (L.) Spreng.)	India	India, Burma	Leaf	Murrayacine, koenigine, α-pinene, β-phellandrene	Antidiabetic, Antioxidant, Anti-inflammatory, Antimicrobial
16.	**Dill** [20, 21, 23] (*Anethum graveolens* L.)	Europe	India	Fruit	Dillapiole	Antimicrobial
17.	**Fennel** [20, 21, 23] (*Foeniculum vulgare* Mill.)	Europe and Asia Minor	India, Syria, Egypt, Turkey	Fruit	Anethole, estragol	Acaricidal, Anticancer, Antimicrobial, Antioxidant, Hepatoprotective
18.	**Fenugreek** [2, 20, 21, 23] (*Trigonella foenum-graecum* L.)	South Eastern Europe and West Asia	India	Leaves, Fruit, Seeds	Diosgenin	Anticarcinogenic, Antifertility, Antioxidant, Hypocholesterolemia, Hypoglycaemic, Immunomodulatory

S.N.	Common name (Botanical name)	Native range	Production rank in the world	Parts use	Principle phytochemical compound	Pharmacological activity
19.	**Garlic** [20, 21, 23] (*Allium sativum* L.)	Central Asia to NE. Iran	China, India, Bangladesh	Bulb/clove	Organosulfur	Anti-atherosclerotic, Antibacterial, Anticarcinogenic, Antifungal, Antihypertensive, Antioxidant, Antidiabetic, Renoprotective,
20.	**Garcinia** [20, 21] (*Garcinia gummi-gutta* (L.) Roxb.)	India	India	Fruit	a-Humelene, valencene, b-caryophyllene	Analgesic, Antibacterial, Anti-HIV, Anti-inflammatory, Antiobesity, Antioxidant, Astringent, Cancer suppressant, Hepatotic tonic,
21.	**Ginger** [20, 21, 23] (*Zingiber officinale* Roscoe)	India to S. Central China	India, Indonesia, Nigeria, China	Rhizome	Gingerol, shogoal, citral, zingiberene, ar-curcumene	Anticancer, Anticonvulsive, Anti-inflammatory, Antioxidant, Antiplatelet, Anti-ulcer, Cardiovascular
22.	**Mint** [20, 21, 23] (*Mentha* × *piperita* L.)	Europe to Central Asia	India, China, Brazil	Leaf/ terminal shoot	Menthol and Menthone	Anticancer, Anti-diabetic, Anti-inflammatory, Antimicrobial, Anti-obesity, Cardioprotective effects
23.	**Mustard/Indian mustard** [20, 21] (*Brassica juncea* L.Czern)	Southern and eastern Asia	—	Seeds	Sinigrin, Allyl isothiocyanate	Antibacterial/Fungicidal, Anticancer, Anti-inflammation, Anti-oxidation, Anti-tumor
24.	**Mustard (Black)** [20, 21, 23] (*Brassica nigra* (L.) Koch)	Eurasia	Canada, Denmark, Ethiopia, UK, India	Seeds	Sinigrin, Allyl-isothiocyanate	Antibacterial/Fungicidal, Anticancer, Anti-inflammation, Anti-oxidation, Anti-tumor
25.	**Nigella** [2, 21, 23, 25] (*Nigella sativa* L.)	Romania to W. & SW. Iran	India, Sri Lanka, Bangladesh	Seeds	Thymoquinone	Anticancer, Antidiabetic, Antihyperlipidemic, Antihypertensive, Anti-inflammatory, Antimicrobial, Antioxidant,
26.	**Nutmeg** [20, 21, 23] (*Myristica fragrans* Houtt.)	Maluku (Banda Islands)	India	Aril/seed kernel	Myristicin, eugenol	Antiamoebic, Anticancer, Antimicrobial, Antioxidant, Antibacterial, Hypolipidaemic, Insecticidal,

S.N.	Common name (Botanical name)	Native range	Production rank in the world	Parts use	Principle phytochemical compound	Pharmacological activity
27.	**Onion** [20, 21, 23] (*Allium cepa* L.)	Central Asia	China and India	Bulb	Organosulfur	Antihyperglycemic, Antimicrobial, Anti-mutagenic, Antioxidant, Cardiovascular protectives
28.	**Oregano** [20, 21, 23] (*Origanum vulgare* L.)	Mediterranean region	China and India	Leaf	Carvacrol, β-fenchyl alcohol, thymol, and γ-terpinene	Antidiabetic, Anti-inflammatory, Antimicrobial, Antioxidant
29.	**Paprika** [20, 21, 23] (*Capsicum annuum* L.)	Mexico to Guatemala	India, China	Fruit	Capsanthin, capsorubin	Aflatoxigenic Anthelmintic, Anticancerous, Anti-inflammation, Antioxidant, Insecticidal
30.	**Turmeric** [2, 20, 21, 23] (*Curcuma longa* L.)	India	India, China, Myanmar	Rhizome	Curcumin, Zingeberene	Anticancer, Anti-inflammatory, Antimicrobial, Antimutagenic, Antiobesity, Antioxidant, Cardioprotective, Neuroprotective
31.	**Vanilla** [20, 21] (*Vanilla planifolia* Andrews)	S. Mexico to Brazil	Indonesia, Madagascar, Mexico, India	Fruit/ beans	Vanillin	Anticarcinogenic, Antioxidant, Neuroprotection, Sedative

Table 1.
Status of major spices and condiments with their pharmacological content [16–19].

flavor i.e., pepper, cardamom, clove, nutmeg, cinnamon, etc., while condiments are also parts of plants which are used as food ingredients to enhance taste and flavor [12, 15]. So, spices and condiments are used for taste or flavoring, as well as preservatives, essential oils and coloring agents in many pharmaceutical and chemical industries (**Figure 2**). Along with being a taste enhancer, they are also known for rich nutraceutical properties which maintain the healthy immune system of the body. Specific phytochemical compounds are responsible for the aromatic, pungent, and coloring qualities of spice and condiments. These phytochemical compounds possess medicinal properties such as antioxidant, anti-inflammatory, anti-diabetic, anti-mutagenic, anti-carcinogenic, anti-microbial, anti-arthritic, and hypoglycemic activity which are beneficial in the prevention of many diseases like diabetes, inflammatory, cardiovascular, cancer, and neurodegenerative disorders. Some popular spices which are famous for their taste in every kitchen of the world and healing aid remedy are as follow- asfoetida, black paper, bay-leaf, carom seeds, capsicum, cardamom (small & large), coriander, cinnamon, clove, cumin, curry leaves, dill, fennel, fenugreek, ginger, garlic, mint, mustard, Nigella, nutmeg, onion, paprika, turmeric and vanilla, etc. International Organization for Standardization (ISO) listed 109 spices in the world of which 63 spices are grown in India. The list of major spice & condiments belonging to the land of India with their uses, principle phyto-constituents, and nutrient components are mentioned in **Table 1** [3, 15, 16, 20, 21, 25–28].

4. Nutraceutical

Nutraceutical is driven by "nutrition" and "pharmaceutics". Which referred to natural plant products or food-based substances such as cereals, fruits, vegetables, spices, and beverages that are used for nutrition as well as therapeutic purpose. Nutraceuticals are grouped into three categories such as nutrients, herbal and dietary supplements. Spices and condiments are also special plant products that have both rich nutritional and medicinal properties. Nutritional components help to nourish

Spice & condiments	Nutritional value (100gms)	Common uses	Health benefits
Asafoetida (*Ferula assa-foetida* L.) [2, 22, 23]	Moisture: 16.0% Carbohydrate:7.8% Protein: 4.0% Fat: 1.1% Fiber: 4.1%	Seasoning food especially snacks and various types of pickles	asthma, epilepsy, stomach-ache, flatulence, intestinal parasites, weak digestion and influenza Help to cure asthma, bronchitis, whooping cough, epilepsy, stomachache, flatulence, intestinal parasites, weak digestion, and influenza
Indian bay-leaf (*Cinnamomum tamala* (Buch.-Ham.) T.Nees & C.H.Eberm.) [2, 21, 23]	Carbohydrate (g): 74.96 Protein (g): 7.61 Fat (g): 8.36 Ca (g) 0.83 Fe (mg): 43.0 Ascorbic acid (mg): 46.53	Flavoring food, meat products, soups, and fish	Reduced the risk of bacterial and fungal infections

Spice & condiments	Nutritional value (100gms)	Common uses	Health benefits
Black pepper (*Piper nigrum* L.) [2, 21, 23]	Carbohydrates (g): 66.5 Protein (g): 10.0 Fat (g) 10.2 Ca (g): 0.4 P (mg) 160.0 K (mg): 1200.0 Fe (mg): 17.0 Thiamine (mg): 0.07 Riboflavin (mg): 0.210 Niacin (mg): 0.8	Flavoring food, soups, and preservative	Help to cure flu, colds, fevers, rheumatism, chills, exhaustion, muscular aches, physical and emotional coldness, and as a nerve tonic
Carom seed/ Bishop's weed/Ajwain (*Trachyspermum ammi* (L.) Sprague) [21, 23, 28, 29]	Carbohydrate (g): 24.6 Protein (g): 17.1 Fiber (g): 21.2 Ca (g): 1.525 P (g): 0.443 Na (mg): 56 K (mg): 1.38 Fe (mg): 27.7	Use in curry dish for the aromatic and pungent taste	Digestive aid, colds, and flu, for relieving flatulence, dyspepsia and spasmodic disorders
Cardamom (Small) (*Elettaria cardamomum* (L.) Maton) [2, 21, 23, 28]	Carbohydrate (g): 68.47 Protein (g): 10.76 Fat (g): 6.70 Ca (g): 0.383 P (g): 178 Na (mg): 18 K (mg): 1119 Fe (mg): 13.97 Volatile oil: 2.80%	Sweet/savory flavor to desserts, main dishes, and beverages	Reduce bad breath, digestive disorders, relieving flatulence, and constipation
Cardamom (Large) (*Amomum subulatum* Roxb.) [21, 23, 28]	Carbohydrate (g): 68.47 Protein (g): 10.76 Fat (g): 6.70 Ca (g): 0.383 P (g): 178 Na (mg): 18 K (mg): 1119 Fe (mg): 13.97 Volatile oil: 8.30%	Rice preparation, meat dishes, desserts, and beverages	Help to cure mouth infections, digestive disorders, abdominal pains, heart and liver problems
Chili and paprika (*Capsicum frutescens* L.) [2, 21, 23, 28]	Carbohydrate (g): 58.20 Protein (g): 14.0 Fat (g): 6.70 Ca (g): 0.10 P (g): 0.32 Na (mg): 0.01 K (mg): 2.10 Fe (mg): 9.90 Niacin (mg): 14.20 Ascorbic acid (mg): 63.70	Pungent and hot flavor to the food	Help to cure asthma, coughs, and sore throats
Cinnamon (*Cinnamomum verum* J.Presl) [2, 3, 21, 23, 28]	Carbohydrates (g): 79.85 Protein (g): 3.89 Fat (g): 3.18 Ca (g): 1.23 Fe (mg): 38.07 Ascorbic acid (mg): 28.46	Seasoning food and preparing masalas	Help in insulin production and lowering blood cholesterol

Spice & condiments	Nutritional value (100gms)	Common uses	Health benefits
Clove (*Syzygium aromaticum* (L.) Merr. & L.M.Perry) [2, 3, 21, 23, 28]	Carbohydrates (g): 61.22 Protein (g): 5.98 Fat (g): 20.06 Ca (g): 0.646 P (mg): 105 Fe (mg): 8.68 Ascorbic acid (mg): 80.81	Flavoring food and masalas	Help to cure toothache, sore gums, fever, digestive problems, cough, cold, and chest pains
Coriander (*Coriandrum sativum* L.) [2, 21, 23, 28]	Carbohydrates (g): 64.99 Protein (g): 12.37 Fat (g): 17.77 Ash (g): 6.02 Ca (g): 0.709 P (mg): 409 Fe (mg): 16.32 Niacin (mg): 2.130	Leaves and seeds used in cooking	Help to cure sore throat, allergies, digestion problems, hay fever, joint pain, and rheumatism
Cumin (*Cuminum cyminum* L.) [2, 23, 28]	Carbohydrates (g): 0.88 Protein (g): 0.36 Fat (g): 0.44 Ash (g): 0.16 Ca (g): 18.62 P (mg): 9.98 Fe (mg): 1.37 Ascorbic acid (mg): 0.16	Used for cooking	Keeps the immune system healthy
Curry leaves (*Murraya koenigii* (L.) Spreng.) [2, 3, 21, 23, 30]	Moisture (g): 63 Carbohydrates (g): 18 Protein (g): 6.1 Fat (g): 1 Fiber (g): 6 Ca (mg): 830 P (mg): 57 Fe (mg): 0.93 Ascorbic acid (mg): 4	Used as an ingredient for seasoning	Lowering blood sugar, bacterial and fungal infections, febrile disorders, dysentery, diarrhea, and inflammation of the gums
Ginger (*Zingiber officinale* Roscoe) [3, 21, 23]	Carbohydrates (g): 70.70 Protein (g): 9.12 Fat (g): 5.95 Ash (g): 4.77 Ca (g): 0.116 P (mg): 148 Fe (mg): 11.52 Ascorbic acid (mg): ---	Used for giving specific flavor to food	Help to cure cough, cold and digestive disorders
Garlic (*Allium sativum* L.) [2, 21, 23, 28, 31]	Carbohydrates (g): 33.06 Protein (g): 6.36 Fat (g): 0.5 Ca (mg): 181 P (mg): 153 Fe (mg): 1.7 Ascorbic acid (mg): 31.2	Used for cooking and in the preparation of pickles	Help to cure cough, cold, and lowering of blood cholesterol
Fennel (*Foeniculum vulgare* Mill.) [21, 23]	Carbohydrates (g): 52.29 Protein (g): 15.80 Fat (g): 14.87 Ash (g): 8.22 Ca (g): 1.96 P (mg): 487 Fe (mg): 18.54 Ascorbic acid (mg): ---	Flavoring to food, pudding, and snack	Digestive stimulant action and reduces bloating, gas and heaviness,

Spice & condiments	Nutritional value (100gms)	Common uses	Health benefits
Fenugreek (*Trigonella foenum-graecum* L.) [2, 21, 23, 28]	Carbohydrates (g): 58.35 Protein (g): 23.00 Fat (g): 6.41 Ash (g): 3.40 Ca (g): 0.176 P (mg): 296 Fe (mg): 33.53 Ascorbic acid (mg): 3.00	Leaves use as green leafy vegetables and seeds for seasoning and preparing masalas	Lowering blood cholesterol, diabetes and helps to cure fever, vomiting, anorexia, cough, bronchitis
Mustard (*Brassica juncea* L.Czern) [2, 23]	Fat (total) (g): 28.76 Dietary fiber (g): 14.7 Protein (g): 1.88 Ca (g): 521 P (mg): 841 Mg (mg): 298 Fe (mg): 9.98 Ascorbic acid (mg): 3	Use as green leafy vegetables and seeds for cooking	Help in good blood circulation and reduces the risk of bacterial and fungal infections
Onion (*Allium cepa* L.) [23, 32, 33]	Carbohydrates (g): 11 Protein (g): 1.5 Fiber (g): 0.5 Ca (mg): 30 P (mg): --- Fe (mg): 0.5 Ascorbic acid (mg): 10	Used for cooking and eaten raw as salad	Prevent bacterial and fungal infections, stimulate hair growth
Saffron (*Crocus sativus* L.) [2, 3, 21, 23, 28, 34]	Carbohydrates (g): 65.37 Protein (g): 11.43 Fat (g): 5.85 Dietary fiber (g): 3.9 Ca (mg): 111 P (mg): 252 Fe (mg): 11.10 Ascorbic acid (mg): 80.8 mg	Used for cooking or coloring agent in many sweet dishes, also used in beauty products	Reduce the risk of skin diseases, cough, cold, and asthma
Turmeric (*Curcuma longa* L.) [2, 3, 21, 23, 28]	Carbohydrates (g): 64.93 Protein (g): 7.83 Fat (g): 9.88 Ca (g): 0.182 mg P (mg): 268 mg Fe (mg): 41.42 mg Ascorbic acid (mg): 25.85 mg	Used for cooking and as a coloring agent, and also used in skincare products	Reduce the risk of skin diseases, microbial infections, healing cuts, and wounds

Table 2.
Nutritional profile, uses, and health benefits [16–19].

the body, improve health and give energy to work such as carbohydrates, proteins, vitamins-A, B, C, minerals, amino acids and fatty acids in which antioxidants, vitamins, and essential minerals are the most common nutrient found in many plants. Phytoconstituents are unique compound that occurs naturally in plant and plays a significant role in human health. It is responsible for the unique taste, color, and bio-activity to protect from many chronic diseases such as cancer, cardiovascular, neuro-degenerative, diabetes, inflammation, and liver disorder. Spices and condiments act as major nutraceutical agents and have both essential and nonessential phytonutrients which play a significant role in our daily lifestyle beyond making our food tasty. Both **Tables 1** and **2** combinedly explains nutritional and pharmacological properties with their common uses and health benefits.

5. Indian spice scenario

The diversity of spices has different origins therefore their use and taste are famous in the world. The Mediterranean region, South Europe and Asia have historically recorded lands from where many types of spices originate and distributed in many countries. At present spices are growing in many countries such as Bangladesh, Brazil, China, Ethiopia, Germany, Guatemala, India, Indonesia, Japan, Madagascar, Nepal, Pakistan, Sri Lanka, Turkey, and Vietnam. Among these countries, India is the leading spice-producing country with a 70% contribution of spices in the world's production and retaining a large quantity of its supply for national consumption, that's why India is known as the 'land of spices' [25, 35, 36].

In India, spices are cultivated in the regions of Bihar, Karnataka, Kerala, Madhya Pradesh, Odisha, Punjab, Rajasthan, Tamil Nadu Uttar Pradesh and West Bengal. Among them, Kerala is the leading state in the production of black pepper and small cardamom, whereas Andhra Pradesh is the leading producer of chilies, turmeric, and several spice seeds, and Madhya Pradesh and Gujarat are famous for ginger production. Rajasthan and Gujarat are famous seed spices producing states that's why they are known as the seed spices bowl of India. The area and production of spices in

Spices	2018–2019		2019–2020		2020–2021	
	Area (000'Ha)	Production (000'MT)	Area (000'Ha)	Production (000'MT)	Area (000'Ha)	Production (000'MT)
Ajwain	35	22	41	29	29	22
Cardamom	81	23	85	21	84	34
Chillies (Dried)	780	1743	626	1835	729	2092
Cinnamon/ Tejpata	2	5	3	8	2	5
Celery, Dill & Poppy	30	30	33	35	31	31
Clove	2	1	2	1	2	1
Coriander	470	592	529	701	662	832
Cumin	1027	699	1276	912	1241	856
Fenugreek	122	192	126	182	121	203
Fennel	90	157	83	140	79	127
Garlic	358	2910	352	2925	391	3185
Nutmeg	24	15	24	16	23	15
Pepper	245	137	259	104	260	120
Vanilla	0	0	0	0	0	0
Saffron	3	0	4	0	4	0
Turmeric	253	961	296	1153	291	1064
Mint (Mentha)	334	34	328	44	359	47
Total spices	**4067**	**9500**	**4291**	**10,137**	**4528**	**10,679**

Table 3.
Area and production of Indian spices [37].

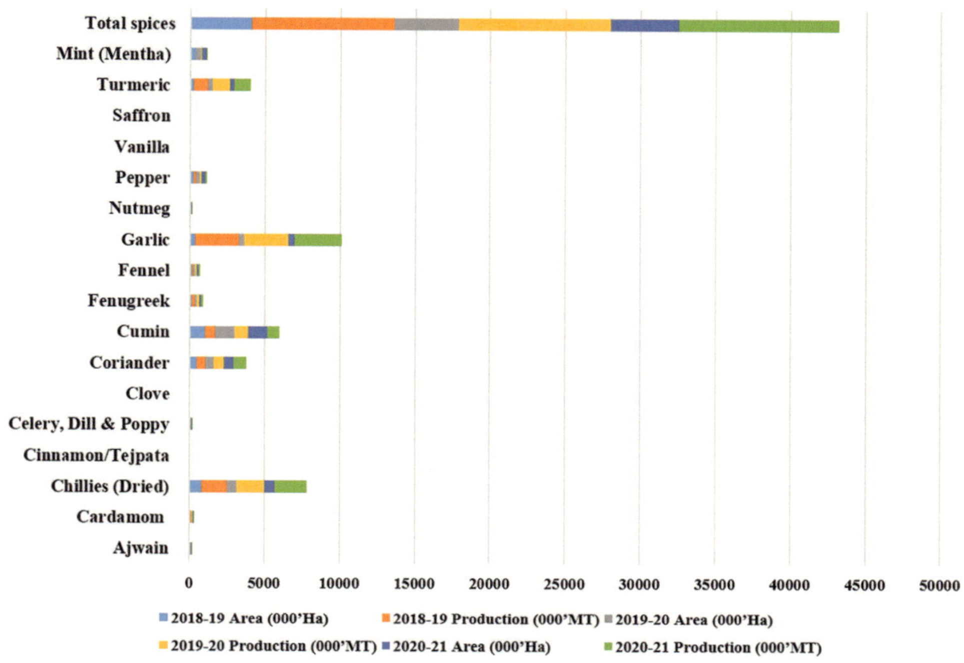

Figure 3.
Area and production of Indian spices chart.

2018–2019 was 4067Mha and production 9500MT and in 2020–2021 both slightly increase by area of 4528 Mha and production of 10679MT, as given in the **Table 3** and area & production for each spices are shown in **Figure 3** [25, 35, 37, 38].

6. Conclusion

India's vegetation is rich with many spices and condiments species on which various occupations are dependent. Since ancient India's food was very popular for its taste and fragrance in the world, therefore it became a point of attraction for many explorers or traders for coming to India. Spice & condiments are an essential part of our daily life from the morning with tea or herbal beverages to a good night drink with turmeric milk. They play the biggest role in the nourishment and refreshment of the body. The ancient literature also reveals that dried parts of the plant are very popular for their use to cure various types of diseases beyond enhancing the taste of food. Unique phytochemical compounds found in particular spices not only enhances the taste of food but also helps to enhance the nutrients present in vegetables or fruits or other food preparation in which they are used, beyond this goodness they are also helpful to suppress the worse effect of another chemical in our body. They strongly fight bacterial and viral infections and make our immune system healthy. Some spices are very popular in the world for their use in every culinary and medicinal practice to cure diseases. The specific phytochemicals such as curcumin in turmeric, piperine in black pepper, gingerol in ginger, eugenol in clove, eugenol, and cinnamaldehyde in cinnamon, linalool in coriander, cuminaldehyde in cumin, diosgenin in fenugreek, thymol in carom seeds and murrayacine in curry leaves possess antioxidant, anticancer, anti-inflammatory, anti-diabetic, anti-mutagenic, anti-microbial, anti-arthritic, and hypoglycemic activities against many diseases. Our farmers are very intelligent and they know every particular effect of these spices on health and they are using them for ages but the over-chemical fertilizer use in the cultivation of these nutraceutical crops reduce their nutritional qualities and that is the biggest reason, they are notable to fight against all the diseases. Another biggest reason is food adulteration, which is a severe problem nowadays with many food supplements. The common adulterants of spices such as sand, dirt, earth gritty matter, artificial color, starch, chalk powder, bark, and papaya seeds are used to increase the quantity of various powder spices. These adulterants degrade the quality of spices and can lead to serious health complications. The safest way to avoid adulterated spices is to purchase raw spices and otherwise fully packed approved spice powders. Promote organic cultivation to retain the nutraceutical values of plants and create awareness among the farmers about harmful chemical effects. Proper planning and intensive research should be initiated for the conservation of spices & condiments for future health.

Author details

Acharya Balkrishna[1,2], Bhasker Joshi[1,2], Anupam Srivastava[2] and Seema Bisht[2*]

1 Department of Allied Sciences, University of Patanjali, Haridwar, India

2 Patanjali Herbal Research Department, Patanjali Research Institute, Haridwar, India

*Address all correspondence to: seema.bisht@prft.co.in

References

[1] Khan NR. The spice route: A historical survey. International Journal of Applied Research. 2018;**4**(12):131-133

[2] Sachan AK, Kumar S, Kumari K, Singh D. Medicinal uses of spices used in our traditional culture: Worldwide. Journal of Medicinal Plants Studies. 2018;**6**(3):116-122

[3] Shukla A, Yadav N. Role of Indian spices in Indian history. International Journal of Management Research and Reviews. 2018;**8**(11):1-6

[4] Schou C. (n.d.). Garlic: A Taste for Health. Ethnobotanical Leaflets. SIUC. Available from: http://www.siu.edu/~ebl/ [Accessed: September 9, 2022]

[5] Tapsell LC, Hemphill I, Cobiac L, Sullivan DR, Fenech M, Patch CS, et al. Health benefits of herbs and spices: The past, the present, the future. The Medical Journal Australia. 2006;**185**(4):1-24

[6] Balasasirekha R. Spices-the spice of life. European Journal of Food Science and Technology. 2014;**2**(1):29-40

[7] Dattatray S, Bhingardive K, Jaiswal M. The queen of spices and ayurveda: A brief review. International Journal of Research Ayurveda Pharmacy. 2016;**7**(4):1-7

[8] Asthana AK, Monika MA, Sahu R. Significance of Doshas in management of various disease. Asian Journal of Pharmaceutical Research and Development. 2018;**6**(5):41-45

[9] Singh MMM, Bhatnagar S. Concept and significance of use of spices as per Ayurveda. International Journal of Health Sciences & Research. 2019;**9**(4):250-254

[10] Joshi K, Thapliyal A, Singh V. The Tridosha theory according to Ayurveda. International Journal for Modern Trends in Science and Technology. 2021;**7**(8):120-124

[11] Savita S, AK. Concept of Tridosha theory: A critical review. International Journal of Creative Research Thoughts. 2021;**9**(1):2184-2190

[12] D'Souza SP, Chavannavar SV, Kanchanashri B, Niveditha SB. Pharmaceutical perspectives of spices and condiments as alternative antimicrobial remedy. Journal of Evidence-Based Complementary & Alternative Medicine. 2017;**22**(4):1002-1010

[13] Patel MR. Applying the Knowledge of Ayurveda to Appraise the US Nutritional Paradigm. Nevada City, CA: California College of Ayurveda; 2010

[14] Shukla V, Tripathi R. Charaka Samhita. Delhi: Chaukhamba Sanskrit Pratishthan; 2017

[15] Reddy IVS. Production Technology of Spices, Aromatic, Medicinal, and Plantation Crops. Andhra Pradesh: Acharya N.G Ranga Agricultural University; n.d.

[16] Srinivasan K. Role of spices beyond food flavoring: Nutraceuticals with multiple health effects. Food Reviews International. 2005;**21**(2):167-188

[17] Pandey N, Meena RP, Rai SK, Pandey-Rai S. Medicinal plants derived nutraceuticals: A re-emerging health aid. International Journal of Pharma and Bio Sciences. 2011;**2**(4):420-441

[18] Jhansi D, Manjula K. Functional and nutraceutical properties of herbals and its applications in food. International Journal of Science and Research. 2016;**5**:196-198

[19] POWO. Plants of the World Online. Facilitated by the Royal Botanic Gardens, Kew. Published on the Internet http://www.plantsoftheworldonline.org/ [Retrieved 22 October 2022]

[20] Peter KV. Handbook of Herbs and Spices. Vol. 3. Cambridge: Woodhead Publishing Limited; 2001. pp. 1-311

[21] Parthasarathy VA, Chempakam B, Zachariah TJ, editors. Chemistry of Spices. Wallingford, Oxfordshire, England: CABI; 2008. p. 445

[22] Mahendra P, Bisht S. Ferula asafoetida: Traditional uses and pharmacological activity. Pharmacognosy Reviews. 2012;**6**(12):141

[23] SBI. Spice Catalogue-Spice Board of India [Internet]. 2019. Available from: http://www.indianspices.com/spices-development/spice-catalogue.html [Accessed: September 20, 2022]

[24] Poonkodi K. Chemical composition of essential oil of Ocimum basilicum L. (basil) and its biological activities-an overview. Journal of Critical Reviews. 2016;**3**(3):56-62

[25] Lal G. Scenario, importance and prospects of seed spices: A review. Current Investigations in Agriculture and Current Research. 2018;**4**(2):491-498

[26] Srinivasan K. Spices for Taste and Flavour: Nutraceuticals for Human Health. London: Spices: The Elixir of Life; 2011. pp. 29-48

[27] Fasoyiro S. The Value of Spices; Uses, Nutritional and Health Benefits. Chisinau, MD: LAP Lambert Academic Publishing; 2015. p. 54

[28] Dubey S. Indian spices and their medicinal value. Indian Journal of Pharmaceutical Education and Research. 2017;**51**(3):330-331

[29] Dwivedi SN, Mishra RP, Alava S. Phytochemistry, pharmacological studies and traditional benefits of Trachyspermum ammi (Linn.) Sprague. International journal of pharmacy & life sciences. 2012;**3**(5):1705-1709

[30] Disegha GC, Izionworu VO. Antifungal activities of curry leaf (Murraya koengii) extract on some selected fungi. Chemistry and Materials Research. 2014;**6**(11):2224-3224

[31] Upadhyay RK. Garlic: A potential source of pharmaceuticals and pesticides: A review. International Journal of Green Pharmacy. 2016;**10**(1):1-28

[32] Kumar KS, Bhowmik D, Chiranjib B, Tiwari P. Allium cepa: A traditional medicinal herb and its health benefits. Journal of Chemical and Pharmaceutical Research. 2010;**2**(1):283-291

[33] John V, Murmu R, Maurya A, Pant H. Eco-friendly management of pre and post-harvest diseases of onion (Allium cepa L.). In: Singh HK, editor. Current Research and Innovations in Plant Pathology. New Delhi: AkiNik Publications; 2020. pp. 115-131

[34] Bilal AW, Hamza AKR, Mohiddin FA. Saffron: A repository of medicinal properties. Journal of Medicinal Plants Research. 2011;**5**(11):2131-2135

[35] Jaffee S. Delivering and taking the heat: Indian spices and evolving product and process standards. In: The International Bank for Reconstruction and Development. The World Bank; 2005. pp. 1-42

[36] Sahu PK, Mishra P. Modelling and forecasting production behaviour and import-export of total spices in two most populous countries of the world. Journal of Agricultural Research. 2013;**51**(1):81-97

[37] Anonymous. Agricultural Statistics at a Glance, 2021- Department of Agriculture & Farmers Welfare Ministry of Agriculture & Farmers Welfare. Krishi Bhawan, New Delhi: Government of India; 2021. pp. 1-431

[38] Malhotra SK, Cheriyan H, Meena B, Manojkumar K, Sreekumar S. Spices Statistics at a Glance 2021. Calicut, Kerala: Directorate of Arecanut and Spices Development; 2021

Chapter 3

Bioaccessibility, Bioavailability, Antioxidant Activities and Health Beneficial Properties of Some Selected Spices

Boris Nemzer and Diganta Kalita

Abstract

Herbs and spices have been used as therapeutic agents in traditional medicine due to the presence of bioactive compounds including flavonoids, polyphenols, alkaloids, carotenoids, organosulfur compounds, glucosinolates etc. As a result, they are associated with various functional properties such as digestive stimulant, antioxidant, anti-inflammatory anticancer, anti-diabetic, cardioprotective, neuroprotective, and antimicrobial activities. However, the bioefficacy of different spices are affected by the bioavailabilties of their bioactive compounds and depends on various factors such bioaccessibility, molecular structures, composition of food matrices, and metabolizing enzymes. In this chapter we discuss on major phytochemical compounds of some selected spices including turmeric, garlic, ginger, onion, cinnamon, chili pepper, and black pepper including their bio accessibilities, bioavailabilities and their health beneficial effects. The knowledge of bioaccessibility and bioavailability of spices bioactive compounds will give a better understanding towards the development of strategies to optimize the positive health benefits of spices.

Keywords: spices, phytochemicals, polyphenols, nutrients, bioavailability, bioactive compounds, antioxidant activities, anti-inflammatory activities, anticancer properties

1. Introduction

Herbs and spices from leaves, seeds, bark, roots, rhizomes, or buds of aromatic plants have long been used for ages in food and medicine. Although herbs and spices are used to enhance flavor, taste, and color of foods, they also supply basic nutrients, promote health, and prevent from the risk of development of chronic diseases [1–5]. There are numerous groups of bioactive compounds present in herbs and spices due to which they are gaining continuous interest over time from scientific and health perspectives [3–7]. Several phytochemicals comprising carotenoids, phenolic compounds (flavonoids, flavonol, flavanols, anthocyanins, proanthocynains, and phenolic acids), phytosterols, phytostanols, tocotrienols, organosulfur compounds, alkaloids, dietary fibers, prebiotics, protein, amino acids, and minerals contribute to the potential health benefits [3, 4, 7]. In general, the spices phytochemicals are safe to humans and recognized as GRAS (Generally Recognized As Safe) by USFDA (United State Food and Drug Administration) except some cases with age, and medical conditions. The spices are consumed as fresh, processed, or cooked where it could undergo physical and chemical transformation from the original sources and could affect their levels of content and efficacy [4–7]. Numerous research reports supported the potential role of spices phytochemicals in reducing and curing form diseases such as coronary heart disease, hypercholesterolemia, high blood pressure, diabetes, inflammation, cancers, arthritis, microbial, viral, and parasitic infections [4–10]. Extensive *in vitro* and *in vivo* studies and clinical trial investigations confirmed the correlations of molecular structures of these phytochemicals and their biochemical activities [4–10]. However, most of their mechanisms of actions are still not completely understood to underscore their corresponding health benefits. One of the major pathways of these protective roles of phytochemicals are associated with their antioxidant activities by reducing activities of reactive oxidants which cause oxidative stress related chronic diseases like cancer, diabetes, cardiovascular diseases and other pathogenic conditions [8, 9]. In order to exert the biological benefits of spices chemical compounds it needs to bioavailable which depends various factors like nature and composition of food matrices and health status of human being [11, 12]. However, one of the major challenges of most of the spice phytochemicals is poor oral bioavailability. Several strategies such as nanoparticles, polymers, and liposomes inclusion have been adopted to improve the bioavailabilities of phytochemicals. Moreover, in most of the cases the health benefits of spices are attributed to the isolated and/or synergistic biological activities of phytochemicals present in the spices [13, 14]. Novel formulations and supplements have been developed using the extracts of spice phytochemicals for multiple health benefits following synergistic effect. This chapter gives and overview of bioactive compounds and their potential health benefits such as antioxidant activities, anti-inflammatory activities, antidiabetic, and anticancer activities by some selective spices such as turmeric, garlic, ginger, onion, chili, cinnamon, and black peppers.

2. Bioactive compounds and health benefits of spices

2.1 Turmeric (*Curcuma longa* L)

2.1.1 Bioactive compounds

Turmeric is an orange-yellow-colored rhizomes which has been used as spice and health care additives since the ancient times. Turmeric is rich in polyphenolic compounds. Curcumin is the major polyphenolic compounds in turmeric followed by demethoxycurcumin and bisdemethoxycurcumin. Some other bioactive compounds found in the rhizome of turmeric are α-turmerone, and β-turmerone [15, 16]. Moreover, turmeric contains volatile compounds like camphor, eucalyptol, β-pinene phenyl propionoids, monoterpenes, sesquiterpenes, α-pinene, camphene, α-phellandrene, 3-carene, β-cymene, β-elemene, α-santalene, caryophyllene, α-farnesene, zingiberene, β-cedrene, α-bisabolol, and β-sesquiphellandrene [15, 16].

2.1.2 Antioxidant activities

Various research studies indicated that turmeric possesses moderate to strong antioxidant activities due to the presence of curcuminoids. The antioxidant potential of curcuminoids arises from its structural composition with functional groups including the β-diketo group and phenyl rings containing varying amounts of hydroxyl and methoxy substituents [15, 16]. Due to its potential antioxidant activities curcumins have been reported to have significant role in maintaining oxidative stress mediated pathological conditions [15–17]. It also protects biomembranes against peroxidative damage via scavenging of free radical activities involved in the peroxidation [15–17]. For very long-time number research is carried out to oversee the mechanism of antioxidant activities of curcumin. Jovanovic et al. reported that the central methylenic group of curcumin can donate H- rather than from the phenolic group [18]. However, some other studies proposed that phenolic group of curcumin better H donor to act as strong free radical scavenger [19, 20]. In addition to the free radical scavenging pathways curcuminoids displayed antioxidant activities stimulating the activities of antioxidant enzymes such as glutathione peroxidase, superoxide dismutase, and catalase [15, 16, 21]. Moreover, curcumin displayed antioxidant activities by preventing the inhibition of Nrf2, NFκB translocation and IκB degradation which are involved in regulating antioxidant activity [15–17].

2.1.3 Anti-inflammatory activities

Numerous *in vitro* and *in vivo* research studies on anti-inflammatory activity of curcumin derivatives reported that curcumin exhibited anti-inflammatory activities by interacting with various biomolecules related to inflammation such as cyclooxygenase 2, phospholipase, lipoxygenase, leukotrienes, thromboxane, prostaglandins, nitric oxide, collagenase, elastase, hyaluronidase, monocyte chemoattractant protein-1 (MCP-1), interferon-inducible protein, tumor necrosis factor (TNF), and interleukin-12 (IL-12) [15, 16, 21, 22]. Curcumin suppresses the regulation of proinflammatory interleukins (IL-1, −2, −6, −8, and − 12), cytokines (tumor necrosis factor-alpha (TNF-α), monocyte chemoattractant protein-1) by causing down-regulation of janus kinase and signal transducer and activator of transcription (JAK/STAT) signaling pathway which can contribute to the anti-inflammatory activity in the brain [15, 16, 21–23].

2.1.4 Anticancer activities

Curcumins have been shown to prevent carcinogenesis by affecting many phases of cancer including development, transformation, invasion, angiogenesis, and metastasis [15, 24]. It is effective for decreasing or preventing various cancer types such as colon, pancreas, breast, prostates, and lung cancers [15, 24–28]. Curcumin has been reported to suppress the growth of tumor cells via cell proliferation pathway (cyclin D1, c-myc), cell survival pathway (Bcl-2, Bcl-xL, cFLIP, XIAP, and cIAP1), caspase activation pathway (caspase -8, -3, and -9), tumor suppressor pathway (p53, p21), death receptor pathway (DR4, DR5), protein kinase pathway, adenosine monophosphate-activated protein kinase (AMPK) pathway [27–30].

2.1.5 Antidiabetic effect

Curcumin exhibited antidiabetic activities by decreasing hepatic glucose production, suppressing inflammatory response stemming from hyperglycemia, increasing

GLUT2, GLUT3, and GLUT4 gene expression, increasing glucose intake of cells, and activating AMPK [31]. It could decrease blood glucose decreasing insulin resistance. Curcumin also played significant role to control of hyperglycemia by downregulating alpha-glucosidase and alpha-amylase activity [32]. After being treated diabetic rats with curcumin the glucose tolerance and insulin sensitivity of diabetic rats were enhanced [33].

2.1.6 Gastrointestinal effect

Research study showed that abdominal pain or irritation and Irritable Bowel Syndrome (IBS) are reduced by the administration of *C. longa* extract [34]. Curcumin could ameliorate the gastric damage, recover from gastric mucosal injury, reduce the leucocyte adherences, intracellular adherence molecule1, and tumor necrosis factor (TNF)-α formation in nonsteroidal anti-inflammatory drugs (NSAIDs)-induced gastropathy in rats [28].

2.1.7 Cardiovascular health

Administration of curcuminoids regulate triglycerides, cholesterol, and other lipids in the bloodstream which are the risk factors for cardiovascular disorders [15, 35, 36]. In an animal model study mice fed with the turmeric added diet possessed 20% less blockage of the arteries in comparison with that mouse fed with the American diet [37]. In another investigation, rabbits fed with turmeric enriched diet to treat the atherosclerosis disease. It has been reported that the cholesterol, and triglycerides levels have been reduced in the turmeric treated rabbits [38]. Turmeric contains antioxidants that inhibit damage to cholesterol and thus provided a protective activity against atherosclerosis [38].

2.2 Garlic (*Allium sativum* L.)

2.2.1 Bioactive compounds

Garlic is composed of various bioactive compounds covering polysaccharides, organosulfur compounds, saponins, and phenolic compounds [39–42]. Among them the major bioactive compound of garlic are organosulfur compounds, such as diallyl thiosulfonate (allicin), diallyl sulfide (DAS), diallyl disulfide (DADS), diallyl trisulfide (DATS), E/Z-ajoene, S-allyl-cysteine (SAC), and S-allyl-cysteine sulfoxide (alliin) which are responsible for numerous health benefits [43]. Several phenolic compounds such as resorcylic acid, pyrogallol, gallic acid, rutin, protocatechuic acid, as well as quercetin are significant bioactive compounds contribute to biochemical properties [39–43].

2.2.2 Antioxidant activity

Various in vitro studies revealed that garlic extract exhibited antioxidant activities in DPPH, ABTS, FRAP, H_2O_2 scavenging assay, and Fe^{2+} chelating assays [42–44]. It was reported that storage of garlic for long days accumulated higher level of antioxidant than the fresh ones and shows higher antioxidant activities. However, the postharvest conditions and storage time garlic affect the extent of their antioxidant activities. Usually, fresh garlic had a stronger antioxidant activity than cooked and fermented garlic [45]. Other than radical scavenging activities earlier studies of garlic extract showed that antioxidant activities of garlic compounds resulted the expression of some antioxidant enzymes, such as heme oxygenase-1 (HO-1), stimulating the activities of antioxidant enzyme activities, and the regulation of the Nrf2-ARE pathway [46]. Earlier studies indicated that garlic saponins scavenge intracellular reactive oxygen species (ROS) and also protect DNA damage induced by H_2O_2.

2.2.3 Anti-inflammatory activities

Garlic offers anti-inflammatory benefits because of the presence of various diallyl disulfide compound that controls the effects of pro-inflammatory cytokines [47, 48]. Garlic has great potential to treat inflammatory diseases including arthritis in humans [49]. *In vitro* and *in vivo* experiments studies reported that garlic could inhibit inflammation mainly by inhibiting inflammatory mediators, such as NO, TNF-α, and IL-1 [47].

2.2.4 Anticancer activities

Several research studies indicated that garlic organosulfur compounds displayed anticancer activities via the inhibiting the cell proliferation and inducing apoptosis of cancer cells both in human culture as well as animal models [50]. Garlic active constituents could protect against diverse cancers, such as colorectal, lung, gastric, and bladder cancers [51–53]. These compounds showed anticancer activities by suppressing cell growth and proliferation and exhibited an anti-proliferative effect on human cancer cell lines, such as liver (HepG2), colon (Caco2), prostate (PC-3), and breast (MCF-7) cancer cells [39]. Moreover, the anticancer properties of garlic occur via the regulation of carcinogen metabolism, induction of apoptosis, suppression of angiogenesis, and inhibition of invasion and migration [39, 44].

2.2.5 Antidiabetic activity

Garlic supplements were effective in the management of type 2 diabetes mellitus. Garlic has been shown to reduce pancreatic cell injury, oxidative stress, and pathological changes in streptomycin-induced type 1 diabetic rats. Results from the meta-analysis performed on 768 patients with type 2 diabetes mellitus in nine randomized controlled trials showed that garlic supplements significantly reduced fructosamine and glycosylated hemoglobin [54]. Fermented garlic products had certain positive effects on obesity by inhibiting lipogenesis and regulating lipid metabolism [55].

2.2.6 Antimicrobial activities

Several research study reported that garlic extract showed antibacterial activities by inhibiting the growth of *Staphylococcus aureus*, *Escherichia coli*, and *Bacillus subtilis* [56]. Garlic extract compounds also showed antifungal activities by inhibiting the growth of fungus *Penicillium funiculosum* [57]. In a clinical trial, the treatment of raw garlic inhibited *Helicobacter pylori* in the stomach of patients with *H. pylori* infection [58].

2.2.7 Cardiovascular protection

Multiple research studies indicated that consumption of garlic and its compounds effectively reduced blood pressure, total cholesterol, low-density lipoprotein cholesterol, and cardiovascular complexities [59]. Garlic derived compounds reduced oxidative stress, increased the regulation of endothelial nitric oxide (NO), and stimulated the production of the vascular gasotransmitter hydrogen sulfide (H_2S), and inhibited the angiotensin converting enzyme [39, 60]. These could affect to induce smooth muscle cell relaxation, vasodilation, and lower hypertension.

2.3 Ginger (*Zingiber officinale* Rosc)

2.3.1 Bioactive compounds

Major bioactive compounds of gingers comprise of phenolic and terpene compounds [61]. Among the phenolic compounds gingerols, shogaols, and paradols are found to be major ones. In fresh ginger gingerols are available in different forms such as 6-gingerol, 8-gingerol, and 10-gingerol [62, 63]. Ginger is dried and stored for long time after harvesting for commercial purpose. During long time storage gingerols are transformed into corresponding shogaols and shogaols transformed into paradols [64]. Ginger contains several phenolic and terpenoids compounds such as quercetin, zingerone, gingerenone-A, 6-dehydrogingerdione, β-bisabolene, α-curcumene, zingiberene, β-farnesene, and β-sesquiphellandrene, which are major part of ginger essential oils [62]. Also, polysaccharides, lipids, organic acids, and raw fibers are other important compounds available in ginger.

2.3.2 Antioxidant activity

Several *in vitro* studies on antioxidant activities of ginger have been investigated using (FRAP), 2,2-diphenyl-1-picrylhydrazyl (DPPH), and 2,2- azinobis-(3-ethylbenzothiazoline-6-sulfonic acid) (ABTS) assays [64]. Number of *in vitro* antioxidant activity assays have also been investigated by using various cell models and provided underlying mechanisms of antioxidant action [62, 64]. For example, ginger extract showed antioxidant effects in human chondrocyte cells, with oxidative stress mediated by interleukin-1β (IL-1β) [65]. It stimulated the expression of several antioxidant enzymes and reduced the generation of ROS and lipid peroxidation [62]. Additionally, ginger extract could reduce the production of ROS in human fibrosarcoma cells with H_2O_2-induced oxidative stress [66]. Ginger and its bioactive compounds (such as 6-shogaol) exhibited antioxidant activity via the nuclear factor erythroid 2-related factor 2 (Nrf2) signaling pathway [67]. 6-shogaol increased intracellular glutathione/glutathione disulfide (GSH/GSSG) and upregulated Nrf2 target gene expression in human colon cancer cells [68].

2.3.3 Anticancer activities

Ginger possessed promising potential for inhibiting the proliferation of multiple cancer cells, such as cancers of the colon, liver, lung, and cervix [62, 69, 70]. Treatment of the human colorectal cancers such as HCT-116, H-1299, and LoVo cells with 6-gingerol and 10-gingerol reduced the cell viability and induced apoptosis in a dose-dependent manner [71, 72]. Ginger extract was responsible for the activating transcription factor 3 (ATF3)-mediated apoptosis induction in human colorectal cancer cells [73]. 6-shogaol and 10-shogaol displayed anti-cancer potentials against human promyelocytic leukemia of HL-60 cells [51]. The anticancer effects of 6-gingerol, 10-gingerol, 6-shogaol, and 10-shogaol acted as prominent bioactive compounds for anticancer activities that used multiple molecular targets such as NF-κB, TNF-α, PI3K, Caspase-3 [62, 69–72].

2.3.4 Antidiabetic activity

Ginger has been examined for blood glucose lowering effect and improvement in metabolic disorders in diabetic animals and humans. Streptozotocin (STZ) is considered as a diabetogenic agent due to its ability to selectively destroy the β-cells of the pancreatic islets. When STZ rat were administered by ginger extract their blood glucose levels were decreased and the body weights was improved [52]. Oral administration of aqueous ginger extract increased the serum insulin levels and insulin sensitivity in the alloxan-induced and insulin-resistant diabetic rats [53]. Wei et al. demonstrated that 6-shogaol, 6-paradol, and 8-paradol showed antidiabetic activities by improving glucose utilization in both the adipocytes and muscle cells in high-fat diet (HFD) fed rats [74].

2.3.5 Gastrointestinal activity

After oral administration of 6-gingerol in rats it showed high tissue partitioning and distribution in the brain, heart, lung, spleen, liver, kidney, stomach, and small intestinal tissue. However, the highest concentration were detected in the gastrointestinal tract [75]. That is why ginger is commonly used to treating gastrointestinal diseases since ancient times and 6-gingerol and its analogues compounds are reported to be responsible for the gastro-intestinal pharmacological activity [62].

2.4 Onion (*Allium cepa* L.)

2.4.1 Bioactive compounds

Quercetin and its glucoside are major compounds found in onions [76]. Other secondary metabolites are saponins, flavonoids, and phytosterols, polysaccharides, organosulfur compounds-onionin A and cysteine sulfoxides and various phenolic compounds [76, 77]. Anthocyanins are also found in onion. Onion contains three types of alkyl cysteine sulfoxides (ACSO), 1 trans- (±S-1-propenyl-L-cysteine sulfOxide (PECSO), 2(±S-methyl-L-cysteine sulfoxide (MCSO), and 3(±S-propyl-L-cysteine sulfoxide (PCS) [76, 78].

2.4.2 Antioxidant activity

Onion is one of the great sources of natural antioxidant comprising quercetin, kaempferol, and anthocyinns, and some other polyphenolic compounds [76, 77]. Numerous in vitro studies adopting DPPH, ABTS, ORAC and TEAC assay suggested the strong antioxidant potential of onion [78]. Several human trial and other animal model studies demonstrated that the antioxidant role against oxidative stress and lipid peroxidation in various body organs [79, 80]. Due to their antioxidant activities onion and its extract compounds reduced risk of neurodegenerative disorders [81]. Onion decreased lipid peroxidation and enhanced activities of antioxidant enzymes such as SOD, (superoxide dismutase), CAT (catalase), GSH (glutathione), GPx(glutathione peroxidase), TrxR (Thioredoxin reductase), SDH, GST and GR [80].

2.4.3 Anti-inflammatory activity

Presence of polyphenolic compounds in onion such as tannin, flavonoids, anthocyanin, saponin contributed to anti-inflammatory activities [76, 81]. Onion exhibited anti-inflammatory activities due to presence of high level of quercetin and some organosulfur compounds [76, 81]. Quercetin exhibited anti-inflammatory activities by reducing the production of inflammatory cytokines such as IL-1, IL-4, and TNF-α and inhibited the proliferation and activity of lymphocytes [82, 83]. Moreover Umoh et al. showed that quercetin enriched red onion decreased inflammation by inhibition of NF-κB, MARK and STAT-1 [83]. Organosulfur compounds such as thiosulfinates and cepaenes exhibited anti-inflammatory properties by inhibiting the actions of COX and LOX enzymes in arachidonic acid metabolic pathways [84].

2.4.4 Anticancer activities

Earlier research studies indicated that moderate consumption of onions may have a role in the prevention of a wide range of different cancers, including colorectal, breast, lung, stomach, liver, brain, renal, bladder, ovarian, esophagus, and laryngeal cancer [61, 85–87]. Several epidemiological studies reported that due to the high level of flavonoids in onion it protect from developing lung cancers [85]. Numerous research studies demonstrated that the organosulfur compounds in onions are responsible for their anticarcinogenic properties in cell experiments, animals and human trials [86]. Another class of anticarcinogenic compounds of highly abundant is organoselenium compounds [76].

2.4.5 Antimicrobial activity

It has been evident form the earlier research that onion extract possesses antibacterial and antifungal properties [87–90]. *In vitro* studies indicated that aqueous extract of onion inhibited growth of *E. coli*, *Serratia marcescens, Steptococcus species, Acetobacillus odontolyticus, Pseudomonas aeruginosa and Salmonella Typhosa, Streptococcus mutans, Streptococcus sobrinus, Porphyromonas gingivalis and Prevotella intermedia* [87–92]. A petroleum ether extract of onion inhibited the in vitro growth of *Clotridium paraputrificum and S. aureus* [76].

2.4.6 Anti-diabetic activity

Several research studies reported that onion and its extract are strongly associated with managing diabetes and reducing diabetic complications [93–95]. Several animal model studies also reported that onions play significant role in lowering blood sugar levels in fasting diabetic rats [94]. Quercetin from onion inhibited the action of digestive enzymes α-glucosidase and induce hypoglycemia [96]. It also reduced insulin resistance by increasing adiponectin which is responsible for carbohydrate digestion [96]. Quercetin also protected pancreatic islets against oxidative damage by acting through phosphorylation of extracellular signal-regulated kinase (ERK) [97]. Quercetin showed a significant increase in protection against DNA damage from hydrogen peroxide on human diabetic lymphocytes [98]. Sulfur containing compounds such as S-methly cysteine sulpoxide and S-allyl cysteine sulpoxide controlled the blood glucose and lipids in serum and tissues and normalized the activities of liver hexokinase, glucose 6-phosphatase and HMG CoA reductase and increase the level of insulin in blood [99]. Earlier study indicated that administration of onion extract to human reduced LDL-C, waist circumference, and total cholesterol in blood [100–102].

2.5 Chili (*Capsicum annuum* L.)

2.5.1 Bioactive compounds

Capsaicinoids, an acid amide of vanillylamine with C9-C12 branched fatty acid chain is the major compound of chili that confers the characteristic pungency [103]. Other major isomers of capsacins are dihydrocapsaicin, nordihydrocapsaicin, homocapsaicin, and homodihydrocapsaicin [103–105]. Other bioactive valuable bioactive compounds such as polyphenols (phenolic acids, apigenin, luteolin, quercetin, catechins, anthocyanins and proanthocyanidins), steroids, saponins, anthroquinones, carotenoids, terpenoids and alkaloids are highly abundant in chili peppers [103–106].

2.5.2 Antioxidant activity

As chili pepper contains high level of vitamin C, E, anthocyanin, and phenolic compounds it showed strong antioxidant activities *in vitro, in vivo,* and clinical studies [103–107]. From earlier research studies it was demonstrated a positive correlation between phenolic content and antioxidant potential with strong radical scavenging activities in ABTS, DPPH, and FRAP assays [103]. Various *in vivo* studies indicated antioxidant activities by mitigating oxidative stress in various tissues or organs [104–106].

2.5.3 Anti-inflammatory activity

It has been shown that capsaicin could reduce inflammations in different animal models and human trials. Capsacin has been reported to have anti-inflammatory activities by inhibiting the NO, IL-6, and TNF-α in LPS-induced in RAW 264.7 cells [107, 108]. Capsaicin reduced the inflammatory responses by inhibiting the pro-inflammatory cytokines such as interleukin 1β (IL-1β) and tumor nuclear factor-kappa (NF-κ) [109]. Capsaicin could be used as analgesic since it could induce inflammatory effects in adipose tissues [110].

2.5.4 Anticancer properties

Chili phytochemicals has been reported to trigger apoptosis of various cancerous cell lines including skin cancer, colon cancer, bladder cancer, breast cancer, prostate cancer and lung cancer in human and some other experimental animal models [111–120]. Capsaicin exhibited inhibitory effects against cancer initiation, promotion, progression, and metastasis. It has been found that capsaicin could inhibit nuclear factor-kappa (NF-κ) activation in prostate cancer cells. In some cases, capsaicin could alter the expression of several genes involved in cancer growth process. For example, capsaicin down-regulated Bcl-2 (B-cell lymphoma 2) expression during the growth of skin cancer in mouse [113, 115]. Capsaicin induced p53 phosphorylation at the Ser-15 residue and activated the apoptosis of cancer cells [119]. In vitro studies revealed that capsaicin could inhibit the growth of blood cancer by inhibiting human T-cell leukemia virus type 1 [120].

2.5.5 Antimicrobial activity

It has been demonstrated that capsaicinoids and other phenolic compounds inhibited growth of microorganism like bacteria, yeasts, and fungi [121]. Capsaicin could inactivate the virus binding proteins and prevent their replication [121]. Previous reports supported that capsaicin showed strong antimicrobial activities against *Streptococcus pyogenes, E. coli, S. aureus, Proteus mirabilis, Proteus vulgaris, P. aeruginosa, Enterobacter aerogenes and S. mutans*. Bell pepper extract inhibited the *Listeria monocytogenes, Salmonella typhimurium, S. aureus,* and *Bacillus cereus* including few foodborne bacteria *Salmonella typgimurium* [122].

2.5.6 Anti-diabetic activity

Chili pepper imparted antidiabetic activity by their potential inhibition capacities of α-amylase and α-glucosidase activities which has a significant effect in carbohydrate metabolism [123]. It has been reported that consumption of chili pepper reduces the glucose absorption in the intestine and controls post-prandial rise of glucose [124]. Administration of capsaicin to rats lowered blood glucose levels and increased blood insulin level [125].

2.5.7 Cardiovascular activity

Capsaicin promoted vascular health by increasing nitric oxide (NO) production and reducing inflammatory responses. It also reduced low-density lipoprotein (LDL) levels, increased high-density lipoprotein (HDL) levels, and reduced oxidative stress levels in various tissues [126]. Capsaicin could lower low-density lipoprotein cholesterol (LDL-C), plasma cholesterol, and inhibits LPS-induced IL-1β, IL-6 and TNF-α production in a time- and dose-dependent [127–129].

2.6 Cinnamon bark (*Cinnamomum cassia*)

2.6.1 Bioactive compounds

The major phytochemical in cinnamon bark is cinnamaldehyde. Some other bioactive compounds of essential oils in cinnamon bark are cinnamic acid, coumarin, cinnamyl alcohol, and 2-methoxycinnamaldehyde [130]. Cinnamon bark also contain terpenoids such as oxygenated sesquiterpenes, oxygenated monoterpenes, sesquiterpene hydrocarbon [130–132]. In addition to essential oils and terpenoids cinnamon bark consist of guaiacol, benzenepropanal, cis-cinnamaldehyde, bornyl acetate, acetophenone, geranyl acetate, tetradecanal. Oxygenated monoterpenes are eucalyptol, linalool, borneol, L-α-terpineol, benzaldehyde, anethole, and eugenol. Some of the sesquiterpene hydrocarbons are α-cubebene, copaene, β-caryophyllene, α-muurolene, trans-α-bergamotene, α-humulene, α-amorphene, 1 s-cis-calamenene, calarene, cedrene, and β-cadinene [130–132].

2.6.2 Antioxidant activity

Cinnamon is considered as one of the most important flavored spices with strong antioxidant activity [133]. Different extraction method has been applied to investigate the antioxidant activities of cinnamon bark extract. For example Yang et al. [134]

investigated the antioxidant activity of ethanol and aqueous extracts of cassia bark to evaluate its antioxidant activity by the DPPH and ABTS radical scavenging activity. Both extracts reported to possess strong antioxidant activities however ethanolic extract possessed higher than the aqueous extract [134]. The polyphenolic extracts of cinnamon bark reduced oxidative stress in a dose-dependent manner through inhibition of 5-lipooxygenase enzyme [135].

2.6.3 Anti-inflammatory activities

Numerous research studies reported that cinnamon essential oil possess anti-inflammatory activities and have been used in soothing and numbing for joint aches and pain [136, 137]. On human dermal fibroblast system, a model of chronic inflammation and fibrosis, cinnamon (*Cinnamomum zeylanicum*) bark essential oil (CBEO) significantly inhibited the production of several inflammatory biomarkers such as vascular cell adhesion molecule-1, intercellular cell adhesion molecule-1, monocyte chemoattractant protein-1, interferon gamma induced protein 10 [138]. Cinnamon extract also showed significant reduction in both IL-6 and TNF-α level on Lipopolysaccharide (LPS)-induced Interlukin-6 (IL-6) and Tumor Necrosis Factor-α (TNF-α) which indicates anti-inflammatory effect [136–138].

2.6.4 Antidiabetic effect

Available *in vitro* and *in vivo* evidence demonstrated that cinnamon confers health benefits in relation to hypoglycaemic activity [139, 140]. Consumption of cinnamon bark reported to have antidiabetic activities as it showed improvements in fasting blood glucose and lipid profile after consumption [139]. *In vivo* studies on cinnamon extract showed that it could improve insulin action via enhancing glucose uptake [141]. The cinnamon bark extract could reduce the blood glucose level by decreasing the carbohydrate absorption in the small intestine [142]. Another *in vivo* study demonstrated that administration of cassia bark extracts the intestinal glycosidase activity was reduced, whereas the serum insulin level and HDL-cholesterol level are increased [142]. Compiling the human studies of 2003–2018 concerning the glycemic profiles of individuals with type II diabetes mellitus showed that fasting blood glucose reduced from 12.9 to 52.2 mg/dL and HbA1c from 0.27 to 0.83%, after moderate consumption of cinnamon extract [143]. Some meta-analysis also indicated that cinnamon powder intake decreased fasting blood glucose and HbA1c [144]. Methylhydroxychalcone polymer (MHCP) in cinnamon bark reported as effective mimetic of insulin which could activate glycogen synthase and inhibit actions of glycogen synthase kinase-3b as well as insulin receptor phosphorylation homologous [145].

2.6.5 Cardiovascular health

Previous research studies reported that cinnamon could reduce the risk of cardiovascular diseases and its complications such as cardiac ischemia, cardiac hypertrophy, and myocardial infarction [130]. Cinnamaldehyde and cinnamic acid are among the main cinnamon compounds with protective effects on cardiovascular diseases through different molecular mechanisms [130]. Cinnamaldehyde played crucial role in the cardiovascular system like vasorelaxation and reduction in blood pressure [146]. Cinnamaldehyde could protect human umbilical vein endothelial cells from the oxidative stress via stimulation of the nuclear factor erythroid

2-related factor signaling pathway [147]. Cinnamaldehyde prevents the progression of hypertension in insulin deficiency and insulin resistance due to its insulinotropic properties [148]. Using Wistar rats of induced metabolic syndrome it was found that cinnamon altered the body composition in association with improved insulin sensitivity [149].

2.7 Black pepper (*Piper nigrum*)

2.7.1 Bioactive compounds

Black pepper is composed of carbohydrate, proteins, fibers, fats, minerals, and aromatic phytochemicals. Among the phytochemicals piperine is the major bioactive compound that gives the pungent flavor to black pepper [150]. Other volatile flavor compounds in black pepper are terpenes, α- and β-pinene, myrcene, α-phellandrene, limonene, linalool, methyl propanal, methylbutanal, butyric acid, methylpyrazine and methoxypyrazines [150–153].

2.7.2 Antioxidant activity

It is evident from earlier research investigations that piperine from black pepper exhibited antioxidant potential and reduce lipid peroxidation [150, 151]. and *in vitro* study demonstrated that the antioxidant potential of piperine could be resulted by trapping superoxide and hydroxyl free radicals, retarding lipid peroxidation, and inhibiting human lipoxygenase activities [151]. Piperine acted as potent antioxidant by reducing thiobarbituric acid-reactive substances and maintaining superoxide dismutase, catalase, glutathione peroxidase, glutathione- S-transferase, and glutathione levels [153].

2.7.3 Anti-inflammatory activities

Number research studies demonstrated analgesic and anti-inflammatory activity of piperine and black pepper extracts using various animal model and clinical studies [154]. Piperine also acted as useful gastrointestinal anti-inflammatory agent. Moreover, it showed anti-inflammatory effects on interleukin 1β (IL-1β)-stimulated fibroblast-like synoviocytes [155]. Piperine effectively treated asthma by inhibiting airway inflammation due to suppression of cytokines (IL-4, IL-5, IL-13) and enhanced TGF-β gene expression in the lungs in a murine model system [156].

2.7.4 Antidiabetic activity

Various animal model and human trial studies reported hypoglycemic effect of piperine. Administration of peiperine to hyperglycemic rats reported that it could reduce lipid peroxidation, hyperglycemic activities, and showed antioxidant activities. With Alloxan-induced diabetic rats it was reported piperine could reduce the blood glucose level [157]. Also, it was reported to enhance the serum cholesterol, serum liver cholesterol concentration, and hepatic cholesterol-7α-hydroxylase level after administration of piperine. Several research studies demonstrated that piperine could be used as bioavailability enhancer for other phytochemicals to receive better health beneficial properties. For examples, co-administration of curcumin with piperine was found to decrease the levels of total cholesterol (TC), triglyceride (TG) and low-density lipoprotein cholesterol in the serum and liver in higher extent compared with administration of curcumin alone [158].

2.7.5 Cardiovascular health

Piperine played critical role on cardiovascular disease by mediating oxidation status, lipid metabolism, and inflammation [150]. Piperine inhibited development of lipid droplet, oxidized low density lipoprotein uptake in macrophages, retarded lipid peroxidation, induce cholesterol efflux from macrophages [159]. It has been reported to show antihypertensive, antithrombosis effect, and protect arterial stenosis through retarding vascular smooth muscle cell proliferation [150].

3. Bioaccebilities and bioavailabilities of bioactive compounds

In order to receive optimum health benefits from the bioactive compounds of foods, they have to be released from the food matrix and be bioaccessible in the gastrointestinal tract, then undergo metabolism and reach the target tissue of action. Finally, this phenomenon determines the bioavailability of the biomolecules before showing its bioefficacy [11]. Bioavailability is a complex process that involves several different phases like liberation, absorption, distribution, metabolism, and elimination. There are several factors that could affect bioavailability of bioactive compounds such as nature of food matrices, molecular structures, metabolizing enzymes, type of food processing and cooking methods [160]. Improvement in the bioavailability of food component could enhance bioefficacy of bioactive compounds. Several technologies have been developed to improve the bioavailability such as structural modifications, colloidal systems, entrapped in liposome, inclusion complexation, nanoencapsulation polymer encapsulation, and emulsion [161].

As aforementioned curcumin has many potential health benefits such as anti-inflammatory, antioxidant, anticancer, antiviral, and neurotrophic activity. However, due to its insolubility in water, the poor intestinal absorption, structural instability limits the potential therapeutic and nutritional benefits [24]. Therefore, efforts have been directed to develop curcumin formulations with greater bioavailability and systemic tissue distribution [162]. Among them modification of curcumin's chemical structure, conjugation of curcumin with lipid molecules, nanoparticle encapsulated curcumin, additive matrices with piperine are some of major approaches [162]. In a study polylactic-co-glycolic acid (PLGA) and PLGA-polyethylene glycol (PEG) (PLGA-PEG) blend nanoparticles containing curcumin in rats and it was found that compared to the curcumin aqueous suspension, the PLGA and PLGA-PEG nanoparticles increased the curcumin bioavailability by 15.6- and 55.4-fold, respectively [163]. Yu et al. [164] developed a food grade curcuminoid organogel using Span 20 and medium chain triacylglycerols with high bioaccessibility and high loading of curcumin. Among the biological active components of garlic, sulfur compounds especially allicin have antioxidant, anticancer and antibacterial functions and thus are considered as the main pharmacological active components in garlic. However, it was demonstrated it suffers from instability, low aqueous solubility, strong gastro-intestinal irritation and low bioavailability. To circumvent this issue nanotechnology and other embedding technology have been used. The bioactive compounds extracted from garlic were incorporated into biodegradable and biocompatible nanoparticles such as liposomes, nano-emulsions, solid lipid nanoparticles (SLN), micelles, nano-spheres and nano-capsules, protein-based nanoparticles, biopolymeric particles, and phyto-phospholipid complexes [165]. These techniques could enhance their stability, aqueous solubility, bioavailability, target specificity and circulation time. Garlic oil nanoemulsion generated with ultrasonic emulsification could improve efficacy and reduce toxicity in treating or preventing dyslipidemia [166]. Garlic Essential Oil (GEO) have been nanoencapsulated with chitosan and persian gum as wall materials which improved stability and dispersibility [167]. GEO have been embedded in liposomes formed by lecithin (LT) and β-sitosterol (β-S) and improved the bioavailability upto 51% [168]. [6]-gingerol is the key component of ginger that provides several health benefits. However due to its poor solubility in water coupled it results in low bioavailability. Several strategies such as gingerol incorporated nanoparticles, micelles, emulsions, solid dispersion, liposomes have been prepared to improve the bioavailability. The formulation of [6]-gingerol like proliposomes prepared through modified thin-film dispersion method, which were physicochemically stable with narrow size distribution and improved bioavailability and antitumor activity [169]. Another formulation was prepared by using solid dispersion of ginger extract with hydrophilic polymer, hydroxypropyl cellulose that improved 5 fold higher gingerol bioavailability [170, 171]. Quercetin, the major compound of onion also suffers low availability due to its poor solubility [172]. Several formulations been prepared to improve the poor solubility of quercetin. For example, β-cyclodextrin inclusion complex of quercetin, nano-system quercetin prepared using Eudragit®E and polyvinyl alcohol (PVA), solid lipid nanoparticles of quercetin using soybean lecithin, Tween 80, and PEG 400 increased the poor solubility and good dispersion of quercetin [173–176]. Similarly, capsaicin the major bioactive compounds of pepper suffer some limitations for the short half-life, low bioavailability, burning sensation and skin irritation etc. Several strategies have been applied to improve the delivery of capsaicin such as emerging micro and nanotechnologies to encapsulate capsaicin to liposomes eg: phosphatidylcholine (PC) liposomes, microemulsion, solid-lipid nanoparticle, polymeric carriers such as micelle (eg capsaicin with polyvinylpyrrolidone (PVP)/sodium cholate/phospholipid mixed micellar system, dendrimers (dendrimers formed from oleoyl chloride, Polyethylene glycol (PEG) 400, and triethylamine, and polymersome), Inorganic carriers (metal nanoparticles egcapsaicin-capped silver nanoparticles, carbon spheres) [177–180].

4. Conclusions

Herb and spices are receiving continued interest in food industry because of their numerous health benefits from providing nutrition and maintaining healthy lives. Due to the presence several group of phytochemicals comprising diverse group of phytochemicals including polyphenols, carotenoids, alkaloids, terpenoids, phytosterols, glucosinolates, and many others it protects from chronic diseases like inflammation, diabetes, cancer, Alzheimers, cardiovascular diseases, dementia, and obesities. *In vtro*, *in vivo*, cell culture, and clinical research studies have uncovered the role of these phytochemicals in most of the heath beneficial properties. However, in most of the cases the detail mechanisms are not completely understood. Moreover, depending on the nature of food ingredients and processing of food, nature of eating style greatly affects the bioavailability of active components of spices which in turn affect its bioefficacy. Significant studies indicated the existence of positive health effects from the isolated compounds, e.g. curcumin, quercetin, allicin, gingerol, piperine etc. In some cases, the isolated compounds may not work effectively but combination of one phytochemical with others in food matrices leads to the synergistic effects in biological properties. Thus, combinations of selective phytochemicals may exert multiple functions in the human body after consumption. Using emerging technology of formulation sciences would lead to the development of novel formulations and nutrient supplements to improve the bioefficacy and synergistic effect of spices phytochemicals after consumption.

Author details

Boris Nemzer and Diganta Kalita*
VDF FutureCeuticals, Inc, Momence, IL, USA

*Address all correspondence to: diganta.kalita@futureceuticals.com

References

[1] Tapsell LC, Hemphill I, Cobiac L, Patch CS, Sullivan DR, Fenech M, et al. Health benefits of herbs and spices: The past, the present, the future. Medicinal Journal of Australlia. 2006;**185**:1-24. DOI: 10.5694/j.1326-5377.2006.tb00548.x

[2] Viuda-Martos M, Ruiz-Navajas Y, Fernández-López J, Pérez-Alvarez JA. Spices as functional foods. Critical Reviews in Food Science and Nutrition. 2011;**51**:13-28. DOI: 10.1080/10408390903044271

[3] Achinewhu SC, Ogbonna CC, Hart AD. Chemical composition of indigenous wild herbs, spices, fruits, nuts and leafy vegetables used as food. Plant Foods for Human Nutrition. 1995;**48**(4):341-348. DOI: 10.1007/BF01088493

[4] Guldiken B, Ozkan G, Catalkaya G, Ceylan FD, Ekin Yalcinkaya I, Capanoglu E. Phytochemicals of herbs and spices: Health versus toxicological effects. Food and Chemical Toxicology. 2018;**119**:37-49. DOI: 10.1016/j.fct.2018.05.050

[5] Langhans W. Food components in health promotion and disease prevention. Journal of Agricultural and Food Chemistry. 2018;**66**:2287-2294. DOI: 10.1021/acs.jafc.7b02121

[6] Mandal D, Sarkar T, Chakraborty R. Critical review on nutritional, bioactive, and medicinal potential of spices and herbs and their application in food fortification and nanotechnology. Applied Biochemistry and Biotechnology. 2022;**11**:1-195. DOI: 10.1007/s12010-022-04132-y

[7] Jiang TA. Health benefits of culinary herbs and spices. Journal of AOAC International. 2019;**102**:395

[8] Ahangarpour A, Sayahi M, Sayahi M. The antidiabetic and antioxidant properties of some phenolic phytochemicals: A review study. Diabetes and Metabolic Syndrome. 2019;**13**:854-857. DOI: 10.1016/j.dsx.2018.11.051

[9] Yashin A, Yashin Y, Xia X, Nemzer B. Antioxidant activity of spices and their impact on human health: A review. Antioxidants. 2017;**6**:70. DOI: 10.3390/antiox6030070

[10] Jaime L, Santoyo S. The health benefits of the bioactive compounds in foods. Food. 2021;**10**:325. DOI: 10.3390/foods10020325

[11] Platel K, Srinivasan K. Bioavailability of micronutrients from plant foods: An update. Critical Reviews in Food Science and Nutrition. 2016;**56**:1608-1619. DOI: 10.1080/10408398.2013.781011

[12] Anand P, Kunnumakkara AB, Newman RA, Aggarwal BB. Bioavailability of curcumin: Problems and promises. Molecular Pharmaceutics. 2007;**4**:807-818. DOI: 10.1021/mp700113r

[13] Bag A, Chattopadhyay RR. Evaluation of synergistic antibacterial and antioxidant efficacy of essential oils of spices and herbs in combination. PLoS One. 2015;**10**:e0131321. DOI: 10.1371/journal.pone.0131321

[14] Clark R, Lee J, Seong-Ho L. Synergistic anticancer activity of capsaicin and 3,3′-diindolylmethane in human colorectal cancer. Journal of Agricultural and Food Chemistry. 2015;**63**:4297-4304. DOI: 10.1021/jf506098s

[15] Sharifi-Rad J, El Rayess Y, Rizk AA, Sadaka C, Zgheib R, Zam W,

et al. Turmeric and its major compound curcumin on health: Bioactive effects and safety profiles for food, pharmaceutical, biotechnological and medicinal applications. Frontiers in Pharmacology. 2020;**11**:01021. DOI: 10.3389/fphar.2020.01021

[16] Kocaadam B, Sanlier N. Curcumin, an active component of turmeric (*Curcuma longa*), and its effects on health. Critical Reviews in Food Science and Nutrition. 2017;**57**:2889-2895. DOI: 10.1080/10408398.2015.1077195

[17] Raufa A, Imranb M, Orhanc IE, Bawazeer S. Health perspectives of a bioactive compound curcumin: A review. Trends in Food Science & Technology. 2018;**74**:33-45. DOI: 10.1016/j.tifs.2018.01.016

[18] Jovanovic SV, Steenken S, Boone CW, Simic MG. H-atom transfer is a preferred antioxidant mechanism of curcumin. Journal of American Chemical Society. 1999;**121**:9677-9681. DOI: 10.1021/ja991446m

[19] Priyadarsini KI, Maity DK, Naik GH, Kumar MS, Unnikrishnan MK, Satav JG, et al. Role of phenolic O-H and methylene hydrogen on the free radical reactions and antioxidant activity of curcumin. Free Radical Biology and Medicine. 2003;**35**:475-484. DOI: 10.1016/S0891-5849(03)00325-3

[20] Ak T, Gulcin I. Antioxidant and radical scavenging properties of curcumin. Chemical-Biological Interactions. 2008;**174**:27-37. DOI: 10.1016/j.cbi.2008.05.003

[21] Aggarwal BB, Sung B. Pharmacological basis for the role of curcumin in chronic diseases: An age-old spice with modern targets. Trends in Pharmacological Sciences. 2009;**30**:85-94. DOI: 10.1016/j.tips.2008.11.002

[22] Ghosh S, Banerjee S, Sil PC. The beneficial role of curcumin on inflammation, diabetes and neurodegenerative disease: A recent update. Food and Chemical Toxicology. 2015;**83**:111-124

[23] Kim HY, Park EJ, Joe EH, Jou I. Curcumin suppresses Janus kinase-STAT inflammatory signaling through activation of Src homology 2 domain-containing tyrosine phosphatase 2 in brain microglia. Journal of Immunology. 2003;**171**(11):6072-6079. DOI: 10.4049/jimmunol.171.11.6072

[24] Lopresti AL. The problem of curcumin and its bioavailability: Could its gastrointestinal influence contribute to its overall health-enhancing effects? Advanced Nutrition. 2018;**9**:41-50. DOI: 10.1093/advances/nmx011

[25] Sa G, Das T. Anticancer effects of curcumin: Cycle of life and death. Cell Division. 2008;**3**:14. DOI: 10.1186/1747-1028-3-14

[26] He Y, Yue Y, Zheng X, Zhang K, Chen S, Du Z. Curcumin, inflammation, and chronic diseases: How are they linked? Molecules. 2015;**20**:9183-9213. DOI: 10.3390/molecules20059183

[27] Tomeh MA, Hadianamrei R, Zhao X. A review of curcumin and its derivatives as anticancer agents. International Journal of Molecular Sciences. 2019;**20**:1033. DOI: 10.3390/ijms20051033

[28] Kim JH, Gupta SC, Park B, Yadav VR, Aggarwal BB. Turmeric (*Curcuma longa*) inhibits inflammatory nuclear factor (NF)-κB and NF-κB-regulated gene products and induces death receptors leading to suppressed proliferation, induced chemosensitization, and suppressed osteoclastogenesis. Molecular Nutrition and Food Research.

2012;**56**:454-465. DOI: 10.1002/mnfr.201100270

[29] Anto RJ, Mukhopadhyay A, Denning K, Aggarwal BB. Curcumin (diferuloylmethane) induces apoptosis through activation of caspase-8, BID cleavage and cytochrome c release: Its suppression by ectopic expression of Bcl-2 and Bcl-xl. Carcinogenesis. 2002;**23**:143-150. DOI: 10.1093/carcin/23.1.143

[30] Soltani A, Salmaninejad A, Jalili-Nik M, Soleimani A, Javid H, Hashemy SI, et al. 5′-adenosine monophosphate-activated protein kinase: A potential target for disease prevention by curcumin. Journal of Cellular Physiology. 2019;**234**:2241-2251. DOI: 10.1002/jcp.27192

[31] Shehzad A, Qureshi M, Anwar MN, Lee YS. Multifunctional curcumin mediate multitherapeutic effects. Journal of Food Science. 2017;**82**:2006-2015. DOI: 10.1111/1750-3841.13793

[32] Hasaninezhad F, Tavaf Z, Panahi F, Nourisefat M, Khalafi-Nezhad A, Yousefi R. The assessment of antidiabetic properties of novel synthetic curcumin analogues: α-amylase and α-glucosidase as the target enzymes. Journal of Diabetes and Metabolic Disorders. 2020;**19**:1505-1515. DOI: 10.1007/s40200-020-00685-z

[33] Sayeli VK, Shenoy AK. Antidiabetic effect of bio-enhanced preparation of turmeric in streptozotocin-nicotinamide induced type 2 diabetic Wistar rats. Journal of Ayurveda and Integrating Medicine. 2021;**12**:474-479. DOI: 10.1016/j.jaim.2021.04.010

[34] Bundy R, Walker AF, Middleton RW, Booth J. Turmeric extract may improve irritable bowel syndrome symptomology in otherwise healthy adults: A pilot study. Journal of Alternative and Complementary Medicine. 2004;**10**:1015-1018. DOI: 10.1089/acm.2004.10.1015

[35] Panahi Y, Saadat A, Beiraghdar F, Sahebkar A. Adjuvant therapy with bioavailability-boosted curcuminoids suppresses systemic inflammation and improves quality of life in patients with solid tumors: A randomized double-blind placebo-controlled trial. Phytotherapy Research. 2014;**28**:1461-1467. DOI: 10.1002/ptr.5149

[36] Qin S, Huang L, Gong J, Shen S, Huang J, Ren H, et al. Efficacy and safety of turmeric and curcumin in lowering blood lipid levels in patients with cardiovascular risk factors: A meta-analysis of randomized controlled trials. Nutrition Journal. 2017;**16**:68. DOI: 10.1186/s12937-017-0293-y

[37] Miyazawa T, Nakagawa K, Kim SH, Thomas MJ, Paul L, Zingg JM, et al. Curcumin and piperine supplementation of obese mice under caloric restriction modulates body fat and interleukin-1β. Nutritiona and Metabolism. 2018;**15**:12. DOI: 10.1186/s12986-018-0250-6

[38] Ramírez-Tortosa MC, Mesa MD, Aguilera MC, Quiles JL, Baró L, Ramirez-Tortosa CL, et al. Oral administration of a turmeric extract inhibits LDL oxidation and has hypocholesterolemic effects in rabbits with experimental atherosclerosis. Atherosclerosis. 1999;**147**:371-378. DOI: 10.1016/s0021-9150(99)00207-5

[39] Ao S, Cao SY, Xu XY, Gan RY, Tang GY, Corke H, et al. Bioactive compounds and biological functions of garlic (*Allium sativum L.*). Food. 2019;**8**:246. DOI: 10.3390/foods8070246

[40] Szychowski KA, Rybczynska-Tkaczyk K, Gawel-Beben K, Swieca M, Karas M, Jakubczyk AMM,

et al. Characterization of active compounds of dierent garlic (*Allium sativum L.*) cultivars. Polish Journal of Food and Nutrition Scienc.es. 2018;**68**:73-81

[41] Diretto G, Rubio-Moraga A, Argandona J, Castillo P, Gomez-Gomez L, Ahrazem O. Tissue-specific accumulation of sulfur compounds and saponins in different parts of garlic cloves from purple and white ecotypes. Molecules. 2017;**22**:1359. DOI: 10.3390/molecules22081359

[42] Nagella P, Thiruvengadam M, Ahmad A, Yoon JY, Chung IM. Composition of polyphenols and antioxidant activity of garlic bulbs collected from different locations of Korea. Asian Journal of Chemistry. 2014;**26**:897-902. DOI: 10.14233/ajchem.2014.16143A

[43] Kim S, Kim DB, Jin W, Park J, Yoon W, Lee Y, et al. Comparative studies of bioactive organosulphur compounds and antioxidant activities in garlic (*Allium sativum L.*), elephant garlic (*Allium ampeloprasum L.*) and onion (*Allium cepa L.*). Natural Product Research. 2018;**32**:1193-1197. DOI: 10.1080/14786419.2017.1323211

[44] Farhat Z, Freudenheim JL HPA, Mammen MJ, Blair RH, Aga DS, Mu L. Types of garlic and their anticancer and antioxidant activity: A review of the epidemiologic and experimental evidence. European Journal of Nutrition. 2021;**60**:3585-3609. DOI: 10.1007/s00394-021-02482-7

[45] Locatelli DA, Nazareno MA, Fusari CM, Camargo AB. Cooked garlic and antioxidant activity: Correlation with organosulfur compound composition. Food Chemistry. 2017;**220**:219-224. DOI: 10.1016/j.foodchem.2016.10.001

[46] Hiramatsu K, Tsuneyoshi T, Ogawa T, Morihara N. Aged garlic extract enhances heme oxygenase-1 and glutamate-cysteine ligase modifier subunit expression via the nuclear factor erythroid 2-related factor 2-antioxidant response element signaling pathway in human endothelial cells. Nutrition Research. 2016;**36**:143-149. DOI: 10.1016/j.nutres.2015.09.018

[47] Arreola R, Quintero-Fabián S, López-Roa R, Flores-Gutiérrez EO, Reyes-Grajeda JP, Carrera-Quintanar L, et al. Immunomodulation and anti-inflammatory effects of garlic compounds. Journal of Immunology Research. 2015;**2015**:401630. DOI: 10.1155/2015/401630

[48] Butt MS, Sultan MT, Butt MS, Iqbal J. Garlic: Nature's protection against physiological threats. Critical Reviews in Food Science and Nutrition. 2009;**49**:538-551. DOI: 10.1080/10408390802145344

[49] Ban JO, Oh JH, Kim TM, Kim DJ, Jeong JS, Han SB, et al. Anti-inflammatory and arthritic effects of thiacremonone, a novel sulfurcompound isolated from garlic via inhibition of NF-κB. Arthritis Research and Therapy. 2009;**11**:R145. DOI: 10.1186/ar2819

[50] Bagul M, Kakumanu S, Wilson TA. Crude garlic extract inhibits cell proliferation and induces cell cycle arrest and apoptosis of cancer cells in vitro. Journal of Medicinal Food. 2015;**18**:731-737. DOI: 10.1089/jmf.2014.0064

[51] Ching-Chiung W, Lih-Geeng C, Lain-Tze L, Ling-Ling Y. Effects of 6-gingerol, an antioxidant from ginger, on inducing apoptosis in human leukemic HL-60 cells. In Vivo. 2003;**17**:641-645

[52] Eleazu CO, Iroaganachi M, Okafor PN, Ijeh II, Eleazu KC.

Ameliorative potentials of ginger (*Z. officinale roscoe*) on relative organ weights in Streptozotocin induced diabetic rats. International. Journal of Biomedical Science. 2013;**9**:82-90

[53] Iranloye BO, Arikawe AP, Rotimi G, Sogbade AO. Anti-diabetic and anti-oxidant effects of *Zingiber officinale* on alloxan-induced and insulin-resistant diabetic male rats. Nigereian Journal of Physiological Sciences. 2011;**23**(26):89-96

[54] Wang J, Zhang X, Lan H, Wang W. Effect of garlic supplement in the management of type 2 diabetes mellitus (T2DM): A meta-analysis of randomized controlled trials. Food and Nutrition Research. 2017;**61**(1):1377571. DOI: 10.1080/16546628.2017.1377571

[55] Lee HS, Lim WC, Lee SJ, Lee SH, Lee JH, Cho HY. Antiobesity effect of garlic extract fermented by lactobacillus plantarum BL2 in diet-induced obese mice. Journal of Medicinal Food. 2016;**19**(9):823-829. DOI: 10.1089/jmf.2016.3674

[56] Abidullah M, Jadhav P, Sujan SS, Shrimanikandan AG, Reddy CR, Wasan RK. Potential antibacterial efficacy of garlic extract on *Staphylococcus aureus*, *Escherichia coli*, and *Klebsiella pneumoniae*: An in vitro study. Journal of Pharmacy and Bioallied Science. 2021;**13**:S590-S594. DOI: 10.4103/jpbs.JPBS_681_20

[57] Li WR, Shi QS, Liang Q, Huang XM, Chen YB. Antifungal effect and mechanism of garlic oil on *Penicillium funiculosum*. Applied Microbiology and Biotechnology. 2014;**98**:8337-8346. DOI: 10.1007/s00253-014-5919-9

[58] Sivam GP. Protection against *helicobacter pylori* and other bacterial infections by garlic. Journal of Nutrition. 2001;**131**:1106S-1108S. DOI: 10.1093/jn/131.3.1106S

[59] Ried K, Fakler P. Potential of garlic (Allium sativum) in lowering high blood pressure: Mechanisms of action and clinical relevance. Integrated Blood Pressure Control. 2014;**7**:71-82. DOI: 10.2147/IBPC.S51434

[60] Hosseini M, Shafiee SM, Baluchnejadmojarad T. Garlic extract reduces serum angiotensin converting enzyme (ACE) activity in nondiabetic and streptozotocin-diabetic rats. Pathophysiology. 2007;**14**:109-112. DOI: 10.1016/j.pathophys.2007.07.002

[61] Murayyan AI, Manohar CM, Hayward G, Neethirajan S. Antiproliferative activity of Ontario grown onions against colorectal adenocarcinoma cells. Food Research International. 2017;**96**:12-18. DOI: 10.1016/j.foodres.2017.03.017

[62] Mao QQ, Xu XY, Cao SY, Gan RY, Corke H, Beta T, et al. Bioactive compounds and bioactivities of ginger (*Zingiber ocinale roscoe*). Food. 2019;**8**:185. DOI: 10.3390/foods8060185

[63] Yeh H, Chuang C, Chen H, Wan C, Chen T, Lin L. Bioactive components analysis of two various gingers (*Zingiber ocinale roscoe*) and antioxidant effect of ginger extracts. LWT-Food Science and Technology. 2014;**55**:329-334. DOI: 10.1016/j.lwt.2013.08.003

[64] Li Y, Hong Y, Han Y, Wang Y, Xia L. Chemical characterization and antioxidant activities comparison in fresh, dried, stir-frying and carbonized ginger. Journal of Chromatography B. 2016;**1011**:223-232

[65] Hosseinzadeh A, Juybari KB, Fatemi MJ, Kamarul T, Bagheri A,

Tekiyehmaroof N, et al. Protective effect of ginger (*Zingiber officinale* roscoe) extract against oxidative stress and mitochondrial apoptosis induced by interleukin-1β in cultured chondrocytes. Cells, Tissues, Organs. 2017;**204**(5-6):241-250. DOI: 10.1159/000479789

[66] Ballester P, Cerdá B, Arcusa R, Marhuenda J, Yamedjeu K, Zafrilla P. Effect of ginger on inflammatory diseases. Molecules. 2022;**27**:7223. DOI: 10.3390/molecules27217223

[67] Peng S, Yao J, Liu Y, Duan D, Zhang X, Fang J. Activation of Nrf2 target enzymes conferring protection against oxidative stress in PC12 cells by ginger principal constituent 6-shogaol. Food and Function. 2015;**6**:2813-2823. DOI: 10.1039/c5fo00214a

[68] Chen H, Fu J, Chen H, Hu Y, Soroka DN, Prigge JR, et al. Ginger compound [6]-shogaol and its cysteine-conjugated metabolite (M2) activate Nrf2 in colon epithelial cells in vitro and in vivo. Chemical Research in Toxicology. 2014;**27**:1575-1585. DOI: 10.1021/tx500211x

[69] Lechner JF, Stoner GD. Gingers and their purified components as cancer chemopreventative agents. Molecules. 2019;**24**:2859. DOI: 10.3390/molecules24162859

[70] Lv LS, Chen HD, Soroka D, Chen XX, Leung TC, Sang SM. 6-Gingerdiols as the major metabolites of 6-gingerol in cancer cells and in mice and their cytotoxic effects on human cancer cells. Journal of Agricultural and Food Chemistry. 2012;**60**:11372-11377. DOI: 10.1021/jf303879b

[71] Prasad S, Tyagi AK. Ginger and its constituents: Role in prevention and treatment of gastrointestinal cancer. Gastroenterology Research and Practice. 2015;**2015**:142979. DOI: 10.1155/2015/142979

[72] Lin CB, Lin CC, Tsay GJ. 6-Gingerol inhibits growth of colon cancer cell LoVo via induction of G2/M arrest. Evidance-Based Complementary and Alternative Medicine. 2012;**2012**:326096. DOI: 10.1155/2012/326096

[73] Park G, Park JH, Song HM, Eo H, Kim MK, Lee JW, et al. Anti-cancer activity of ginger (*Zingiber officinale*) leaf through the expression of activating transcription factor 3 in human colorectal cancer cells. BMC Complementary and Alternative Medicine. 2014;**14**:408. DOI: 10.1186/1472-6882-14-408

[74] Wei CK, Tsai YH, Korinek M, Hung PH, El-Shazly M, Cheng YB, et al. 6-Paradol and 6-shogaol, the pungent compounds of ginger, promote glucose utilization in adipocytes and myotubes, and 6-paradol reduces blood glucose in high-fat diet-fed mice. International Journal of Molecular Sciences. 2017;**18**:168. DOI: 10.3390/ijms18010168

[75] Jiang S, Wang N, Mi S. Plasma pharmacokinetics and tissue distribution of [6]-gingerol in rats. Biopharmaceutics and Drug Disposition. 2008;**29**:529-537. DOI: 10.1002/bdd.638

[76] Suleria HAR, Butt MS, Anjum FM, Saeed F, Khalid N. Onion: Nature protection against physiological threats. Critical Reviews in Food Science and Nutrition. 2015;**55**:50-66. DOI: 10.1080/10408398.2011.646364

[77] Zhao XX, Lin FJ, Li H, Li HB, Wu DT, Geng F, et al. Recent advances in bioactive compounds, health functions, and safety concerns of onion (*Allium cepa* L.). Frontiers. Nutrition. 2021;**22**(8):669805. DOI: 10.3389/fnut.2021.669805

[78] Böttcher C, Krähmer A, Stürtz M, Widder S, Schulz H. Effect of cultivar and cultivation year on the metabolite profile of onion bulbs (*Allium cepa L.*). Journal of Agricultural and Food Chemistry. 2018;**28**(66):3229-3238. DOI: 10.1021/acs.jafc.8b00254

[79] Law YY, Chiu HF, Lee HH, Shen YC, Venkatakrishnan K, Wang CK. Consumption of onion juice modulates oxidative stress and attenuates the risk of bone disorders in middle-aged and post-menopausal healthy subjects. Food and Function. 2016;**7**:902-912. DOI: 10.1039/C5FO01251A

[80] Marefati N, Ghorani V, Shakeri F, Boskabady M, Kianiang F, Rezaeeh R, et al. A review of anti-inflammatory, antioxidant, and immunomodulatory effects of *Allium cepa* and its main constituents. Pharmaceutical Biology. 2021;**59**:285-300. DOI: 10.1080/13880209.2021.1874028

[81] Böttcher C, Krähmer A, Stürtz M, Widder S, Schulz H. Health benefits of the flavonoids from onion: Constituents and their pronounced antioxidant and anti-neuroinflammatory capacities. Journal of Agricultural and Food Chemistry. 2020;**68**:799-807. DOI: 10.1021/acs.jafc.9b07418

[82] Jakaria M, Azam S, Cho DY, Haque ME, Kim IS, Choi DK. The methanol extract of *Allium cepa L.* protects inflammatory markers in lps-induced bv-2 microglial cells and upregulates the antiapoptotic gene and antioxidant enzymes in N27-a cells. Antioxidants. 2019;**8**:348. DOI: 10.3390/antiox8090348

[83] Umoh U, Umoh R, Enema O, Ekpo E, Ajibesin K, Eseyin O. Anti-inflammatory constituents of plants: A review. Journal of Chemical and Pharmaceutical Research. 2019;**11**:74-85

[84] Park JB. Effects of typheramide and alfrutamide found in allium species on cyclooxygenases and lipoxygenase. Journal of Medicinal Food. 2011;**14**(3):226-231. DOI: 10.1089/jmf.2009.0198

[85] Fujiwara Y, Horlad H, Shiraishi D, Tsuboki J, Kudo R, Ikeda T, et al. Onionin, a sulfur-containing compound isolated from onions, impairs tumor development and lung metastasis by inhibiting the protumoral and immunosuppressive functions of myeloid cells. Molecular Nutrition and Food Research. 2016;**60**:2467-2480. DOI: 10.1002/mnfr.201500995

[86] Fredotovic Z, Soldo B, Sprung M, Marijanovic Z, Jerkovic I, Puizina J. Comparison of organosulfur and amino acid composition between triploid onion Allium cornutum Clementi ex Visiani, 1842, and common onion *Allium cepa* L., and evidence for antiproliferative activity of their extracts plants. Baseline. 2020;**9**:98. DOI: 10.3390/plants9010098

[87] Jafarpour-Sadegh F, Montazeri V, Adili A, Esfehani A, Rashidi MR, Pirouzpanah S. Consumption of fresh yellow onion ameliorates hyperglycemia and insulin resistance in breast cancer patients during doxorubicin-based chemotherapy: A randomized controlled clinical trial. Integrative Cancer Therapies. 2017;**16**:276-289. DOI: 10.1177/1534735416656915

[88] Pagano C, Marinozzi M, Baiocchi C, Beccari T, Calarco P, Ceccarini MR, et al. Bioadhesive polymeric films based on red onion skins extract for wound treatment: An innovative and eco-friendly formulation. Molecules. 2020;**25**:318. DOI: 10.3390/molecules25020318

[89] Orasan O, Oprean R, Saplontai-Pop A, Filip M, Carpa R, Sarosi C, et al. Antimicrobial activity and thiosulfinates

profile of a formulation based on *Allium cepa* L. extract. Open. Chemistry. 2017;**15**:175-181. DOI: 10.1515/chem-2017-0021

[90] Loredana L, Giuseppina A, FilomenaN,FlorindaF,MarisaD,DonatellaA. Biochemical, antioxidant properties and antimicrobial activity of different onion varieties in the Mediterranean area. Journal of Food Measurement and Characterisation. 2019;**13**:1232-1241. DOI: 10.1007/s11694-019-00038-2

[91] Kocic-Tanackov S, Dimic G, Mojovic L, Gvozdanovic-Varga J, Djukic-Vukovic A, Tomovic V, et al. Antifungal activity of the onion (*Allium cepa* L.) essential oil against aspergillus, fusarium and Penicillium species isolated from food. Journal of Food Processing and Preservation. 2017;**41**:e13050. DOI: 10.1111/jfpp.13050

[92] Benkeblia N. Antimicrobial activity of essential oil extracts of various onions (*Allium cepa*) and garlic (*Allium sativum*). LWT. 2004;**37**:263-268. DOI: 10.1016/j.lwt.2003.09.001

[93] Kang YR, Choi HY, Lee JY, Jang SI, Kang H, Oh JB, et al. Calorie restriction effect of heat-processed onion extract (ONI) using in vitro and in vivo animal models. International Journal of Molecular Science. 2018;**19**:874. DOI: 10.3390/ijms19030874

[94] Yoshinari O, Shiojima Y, Igarashi K. Anti-obesity effects of onion extract in zucker diabetic fatty rats. Nutrients. 2012;**4**:1518-1526. DOI: 10.3390/nu4101518

[95] Ebrahimi-Mamaghani M, Saghafi-Asl M, Niafarc M, Asghari-Jafarabadi M, Mesgari-Abbasi M. Raw red onion intake and insulin resistance markers in overweight or obese patients with polycystic ovary syndrome a randomized controlled-clinical trial. Progressive Nutrition. 2018;**20**:199-208. DOI: 10.23751/pn.v20i1-S.6109

[96] Yen FS, Qin CS, Xuan STS, Ying PJ, Le HY, Darmarajan T, et al. Salvamani S hypoglycemic effects of plant flavonoids: A review. Evidance Based Complementary and Alternative Medicine. 2021;**2021**:2057333. DOI: 10.1155/2021/2057333

[97] Youl E, Bardy G, Magous R, Cros G, Sejalon F, Virsolvy A, et al. Quercetin potentiates insulin secretion and protects INS-1 pancreatic β-cells against oxidative damage via the ERK1/2 pathway. British Journal of Pharmacology. 2010;**161**:799-814. DOI: 10.1111/j.1476-5381.2010.00910.x

[98] Duthie SJ, Collins AR, Duthie GG, Dobson VL. Quercetin and myricetin protect against hydrogen peroxide-induced DNA damage (strand breaks and oxidised pyrimidines) in human lymphocytes. Mutation Research. 1997;**24**(393):223-231. DOI: 10.1016/s1383-5718(97)00107-1

[99] Kumari K, Mathew BC, Augusti KT. Antidiabetic and hypolipidemic effects of S-methyl cysteine sulfoxide isolated from *Allium cepa Linn*. Indian Journal of Biochemistry and Biophysics. 1995;**32**:49-54

[100] Kang HJ, Pichiah BT, Abinaya RV, Sohn HS, Cha YS. Hypocholesterolemic effect of quercetin-rich onion peel extract in C57BL/6J mice fed with high cholesterol diet. Food Science and Biotechnology. 2016;**25**:855-860. DOI: 10.1007/s10068-016-0141-4

[101] Brull V, Burak C, Stoffel-Wagner B, Wolffram S, Nickenig G, Muller C, et al. Acute intake of quercetin from onion skin extract doe not influence postprandial blood pressure and

endothelial function in overweight-to-obese adults with hypertension: A randomized, doubleblind, placebo-controlled, crossover trial. European Journal of Nutrition. 2017;**56**:1347-1357. DOI: 10.1007/s00394-016-1185-1

[102] Wang CK. Health benefits of onion bioactives on hypercholesterolemia, cardiovascular diseases, and bone mineral density. Food Frontiers. 2020;**1**:107-108. DOI: 10.1002/fft2.18

[103] Hamed M, Kalita D, Bartolo ME, Jayanty SS. Capsaicinoids, polyphenols and antioxidant activities of *Capsicum annuum*: Comparative study of the effect of ripening stage and cooking mthods. Antioxidants (Basel). 2019;**8**(9):364. DOI: 10.3390/antiox8090364

[104] Oyagbemi AA, Saba AB, Azeez OI. Capsaicin: A novel chemopreventive molecule and its underlying molecular mechanisms of action. Indian Journal of Cancer. 2010;**47**:53. DOI: 10.4103/0019-509X.58860

[105] Castro-Concha LA, Canche-Chuc I, MirandaHam MDL. Determination of antioxidants in fruit tissues from three accessions of habanero pepper (*Capsicum chinense Jacq*.). Journal of Mexican Chemical Society. 2012;**56**:15-18. DOI: 10.29356/jmcs.v56i1.269

[106] Si W, Man SW, Chenb Z, Chung HY. Stability of capsaicinoid content at raised temperatures. Natural Product. Communications. 2014;**9**:985-988

[107] Bal S, Sharangi AB, Upadhyay TK, Khan F, Pandey P, Siddiqui S, et al. Biomedical and antioxidant potentialities in chilli: Perspectives and way forward. Molecules. 2022;**27**:6380. DOI: 10.3390/molecules27196380

[108] Kim CS, Kawada T, Kim BS, Han IS, Choe SY, Kurata T, et al. Capsaicin exhibits anti-inflammatory property by inhibiting IkB-a degradation in LPS-stimulated peritoneal macrophages. Cellular Signaling. 2003;**15**:299-306. DOI: 10.1016/s0898-6568(02)00086-4

[109] Sancho R, Lucena C, Macho A, Calzado MA, Blanco-Molina M, Minassi A, et al. Immunosuppressive activity of capsaicinoids: Capsiate derived from sweet peppers inhibits NF-kB activation and is a potent anti-inflammatory compound in vivo. European Journal of Immunology. 2002;**32**:1753-1763. DOI: 0.1002/1521-4141(200206)32:6<1753::AID-IMMU1753>3.0.CO;2-2

[110] Kang JH, Kim CS, Han IS, Kawada T, Yu R. Capsaicin, a spicy component of hot peppers, modulates adipokine gene expression and protein release from obese-mouse adipose tissues and isolated adipocytes, and suppresses the inflammatory responses of adipose tissue macrophages. FEBS Letters. 2007;**581**:4389-4396. DOI: 10.1016/j.febslet.2007.07.082

[111] Övey I.S, Güler Y. Apoptotic efficiency of capecitabine and 5-fluorouracil on human cancer cells through TRPV1 channels. Indian Journal of Biochemistry and Biophysics. 2020;**57**:64-72. DOI:10.56042/ijbb.v57i1.27703

[112] Anandakumar P, Kamaraj S, Jagan S, Ramakrishnan G, Asokkumar S, Naveenkumar C, et al. Capsaicin inhibits benzo (a) pyrene-induced lung carcinogenesis in an *in vivo* mouse model. Inflammation Research. 2012;**61**:1169-1175. DOI: 10.1007/s00011-012-0511-1

[113] Tsou MF, Lu HF, Chen SC, Wu LT, Chen YS, Kuo HM, et al. Involvement of Bax, Bcl-2, Ca2+ and caspase-3 in capsaicin-induced apoptosis of human leukemia HL-60 cells. Anticancer Research. 2006;**26**:1965-1971

[114] Huh HC, Lee SY, Lee SK, Park NH, Han IS. Capsaicin induces apoptosis of cisplatin-resistant stomach cancer cells by causing degradation of cisplatin-inducible aurora-a protein. Nutrition and Cancer. 2011;**63**:1095-1103. DOI: 10.1080/01635581.2011.607548

[115] Jun HS, Park T, Lee CK, Kang MK, Park MS, Kang HI, et al. Capsaicin induced apoptosis of B16-F10 melanoma cells through down-regulation of Bcl-2. Food and Chemical Toxicology. 2007;**45**:708-715

[116] Hwang MK, Bode AM, Byun S, Song NR, Lee HJ, Lee KW, et al. Cocarcinogenic effect of capsaicin involves activation of EGFR signaling but not TRPV1EGFR-dependent cocarcinogenic effect of capsaicin. Cancer Research. 2010;**70**:6859-6869. DOI: 10.1158/0008-5472.CAN-09-4393

[117] Pramanik KC, Boreddy SR, Srivastava SK. Role of mitochondrial electron transport chain complexes in capsaicin mediated oxidative stress leading to apoptosis in pancreatic cancer cells. PLoS One. 2011;**6**:e20151. DOI: 10.1371/journal.pone.0020151

[118] Mori A, Lehmann S, O'Kelly J, Kumagai T, Desmond JC, Pervan M, et al. Capsaicin, a component of red peppers, inhibits the growth of androgen-independent, p53 mutant prostate cancer cells. Cancer Research. 2006;**66**:3222-3229. DOI: 10.1158/0008-5472.CAN-05-0087

[119] Ito K, Nakazato T, Yamato K, Miyakawa Y, Yamada T, Hozumi N, et al. Induction of apoptosis in leukemic cells by homovanillic acid derivative, capsaicin, through oxidative stress: Implication of phosphorylation of p53 at Ser-15 residue by reactive oxygen species. Cancer Research. 2004;**64**:1071-1078. DOI: 10.1158/0008-5472.can-03-1670

[120] Zhang J, Nagasaki M, Tanaka Y, Morikawa S. Capsaicin inhibits growth of adult T-cell leukemia cells. Leukomia Research. 2003;**27**:275-283. DOI: 10.1016/s0145-2126(02)00164-9

[121] Romero-Luna HE, Colina J, Guzmán-Rodríguez L, Sierra-Carmona CG, Farías-Campomanes ÁM, García-Pinilla S, et al. Capsicum fruits as functional ingredients with antimicrobial activity: An emphasis on mechanisms of action. Journal of Food Science and Technology. 2022;**1**:11. DOI: 10.1007/s13197-022-05578-y

[122] Koffi-Nevry R, Kouassi KC, Nanga ZY, Koussémon M, Loukou GY. Antibacterial activity of two bell pepper extracts: *Capsicum annuum* L. and *Capsicum frutescens*. International Journal of Food Properties. 2012;**15**:961-971. DOI: 10.1080/10942912.2010.509896

[123] Ahuja KDK, Robertson IK, Geraghty DP, Ball MJ. Effects of chili consumption on postprandial glucose, insulin, and energy metabolism. American Journal of Clinical Nutrition. 2006;**84**:63-69. DOI: 10.1093/ajcn/84.1.63

[124] Islam MS, Choi H. Dietary red chilli (*Capsicum frutescens* L.) is insulinotropic rather than hypoglycemic in type 2 diabetes model of rats. Phytotherapy Research. 2008;**22**:1025-1029. DOI: 10.1002/ptr.2417

[125] Kwon DY, Kim YS, Ryu SY, Cha MR, Yon GH, Yang HJ, et al. Capsiate improves glucose metabolism by improving insulin sensitivity better than capsaicin in diabetic rats. Journal of Nutritional Biochemistry. 2013;**24**:1078-1085. DOI: 10.1016/j.jnutbio.2012.08.006

[126] Jiang Z, Qu H, Lin G, Shi D, Chen K, Gao Z. Lipid-lowering efficacy of the capsaicin in patients with metabolic syndrome: A systematic

review and meta-analysis of randomized controlled trials. Frontiers in Nutrition. 2022;**9**:812294. DOI: 10.3389/fnut.2022.812294

[127] Negulesco JA, Noel SA, Newman HAI, Naber EC, Bhat HB, Witiak DT. Effects of pure capsaicinoids (capsaicin and dihydrocapsaicin) on plasma lipid and lipoprotein concentrations of Turkey poults. Atherosclerosis. 1987;**64**:85-90. DOI: 10.1016/0021-9150(87)90233-4

[128] Qin Y, Ran L, Wang J, Yu L, Lang HD, Wang XL, et al. Capsaicin supplementation improved risk factors of coronary heart disease in individuals with low HDL-C levels. Nutrients. 2017;**9**:1037. DOI: 10.3390/nu9091037

[129] Tang J, Luo K, Li Y, Chen Q, Tang D, Wang D, et al. Capsaicin attenuates LPS-induced inflammatory cytokine production by upregulation of LXRα. International Immunopharmacology. 2015;**28**:264-269. DOI: 10.1016/j.intimp.2015.06.007

[130] Das G, Gonçalves S, Heredia JB, Romano A, Jim'enez-Ortega LA, Guti'errez-Grijalva EP, et al. Cardiovascular protective effect of cinnamon and its major bioactive constituents: An update. Journal of Functional Foods. 2022;**97**:105045. DOI: 10.1016/j.jff.2022.105045

[131] Rao PV, Gan SH. Cinnamon: A multifaceted medicinal plant. Evidence Based Complementary and Alternative Medicine. 2014;**2014**:642942. DOI: 10.1155/2014/642942

[132] Jeyaratnam N, Nour AH, Kanthasamy R, Nour AH, Yuvaraj AR, Akindoyo JO. Essential oil from *Cinnamomum cassia* bark through hydrodistillation and advanced microwave assisted hydrodistillation. Industrial Crops and Products. 2016;**92**:57-66. DOI: 10. 1016/j. indcr op. 2016. 07. 049

[133] Lee YS, Ryu MJ. Antioxidant effects of *Cinnamomum cassia* bark extract and its effectiveness as a cosmetics ingredient. Asian Journal of Beauty and Cosmetology. 2019;**17**:69-80. DOI: 10. 20402/ajbc. 2018. 0262

[134] Yang CH, Li RX, Chuang LY. Antioxidant activity of various parts of *Cinnamomum cassia* extracted with different extraction methods. Molecules. 2012 Jun;**17**(6):7294-7304. DOI: 10.3390/molecules17067294

[135] Borzoei A, Rafraf M, Niromanesh S, Farzadi L, Narimani F, Doostan F. Effects of cinnamon supplementation on antioxidant status and serum lipids in women with polycystic ovary syndrome. Journal of Traditional Complementary Medicine. 2018;**8**:128-133. DOI: 10.1016/j.jtcme.2017.04.008

[136] Liao JC, Deng JS, Chiu CS, Hou WC, Huang SS, Shie PH, et al. Anti-inflammatory activities of *Cinnamomum cassia* constituents in vitro and in vivo. Evidence-Based Complementary and Alternative Medicine. 2012;**2012**:429320. DOI: 10.1155/2012/429320

[137] Song F, Li H, Sun J, Wang S. Protective effects of cinnamic acid and cinnamic aldehyde on isoproterenol-induced acute myocardial ischemia in rats. Journal of Ethnopharmacology. 2013;**150**:125-130. DOI: 10.1016/j.jep.2013.08.019

[138] Han X, Parker TL. Antiinflammatory activity of cinnamon (*Cinnamomum zeylanicum*) bark essential oil in a human skin disease model. Phytotherapy Research. 2017;**31**:1034-1038. DOI: 10.1002/ptr.5822

[139] Costello RB, Dwyer JT, Saldanha L, Bailey RL, Merkel J, Wambogo E. Do cinnamon supplements have a role in glycemic control in type 2 diabetes? A narrative review. Journal of Academy of Nutrition and Dietetics. 2016;**116**:1794-1802. DOI: 10.1016/j.jand.2016.07.015

[140] Medagama AB. The glycaemic outcomes of cinnamon, a review of the experimental evidence and clinical trials. Nutrition Journal. 2015;**14**:108. DOI: 10.1186/s12937-015-0098-9

[141] Qin B, Nagasaki M, Ren M, Bajotto G, Oshida Y, Sato Y. Cinnamon extract (traditional herb) potentiates in vivo insulin-regulated glucose utilization via enhancing insulin signaling in rats. Diabetes Research and Clinical Practice. 2003;**62**:139-148. DOI: 10.1016/s0168-8227(03)00173-6

[142] Hayward NJ, McDougall GJ, Farag SJ, Allwood W, Austin C, Campbell F, et al. Cinnamon shows antidiabetic properties that are species-specific: Effects on enzyme activity inhibition and starch digestion. Plant Foods for Human Nutrition. 2019;**74**(4):544-552. DOI: 10.1007/s11130-019-00760-8

[143] Santos HO, da Silva GAR. To what extent does cinnamon administration improve the glycemic and lipid profiles? Clinical Nutrition ESPEN. 2018;**27**:1-9. DOI: 10.1016/j.clnesp.2018.07.011

[144] Davis PA, Yokoyama W. Cinnamon intake lowers fasting blood glucose: Meta-analysis. Journal of Medicinal Food. 2011;**14**:884-889. DOI: 10.1089/jmf.2010.0180

[145] Jarvill-Taylor KJ, Anderson RA, Graves DJ. A hydroxychalcone derived from cinnamon functions as a mimetic for insulin in 3T3-L1 adipocytes. Journal of the American College Nutrition. 2001;**20**:327-336. DOI: 10.1080/07315724.2001.10719053

[146] Xue YL, Shi HX, Murad F, Bian K. Vasodilatory effects of cinnamaldehyde and its mechanism of action in the rat aorta. Vascular Health Risk Management. 2011;**7**:273-280. DOI: 10.2147/VHRM.S15429

[147] Kim NY, Trinh NT, Ahn SG, Kim SA. Cinnamaldehyde protects against oxidative stress and inhibits the TNF-α-induced inflammatory response in human umbilical vein endothelial cells. International Journal of Molecular Medicine. 2020;**46**:449-457. DOI: 10.3892/ijmm.2020.4582

[148] El-Bassossy HM, Fahmy A, Badawy D. Cinnamaldehyde protects from the hypertension associated with diabetes. Food and Chemical Toxicology. 2011;**49**:3007-3012. DOI: 10.1016/j.fct.2011.07.060

[149] Couturier K, Batandier C, Awada M, Hininger-Favier I, Canini F, Anderson RA, et al. Cinnamon improves insulin sensitivity and alters the body composition in an animal model of the metabolic syndrome. Archives of Biochemistry and Biophysics. 2010;**501**:158-161. DOI: 10.1016/j.abb.2010.05.032

[150] Gorgani L, Mohammadi M, Najafpour GD, Nikzad M. Piperine—The bioactive compound of black pepper: From isolation to medicinal formulations. Comprehensive Reviews in Food Science and Food Safety. 2017;**16**:124-140. DOI: 10.1111/1541-4337.12246

[151] Lee JG, Chae Y, Shin Y, Kim YJ. Chemical composition and antioxidant capacity of black pepper pericarp. Applied Biological Chemistry. 2020;**63**:35. DOI: 10.1186/s13765-020-00521-1

[152] Jagella T, Grosch W. Flavour and offavour compounds of black and white pepper (*Piper nigrum* L.) II. Odour activity values of desirable and undesirable odorants of black pepper. European Food Research and Technology. 1999;**209**:22-26. DOI: 10.1007/s002170050450

[153] Rauscher FM, Sanders RA, Watkins JB. Effects of piperine on antioxidant pathways in tissues from normal and streptozotocin-induced diabetic rats. Journal of Biochemical and Molecular Toxicology. 2000;**14**:329-334. DOI: 10.1002/1099-0461(2000)14:6<329::AID-JBT5>3.0.CO;2-G

[154] Tasleem F, Azhar I, Ali SN, Perveen S, Mahmood ZA. Analgesic and anti-inflammatory activities of *Piper nigrum* L. Asian Pacific Journal of Tropical Medicine. 2014;7:461-468. DOI: 10.1016/S1995-7645(14)60275-3

[155] Bang JS, Choi HM, Sur B-J, Lim S-J, Kim JY, Yang H-I, et al. Anti-inflammatory and antiarthritic effects of piperine in human interleukin 1β-stimulated fibroblast-like synoviocytes and in rat arthritis models. Arthritis Research and Therapy. 2009;**11**:1-9. DOI: 10.1186/ar2662

[156] Seung-Hyung K. Lee young-Cheol Piperine inhibits eosinophil infiltration and airway hyperresponsiveness by suppressing T cell activity and Th2 cytokine production in the ovalbumin-induced asthma model. Journal of Pharmacy and Pharmacology. 2009;**61**:353-359. DOI: 10.1211/jpp/61.03.0010

[157] Atal S, Agrawal RP, Vyas S, Phadnis P, Rai N. Evaluation of the effect of piperine per se on blood glucose level in alloxan-induced diabetic mice. Acta Poloniae Pharmaceutica. 2012;**69**:965-969

[158] Tu Y, Sun D, Zeng X, Yao N, Huang X, Huang D, et al. Piperine potentiates the hypocholesterolemic effect of curcumin in rats fed on a high fat diet. Experimental and Therapeutic Medicine. 2014;**8**:260-266. DOI: 10.3892/etm.2014.1717

[159] Matsuda D, Ohte S, Ohshiro T, Jiang W, Rudel L, Hong B, et al. Molecular target of piperine in the inhibition of lipid droplet accumulation in macrophages. Biological and Pharmaceutical Bulletin. 2008;**31**:1063-1066. DOI: 10.1248/bpb.31.1063

[160] Dima C, Assadpour E, Dima S, Jafari SM. Bioavailability of nutraceuticals: Role of the food matrix, processing conditions, the gastrointestinal tract, and nanodelivery systems. Comprehensive Reviews in Food Science and Food Safety. 2020;**19**:954-994. DOI: 10.1111/1541-4337.12547

[161] Rein MJ, Renouf M, Cruz-Hernandez C, Actis-Goretta L, Thakkar SK, da Pinto MS. Bioavailability of bioactive food compounds: A challenging journey to bioefficacy. British Journal of Clinical Pharmacology. 2013;**75**:588-602. DOI: 10.1111/j.1365-2125.2012.04425.x

[162] Stohs SJ, Chen O, Ray SD, Ji J, Bucci LR, Preuss HG. Highly bioavailable forms of curcumin and promising avenues for curcumin-based research and application: A review. Molecules. 2020;**25**:1397. DOI: 10.3390/molecules25061397

[163] Khalil NM, do Nascimento TCF, Casa DM, Dalmolin LF, de Mattos AC, Hoss I, et al. Pharmacokinetics of curcumin-loaded PLGA and PLGA-PEG blend nanoparticles after oral administration in rats. Colloids and Surfaces. B, Biointerfaces. 2013;**101**:353-360. DOI: 10.1016/j.colsurfb.2012.06.024

[164] Yu H, Shi K, Liu D, Huang Q. Development of a food-grade organogel with high bioaccessibility and loading of curcuminoids. Food Chemistry. 2012;**131**:48-54. DOI: 10.1016/j.foodchem.2011.08.027

[165] Lu X, Wang C, Zhao M, Wu J, Niu Z, Zhang X, et al. Improving the bioavailability and bioactivity of garlic bioactive compounds via nanotechnology. Critical Reviews in Food Science and Nutrition. 2022;**62**:8467-8496. DOI: 10.1080/10408398.2021.1929058

[166] Lawson LD, Gardner CD. Composition, stability, and bioavailability of garlic products used in a clinical trial. Journal of Agricultural and Food Chemistry. 2005;**53**:6254-6261. DOI: 10.1021/jf050536+

[167] Raeisi S, Ojagh SM, Quek SY, Pourashouri P, Salaün F. Nano-encapsulation of fish oil and garlic essential oil by a novel composition of wall material: Persian gum-chitosan. LWT. 2019;**116**:108494. DOI: 10.1016/j.lwt.2019.108494

[168] Daojiu Z, Yujie Z, Yeying G, Yiying L, Chao D, Jiwei Z, et al. Stability, bioavailability, and antimicrobial activity of garlic extract liposomes prepared from lecithin and β-sitosterol. Journal of Food Measurement and Characterization. 2022;**16**:1383-1394. DOI: 10.1007/s11694-022-01284-7

[169] Wang Q, Wei Q, Yang Q, Cao X, Li Q, Shi F, et al. A novel formulation of [6]-gingerol: Proliposomes with enhanced oral bioavailability and antitumor effect. International Journal of Pharmaceutics. 2018;**535**:308-315. DOI: 10.1016/j.ijpharm.2017.11.006

[170] Arcusa R, Villaño D, Marhuenda J, Cano M, Cerdà B, Zafrilla P. Potential role of ginger (*Zingiber officinale* roscoe) in the prevention of neurodegenerative diseases. Frontiers in Nutrition. 2022;**9**:809621. DOI: 10.3389/fnut.2022.809621

[171] Ogino M, Yakushiji K, Suzuki H, Shiokawa K, Kikuchi H, Sato H, et al. Novel ginger extract formulation with enhanced pharmacokinetics and anti-hypothermic action. Drug Metabolism Pharmacokinetics. 2017;**32**:30-31. DOI: 10.1016/j.dmpk.2016.10.138

[172] Dabeek WM, Marra MV. Dietary quercetin and kaempferol: Bioavailability and potential cardiovascular-related bioactivity in humans. Nutrients. 2019;**11**:2288. DOI: 10.3390/nu11102288

[173] Wu T, Yen F, Lin L, et al. Preparation, physicochemical characterization, and antioxidant effects of quercetin nanoparticles. International Journal of Pharmaceutics. 2008;**346**:160-168. DOI: 10.1016/j.ijpharm.2007.06.036

[174] Li H, Zhao X, Ma Y, et al. Enhancement of gastrointestinal absorption of quercetin by solid lipid nanoparticles. Journal of Controlled Release. 2009;**133**:238-244. DOI: 10.1016/j.jconrel.2008.10.002

[175] Kale R, Saraf M, Juvekar A, Tayade P. Decreased B16F10 melanoma growth and impaired tumour vascularization in BDF1 mice withquercetin-cyclodextrin binary system. Journal of Pharmacy and Pharmacology. 2006;**58**:1351-1358. DOI: 10.1211/jpp.58.10.0008

[176] Li H, Li M, Jingxin F, Ao H. Weihua Wang and Xiangtao Wang enhancement of oral bioavailability of quercetin by metabolic inhibitory nanosuspensions compared to conventional nanosuspensions. Drug

Delivery. 2021;**28**:1226-1236. DOI: 10.1080/10717544.2021.1927244

[177] Cirino LMD, Vergne DMC, Santana PF, De Almeida E, Da Costa LP, De Albuquerque-Júnior RLC, et al. Decreased inflammatory response in rat bladder after intravesical administration of capsaicin-loaded liposomes. An. Acad. Brasil. Ciênc. 2016;**88**(3):1539-1547

[178] Zhu Y, Peng W, Zhang J, Wang M, Firempong CK, Feng C, et al. Enhanced oral bioavailability of capsaicin in mixed polymeric micelles: Preparation, in vitro and in vivo evaluation. Journal of Functional Foods. 2014;**8**(1):358-366. DOI: 10.1016/j.jff.2014.04.001

[179] Malar CG. Dendrosomal capsaicin nanoformulation for the invitro anti-cancer effect on hep 2 and mcf-7 cell lines. International Journal on Applied Bioengineering. 2015;**9**(2):30-35. DOI: 10.18000/ijabeg.10133

[180] Amruthraj NJ, Preetam Raj JP, Lebel A. Capsaicin-capped silver nanoparticles: Its kinetics, characterization and biocompatibility assay. Applied Nanoscience. 2015;**5**(4):403-409. DOI: 10.1007/s13204-014-0330-5

Chapter 4

Tasty Spices as Nutraceuticals

Vijaya Rabade, Ashwini Ingole, Purushottam Gangane, Vidya Sabale, Ujwala Mahajan and Yash Kale

Abstract

Spices, food additives, which are the main sources of taste, colour, and perfume in foods and beverages, are becoming more and more important due to their wide range of applications. Spices are consumed as food additives to improve the sensory quality of foods. Traditional systems of medicine have employed spices for centuries since they have been known to have physiological effects that are good for human health. In the past few decades, pioneering experimental research involving both animal studies and human trials has been carried out which proved thatspices have therapeutic effects. The benefits of spices' like nutritional, antioxidant, anti-microbial, and therapeutic characteristics are many. These potentials activities of spices also adds up with their far reaching nutraceutical values. The primary health challenges facing humanity today are diabetes, cardio-vascular illnesses, arthritis, and cancer. Thus the anti-diabetic, anti-hypercholesterolemic, anti-carcinogenic, digestive stimulant action, antilithogenic property, anti-inflammatory property, antimutagenic, and anticarcinogenicand anti-inflammatory actions of spices are of utmost importance in the current situation. The present chapter deals with review of the nutraceutical and health benefits of various spices used in daily diet.

Keywords: nutritional, medicine, antioxidants, health benefits

1. Introduction

Due to the extensive usage of numerous chemicals, heavy metals, electromagnetic waves, and other potentially hazardous man-made things, industrialisation has led to significant soil, water, and food pollution. Due to these issues, the prevalence of diabetes, obesity, different malignancies, vascular illnesses, physiological issues, and other degenerative diseases has increased. The expense of medical treatment has significantly increased due to the rising demand for healthcare. Research into new dietary products with healing properties has created a resurgence in health and nutrition research. Nutraceuticals opens a new era of quality of life research. May reduce the risk of disease by maintaining normal health and boosting immunity [1].

Plants are one of the most important resources in human nutrition and medicine. Increased knowledge of nutrition, medicine and plant biotechnology has drastically changed and revolutionised the concepts of nutrition, health and agriculture [2, 3].

"Food" is a term introduced by Stephen De Felice in 1979 which is defined as "a food or part of a food that has a medical or health benefit, including the prevention and treatment of disease". The motto of nutritional therapy is based on

IntechOpen

complementary therapy with nutraceuticals, because food is not only a source of energy and nutrition, but also has a healing effect. Food detoxifies our body, restores our digestive system and eating habits [4]. Nutrients are sold in concentrated forms such as pills, capsules, powders, and tinctures, either as a single substance or as a combination. Nutrients can be foods rich in natural nutrients such as spirulina, garlic, soybeans, or certain foodstuffs such as omega-3 salmon oil. They are also known as medicinal foods, nutritional supplements, and nutritional supplements. The global demand for herbal and non-herbal extracts is growing all the time. For e.g. green tea is used for weight loss and cancer treatment, while *Ginkgo biloba*L. is widely used as a nutrient to improve cognitive function. The nutrition market has grown in recent years due to the increased attention of researchers and advanced techniques for determining qualitative and quantitative parameters. Consumers are disillusioned with expensive high-tech approaches to disease treatment in modern medicine and looking for useful additions or alternatives to food products [5].

2. Why nutraceuticals?

For many of us, a regular diet does not provide us with enough nutrition. Second, the pollution and pesticides in our surroundings are so poisonous that they prevent our bodies from controlling them. Our culture is being plagued by a variety of new illnesses. High-quality nutritional supplements may be absorbed and utilised by the body, unlike medications, which typically have side effects because they are not natural for the body. They can actually strengthen our bodies and bring energy [6, 7].

2.1 Definition

Nutrient: As coined by Association of American Feed Control Officials (AAFCO) (1996), "a feed constituent in a form and at a level that will help support the life of an animal." Proteins, lipids, carbohydrates, minerals and vitamins are the main categories of feed nutrients.

Feed: As coined by Association of American Feed Control Officials (AAFCO) (1996), "edible materials which are consumed by animals and contribute energy and/or nutrients to the animal's diet."

Food: As coined by the Food, Drug and Cosmetic Act (1968), "an article that provides taste, aroma or nutritive value. Food and Drug Administration (FDA) considers food as 'generally recognized as safe' (GRAS)."

Drug: As coined by Association of American Feed Control Officials (AAFCO) (1996), "a substance intended for use in the diagnosis, cure, mitigation, treatment or prevention of disease in man or other animals. A substance other than food intended to affect the structure or any function of the body of man or other animals."

Dietary Supplement: As coined by the Dietary Supplement Health and Education Act (DSHEA, 1994), "a product that contains one or more of the following dietary ingredients: vitamin, mineral, herb, or other botanical, and amino acid (protein). Includes any possible component of the diet as well as concentrates, constituents, extracts or metabolites of these compounds."

Nutraceutical: As commonly coined by the dietary supplement industry, "any nontoxic food component that has scientifically proven health benefits, including disease treatment and prevention."

Veterinary Nutraceutical: As coined by the newly created North American Veterinarian Nutraceutical Council, Inc. (NAVNC), "a substance which is produced in a purified or extracted form and administered orally to patients to provide agents required for normal body structure and function and administered with the intent of improving the health and well-being of animals" [8].

2.2 Classification

a. Traditional

- Chemical constituents in the form of nutrients and herbals
- Probiotic supplements.
- Enzyme supplements.

b. Non Traditional

- Fortified nutraceuticals.
- Recombinant Nutraceutical.

c. Substance with established nutritional functions

- Vitamins
- Minerals
- Amino acids F
- Fatty acids

d. Herbs (or) Botanical products

e. Reagents derived from other sources

- Pyruvate
- Chondroitin sulphate
- Steroid hormone precursors

f. Functional foods

g. Probiotics and prebiotics

h. Polyunsaturated fatty acids

i. Antioxidant vitamin

j. Polyphenols

k. Spices

2.3 Advantages

- Nutraceuticals have the ability to aid in good eating as well as the diagnosis, treatment, and prevention of diseases.
- There is unquestionably a very large and expanding market, thus many pharmaceutical corporations are now attempting to enter the nutraceutical space.
- Consumers' perception that these foodstuff-like chemicals are less harmful or hazardous than traditional medications [9].

2.4 Dis-advantages

- Companies making unregulated items to generate large profit margins.
- Harder and more expensive than ever to identify new molecules.
- Reduced bioavailability of nutrients [9].

2.5 Traditional nutraceuticals

Foods that do not go through manual modifications fall under this category. The ingredients are all-natural and may actively contribute to health advantages, such as Tomatoes, pink grapes, guava, papaya, and melon water contain lycopene, an antioxidant with anti-cancer properties, notably for the prostate, bladder, cervix, and leukaemia [10].

2.6 Non-traditional nutraceuticals

Nontraditional nutraceuticals are synthetic foods made by adding bioactive ingredients for human health. It can be further broken down into recombinant and fortified nutraceuticals. Nutraceuticals with agricultural breeding or additional nutrients are known as fortified foods. Some examples of fortified nutraceuticals include orange juice with calcium, cereals with extra vitamins or minerals, flour with added folic acid, and milk with cholecalciferol [1].

2.7 Fortified nutraceuticals

Fortification of food components is a technique of enhancing food with micronutrients (vitamins, minerals, and essential elements) increases the food's nutritional worth and effectiveness. Cholecalciferol-enriched breast milk used to treat vitamin D insufficiency is one example [5, 11].

2.8 Recombinant nutraceuticals

In order to produce food like yoghurt and cheese or bioactive extraction components using enzymatic or fermented technology, biotechnology and genetic engineering are applied in this way. Gold Ascorbic acid, carotene, lutein, and zeaxanthin levels in kiwifruit have been increased through genetic modification. For example: Lutin is obtained from corn, avocado, egg yolks, spinach and have potential benefits as an anti-cancer activity [5, 11].

3. Substance with established nutritional functions

3.1 Vitamin

The importance of numerous vitamins in preserving a healthy metabolism and state of wellness cannot be overstated. All vitamin deficiencies can result in distinct clinical signs. As a result, the majority of nutritional supplements or nutraceutical therapy products contain vitamins, often common vitamins like vitamin A, vitamin C, vitamin C, vitamin D, and vitamin E. Humans mostly obtain their vitamins from plant-based meals and plant biotechnology. As a result, it has been utilised to boost the vitamin content of plants [12].

3.2 Herbal (or) botanical products

Extracts and concentrates are the two ways to get herbal or botanical goods. Herbs have been used to treat acute and chronic illnesses for as long as human civilization has existed. The "Ayurveda" natural remedy, which includes numerous efficient means of ensuring health care, has its earliest written heritage in India. The essential elements of herbal medicine contain numerous nutraceuticals.

4. Reagents come from other sources

4.1 Glucosamine and chondroitin

The building and repair of cartilage involve the usage of chemicals known as glycolsaminoglycans, of which glucosamine is a precursor. Bovine or calf cartilage as the source, in certain European nations, glucosamine sulphate is the first line of defence against arthritis. In joint fluid, glucosamine sulphate encourages the formation of hyaluronic acid. Hyaluronic acid improves injured cartilage while reducing discomfort. Proteoglycan dosages were found to rise after glucosamine administration in in vitro tests. It is typically marketed as salt hydrochloride or salt sulphate. Both substances have anti-inflammatory properties. There is a glucosamine and chondroitin supplement available. The most prevalent glycosaminoglycan in cartilage, chondroitin, is what gives cartilage its resilience.

4.2 Flavonoids

Flavonoids are the primary biologically active component of plants. Regarding phenolic compounds, they have anti-inflammatory, hepatoprotective, anti-microbial, antibacterial, antiviral, anti-ulcer, vasorelaxant, anti-atherosclerotic, antithrombogenic, antithrombogenic, cardio added, and anti-Neoplastic properties for profound impacts on the central nervous system [13].

4.3 Food supplements and food fibres

Food supplements are goods that have extra food elements added as medicines for deficiencies or illnesses. Dietary supplements are becoming more and more popular as a way to boost performance, prevent ageing, maintain fitness, and build up the body. One of the growing food and nutritional assessments is of groceries. On the market, there are numerous materials or products with a single ingredient that contain vitamins and minerals as dietary supplements [14]. Other than vitamins and minerals, dietary supplements may also include botanicals, amino acids, pure extracts, concentrates, a combination of glandular extracts, and organ tissue. It wasn't intended to be a staple in the diet or used as a component of traditional or conventional food [15]. Fibre foods and high fibre products are very attractive because of the health benefits signifikan. E.g: rice, bananas, cereals etc.

4.4 Phytochemicals

In today's communication, phytochemicals are also referred to as nutraceuticals and offer medicinal and health benefits. An intriguing reevaluation of conventional diabetes treatment has been made, and one of the key characteristics of phytochemicals is their ability to regulate glucose and insulin. Actually, fewer than a thousand manufacturers have received scientific research despite claims that they offer more unique benefits in the treatment of diabetes. Additionally, the importance of traditional medicines like anticancer, antiviral, and hypolyphical effects have been highlighted, as well as the nature of nutrition, tonic, and mushroom medicine. Lentinan enhances the host's resistance to parasites, viruses, AIDS-causing bacteria and fungus, and other types of infections.

4.5 Functional food

Functional food is a supply of nutrients that is actually required and offers more than what is required for maintenance, growth, and development. Numerous additional subclasses, including cereal, nuts, and fermented foods, are included in the functional food classes [16]. Functional foods, such as cereals like rice, corn, wheat, millet, sorghum, and buckwheat, have been proven to have the ability to lower blood pressure, reduce the incidence of tumours, and remove the risk of coronary heart disease [17]. It has been discovered that kidney beans, almonds, beans, lentils, and soybeans contain potent antioxidants and have preventive effects against diabetes and cardiovascular disease [18]. Additionally, chocolate is a subtype of functional food that is the richest source of protein and a good supply of calcium, iron, magnesium, and riboflavin [19, 20]. Other functional food groups include citrus fruits, which have the potential to boost the immune system and have been shown to have therapeutic benefits as anticancer, antiviral, and antioxidant agents [21]. Other examples of functional foods that have positive effects on digestion are fermented milk and related items. For instance, yoghurt is a very nutrient-dense fermented food with anticancer potential; it has also been linked to the prevention of atherosclerosis and gastrointestinal illnesses. Patients who are lactose intolerant are advised to use it [22].

4.6 Prebiotics and probiotics

Direct microbial foods that are good for your health are under the probiotic group. They adhere to certain parts of the digestive tract and expel infections as a result of their activity [23]. Prebiotics are ingredients that have been specifically or fermented to encourage changes in gastrointestinal bacteria and whose actions have a positive impact on domestic health. They serve as probiotic bacteria's fertilisers in the big intestine. Gastric pH and digestive acid have little effect on this. Examples include insulin, which when subjected to further hydrolysis yields oligo fructose and oligosaccharide from galactose [24, 25].

4.7 Polyunsaturated fatty acids

Omega-3 (N-3) and Omega-6 (N-6) polylist fatty acids (PUFA), which differ in the location of the first double double, are two kinds of polyunsaturated fatty acids (PUFA). Because they cannot be produced by the human body and are crucial for maintaining physiological integrity, two Pufa is known as essential fatty acids. As a result, they need to be consumed with food.

4.8 Anti-oxidant

Free radical-induced cell damage is thought to be a major factor in both the ageing process and the onset of illness. Antioxidants are crucial for preserving our best health and wellbeing because they are our body's first defence against free radical damage. Being a highly reactive element, oxygen can be found in potentially harmful molecules known as free radicals. Healthy bodily cells may be attacked by free radicals, losing their structures and functions. Free radicals can be stabilised or rendered inactive by antioxidants before they damage cells.

4.9 Polyphenols

Natural phytochemicals called polyphenols are found in plant-based foods such fruits, vegetables, grains, cereals, nuts, tea, coffee, wine, and cocoa; All plant meals include more than 8000 polyphenol components, including flavonoids and phenolic acid. These substances are plant secondary metabolites that serve as a line of defence against infections, oxidants, and UV radiation. Based on the amount of phenol rings and the structural components that connect these rings to one another, polyphenols can be divided into a number of types. Berry fruits, kiwis, cherries, apples, pears, chicory, and coffee are foods with high content of this phenolic acid. Phenolic acids constitute around a third of polyphenol compounds in a diet and include two primary types of acid, ferulatic acid, and synapaphic acid.

4.10 Spices

Herbs and spices are seasonings made from plants that are used in cooking. Although the phrases "herbs" and "spices" are sometimes used synonymously, they have distinct meanings in botany. Spices preserve their flavour in their seeds, bark, and roots, whereas herbs store it in their leaves [26]. The word "spice" is derived from the Latin word "species," which denotes a specific kind [27]. Plant parts like clove buds, cinnamon bark, ginger roots, cumin fragrant seeds, and saffron flower stigmas can all be considered spices. Culinary spices have long been used as food preservatives and for their health-improving qualities in addition to improving the taste of food. Additionally, spices pique people's appetites and improve the appearance of food for people all over the world [26]. Spices form the foundation of flavour in food

Sr.no	Name of spice	Biological source	Uses	Health benefits	Contraindications
1.	Turmeric (Haldi)	*Curcuma longa* L.	In addition to cosmetics, it is utilised in food. There are several medical applications for it.	It aids in the treatment of skin issues. Turmeric powder can be used to treat cuts and wounds. It also makes diabetes management simpler.	It is contraindicated in gallstones or a bile duct obstruction.
2.	Star anise (Chakra Phool)	*Illicium verum* Hook.f.	It is useful in both cooking and medicine.	For rheumatism, star anise oil is helpful. Digestive health and breath freshening are benefits.	Pregnant and lactating women, liver disease, alcoholism, hormonal sensitivity, intestinal diseases.
3.	Pepper (Kaali Mirch)	*Piper nigrum* L.	It is frequently used in cooking, particularly as a garnish. It also has a variety of medicinal uses.	It makes it easier to handle illnesses like the common cold, cough, and infections. Both digestion issues and muscle discomfort can be treated with it.	Increase the risk of bleeding in people with bleeding disorders.
4.	Nutmeg (Jaiphal)	*Myristica fragrans* Houtt.	For garnishing and making masala, it is used in powdered form. It is used in soaps, perfumes and shampoos. It can also be used for medicinal purpose.	It helps with the treatment of heart disease, asthma, and foul breath.	It is contraindicated in pregnant women.
5.	Ginger (Adrak)	*Zingiber officinale* Roscoe.	It is used for giving a specific flavour to food and has many medicinal uses.	Helps prevent stomach issues. It helps people deal with coughs and colds.	Contraindicated with aspirin, anticoagulant, antiplatelet, NSAIDS drugs
6.	Garlic (Lassan)	*Allium sativum* L.	In addition to being used medicinally, it is also utilised in cooking.	It helps individuals cope with coughs and colds. Additionally, it possesses antibacterial activities.	Bleeding disorders, surgery within 1–2 weeks.
7.	Coriander (Dhaniya)	*Coriandrum sativum* L.	Both the seeds and the leaves of coriander are used in cooking. It also has a few medical applications.	It can be applied externally to treat rheumatism and achy joints. Additionally, it helps in hay fever, a sore throat, allergies, digestion issues, etc.	—

Sr.no	Name of spice	Biological source	Uses	Health benefits	Contraindications
8.	Cumin (Zeera	*Cuminum cyminum* L.	It has therapeutic qualities in addition to being used in cooking.	It supports a healthy immune system and is a rich source of iron. Dysentery can be treated with water that has been boiled with cumin seeds.	Heavy menstrual bleeding, diabetic patients.
9.	Cinnamon (Dalchini)	*Cinnamomum zeylanicum* Nees	It is widely utilised when making masalas and seasoning food. It also serves medical purposes.	It decreases blood cholesterol and increases insulin production naturally.	Pregnant womens.
10.	Fenugreek (Methi)	*Trigonella foenum* graecum L.	It is typically consumed as a green leafy vegetable, and the seeds are used to make masalas. It can be used medicinally as well.	Tea made from fenugreek seeds or sweet fudge can increase the production of breast milk. It also lowers cholesterol and aids in the treatment of diabetes.	Diabetes and low blood sugar.
11.	Bishop's weed (Ajwain)	*Trachyspermum ammi* L.	It serves a medical benefit in addition to being used as a seasoning and flavouring.	A medication that is applied to treat GI issues like cholera, dyspepsia, flatulence, and diarrhoea. In Ayurvedic medicine, it is utilised as an antiseptic, preservative, and treatment for respiratory and GI problems. As a boost to the body's defence mechanisms, unani medicine.	Contraindicated in diverticulitis, liver diseases and ulcerative colitis.

Table 1.
List of important Indian spices with their uses, health benefits and contraindications [30].

applications. People use spices all around the world to enhance the flavour, texture, and appearance of food as well as to boost hunger. Spices are also prized for their healing abilities as antimicrobials and antioxidants [27].

Essential oils are liquids that are produced when plant parts are steam or water distilled (leaves, stems, bark, seeds, fruits, roots and plant exudates). Citrus oil can only be extracted from fruit peels using expression since heat readily damages the chemical makeup of the oil. Citrus oil production is a substantial byproduct of the juice industry nowadays. Up to several hundred chemical compounds can be found in an essential oil, and it is this complex combination of components that gives the oil its distinctive aroma and flavour. An essential oil can include up to several hundred chemical compounds, and it is this intricate assemblage of ingredients that gives the oil its unique flavour and perfume. In addition to the volatile essential oil, these oleoresins and extracts, which are widely used in the food and pharmaceutical industries, also contain concentrated non-volatile flavour components. The solvent extraction processes are more complex and difficult than steam distillation, and most small-scale producers will not be able to afford them. Selling the raw materials to these extraction facilities, however, might be a good market strategy [28].

The majority of the significant spices that are currently traded internationally are produced in tropical areas. The most notable exceptions to this rule are the capsicums (chilli peppers, paprika, and coriander), which may be cultivated in a far wider variety of tropical and nontropical conditions. In these humid and damp settings, growing spices and essential oils presents unique crop and product management challenges. The crop must be dried in order to produce a stable stored product, which necessitates the use of effective drying techniques in wet, rainy climates [28].

5. Health and medicinal use of spices and herbs of India

Indians employ herbs and spices in their traditional medical practises, much like people from many other cultures do. "Ayurvedic medicine" refers to an Indian medical system that employs herbs and spices. In Indian culture, this all-encompassing method of healing is referred to as the "science of life." In addition to adding flavour to dull dishes, research demonstrates that herbs and spices "have a huge impact on human health because they affect many of the body's metabolic processes." Indian Festival (Rani) Herbs have long been utilised in both Eastern and Western medicine to treat a number of diseases (**Table 1**) [29].

6. Conclusion

Spices are not essential but still have become most important part of our daily routine. The spices makes food attractive and palatable with flavour, colour, taste and aroma. By using healthy and tasty spices, the use of less healthy ingredients can be minimised. Many health problems are prevailing in human being, now a days. The spices are tasty and attractive. In addition, they also possess bioactives which acts as nutraceuticals, and are found to be effective against variety of health problems. The spices like turmeric, nutmeg, pepper, star anise, ginger, garlic, coriander, cumin, cinnamon, fenugreek and Bishop's weed are being using as spices since long. Their medical benefits have been proven. These spices will not only make our food tasty and attractive but their proper use in routine life will keep us healthy.

Author details

Vijaya Rabade[1*], Ashwini Ingole[1], Purushottam Gangane[1], Vidya Sabale[1], Ujwala Mahajan[1] and Yash Kale[2]

1 Dadasaheb Balpande College of Pharmacy, Nagpur, India

2 Kamla Nehru College of Pharmacy, Nagpur, India

*Address all correspondence to: vijayarabade24@gmail.com

References

[1] Rajasekaran A. Nutraceuticals, Comprehensive Medical Chemistry III. Elsevier Science. 2017;**1-8**:107-134

[2] Berger MM, Shenkin A. Vitamins and trace elements: Practical aspects of supplementation. Nutrition. 2006;**22**(9):952-955

[3] Bagchi D. Nutraceuticals and functional foods regulations in the United States and around the world. Toxicology. 2006;**221**(1):1-3

[4] Chauhan B, Kumar G, Kalam N, Ansari SH. Current concepts and prospects of herbal nutraceutical: A review. Journal of Advanced Pharmaceutical Technology & Research. 2013;**4**(1):4-8

[5] Singh J, Sinha S. Classification, regulatory acts and applications of nutraceuticals for health. International Journal of Pharmacy and Biological Sciences. 2012;**2**(1):177-187

[6] Whitman M. Understanding the perceived need for complementary and alternative nutraceuticals: Lifestyle. Clinical Journal of Oncology Nursing. 2001;**5**:190-194

[7] EANN C, Teratogen N, Service I. Over-the-counter products: nonprescription medications, nutraceuticals, and herbal agents. Clinical Obstetrics and Gynecology. 2002;**45**(1):89-98

[8] Baici A, Hörler D, Moser B, Hofer HO, Fehr K, Wagenhäuser FJ. Analysis of glycosaminoglycans in human serum after oral administration of chondroitin sulfate. Rheumatology International. 1992;**12**(3):81-88

[9] Khogali SEO, Harper AA, Lyall JA, Rennie MJ. Effects of L-glutamine on post-ischaemic cardiac function: Protection and rescue. Journal of Molecular and Cellular Cardiology. 1998;**30**(4):819-827

[10] Lokhande SS. Role of nutraceuticals in various diseases: A comprehensive review. Asian Journal of Pharmaceutical Research. 2018;**8**(4):236

[11] Casey CF, Slawson DCNL. VItamin D supplementation in infants, children, and adolescents. American Family Physician. 2010;**81**(6):745-748

[12] Dureja H, Kaushik D, Kumar V. Developments in nutraceuticals. Indian Journal of Pharmacology. 2003;**35**(6): 363-372

[13] Lin JK, Weng MS. Flavonoids as nutraceuticals. Science of Flavonoids. 2006;**7**(September):213-238

[14] Pandey M, Vijayakumar. Nutraceutical supplementation for diabetes: A review. Int. Journal of Pharmacy & Pharmaceutical Sciences. 2011;**3**(SUPPL. 4):33-40

[15] Spano M. Functional foods, beverages, and ingredients in athletics. Strength & Conditioning Journal. 2010;**32**(1):79-86

[16] Gaidhani KA, Harwalkar M, Nirgude PS. Seed extracts. World Journal of Pharmaceutical Research. 2014;**3**(3):5041-5048

[17] Madar Z, Stark AH. New legume sources as therapeutic agents. The British Journal of Nutrition. 2002;**88**(S3):287-292

[18] Preuss HG. Bean amylase inhibitor and other carbohydrate absorption blockers: Effects on diabesity and general health. Journal of the American College of Nutrition. 2009;**28**(3):266-276

[19] Pucciarelli DL, Grivetti LE. The medicinal use of chocolate in early North America. Molecular Nutrition & Food Research. 2008;**52**(10):1215-1227

[20] Cooper KA, Donovan JL, Waterhouse AI, Williamson G. Cocoa and health: A decade of research. The British Journal of Nutrition. 2008;**99**(1):1-11

[21] Okwu DE. Citrus fruits: A rich source of phytochemicals and their roles in human health. International Journal of Chemical Sciences. 2008;**6**(2):451-471

[22] Shiby VK, Mishra HN. Fermented milks and Milk products as functional foods-a review. Critical Reviews in Food Science and Nutrition. 2013;**53**(5):482-496

[23] Gibson GR. Fibre and effects on probiotics (the prebiotic concept). Clinical Nutrition Supplements. 2004;**1**(2):25-31

[24] Ramaa C, Shirode A, Mundada A, Kadam V. Nutraceuticals - an emerging era in the treatment and prevention of cardiovascular diseases. Current Pharmaceutical Biotechnology. 2006;**7**(1):15-23

[25] Venter CS. Prebiotics: An update. Journal of Family Ecology and Consumer Sciences. 2007;**35**:17-25

[26] Ogbunugafor HA, Ugochukwu CG, Kyrian-Ogbonna AE. The role of spices in nutrition and health: A review of three popular spices used in southern Nigeria. Food Quality and Safety. 2017;**1**(3):171-185

[27] Okonkwo C, Ogu A. Nutritional evaluation of some selected spices commonly used in the south-eastern part of Nigeria. Journal of Biology, Agriculture and Healthcare. 2014;**4**(15):97-103

[28] Darriet A. Section II. Flavors. Food processing, product developments, and recent advances: Herbs, spices, and essential oils. In: Handbook of Food Products Manufacturing. Vol. 1. John Wiley & Sons; 2006. pp. 205-220

[29] FCH14-04–Leader's Guide December, 2013

[30] Dubey S. Indian spices and their medicinal value. Indian Journal of Pharmaceutical Education and Research. 2017;**51**(3):S330-S332

Section 2

Medicinal Herbs

Chapter 5

Secondary Metabolites: Alkaloids and Flavonoids in Medicinal Plants

Hamed Zandavar and Mojtaba Afshari Babazad

Abstract

Secondary metabolites (SMs) are natural compounds produced mainly by bacteria, fungi, and plants. They are low molecular weight compounds that have a wide range of chemical structures and biological functions. Secondary metabolites are so named because, unlike primary metabolites such as lipids, amino acids, carbohydrates, and nucleic acids, their synthesis is not required for the organism's development and reproduction. Today, the production of secondary metabolites is an important area of research for organic chemists, molecular biologists, and bioinformaticians. In this research, two types of secondary metabolites produced by plants, such as alkaloids and flavonoids, were studied and information was collected on the types of compounds, structures, biological activities, and commercial applications of these two types of secondary metabolites.

Keywords: secondary metabolites, types of alkaloids, types of flavonoids

1. Introduction

Metabolomics is the study of metabolites in biofluids, cells, tissues, or organisms [1]. Metabolites and their interactions are collectively referred to as the metabolome [2]. Metabolites are tiny molecules formed as a result of metabolic processes; these molecules are either intermediate or final results of metabolic reactions. Natural enzymes found in the cells of organisms accelerate metabolic processes primary and secondary metabolites are compounds that result from primary and secondary metabolism, respectively. Primary metabolites are essential molecules used by organisms for growth, development, and reproduction; these compounds are produced by cells during the growth phase as a result of metabolism. Because of their importance in maintaining normal physiological functions, primary metabolites are called nuclear metabolites. Vitamins (B_2 and B_{12}), lactic acid, amino acids, polyols, alcohols such as ethanol, nucleotides, organic acids, and other substances are examples of primary metabolites [3].

The present chapter examines the meaning and origins or sources of various significant types of secondary metabolites, such as alkaloids, terpenoids, tannins, flavonoids, saponins, cardiac glycosides, phenolic compounds, and others, as well as their impact on human and animal health.

2. Secondary metabolites

Secondary metabolites are organic chemicals created by organisms such as plants, fungi, or bacteria as a result of secondary metabolic processes that result in the creation and accumulation of different chemical compounds known as secondary metabolites. These substances are not essential for the organisms' core metabolic activities [4]. Secondary metabolites are created near the end of the growth phase and hence are not directly engaged in the organism's typical physiologic activities such as growth, development or reproduction. Instead, they boost the organism's survival through the mediation of ecological interaction, which acts as a selection benefit to the organism [4]. Secondary metabolites play crucial roles in interspecies defenses, such as plant defense against herbivory. Secondary metabolites, on the other hand, are used by humans as medications, recreational drugs, flavorings, colors, and so on. Secondary metabolites are generally categorized based on their extensive structural diversity, biosynthesis, and function. Over 2140,000 secondary metabolites have been identified in the literature; secondary metabolites are classified into five types: alkaloids, terpenoids, steroids, polyphenols, fatty-acid-derived compounds, nonribosomal polypeptides, and enzyme cofactors [5].

2.1 Alkaloids

Plants offer a large reservoir of active ingredients with substantial therapeutic uses such as antiviral, anticancer, analgesic, and antitubercular [5]. Alkaloids are significant secondary metabolites that were identified and utilized as early as 4000 years ago and are widely known for their medicinal potential [6]. Alkaloids are categorized into many groups based on their heterocyclic ring system and biosynthetic precursors, such as indole, purine, quinoline, isoquinoline, tropane, and imidazole, among others [7, 8]. Alkaloids contain antiproliferative, antimicrobial, and antioxidant properties that can be exploited in medication development [9]. Alkaloids' medicinal potential expands their industrial applicability. Numerous studies on the medicinal characteristics of various alkaloids derived from plants have been conducted. Alkaloids are naturally occurring chemical composites that often include basic nitrogen atoms. They could also have some neutral or mildly acidic substances in them [10, 11]. Several synthesized substances are also classified as alkaloids [12]. Alkaloids, in addition to carbon, nitrogen, or hydrogen, may include sulfur and, in rare cases, bromine, phosphorus, or chlorine. The term "alkaloid" was coined in 1819 by German scientist Carl F. W. Meissner, who derived it from the Arabic name al-Qali, which is related to the plant from which soda was initially extracted [13]. Alkaloids are low-molecular-weight compounds that account for around 20% of plant-based secondary metabolites [7]. So far, over 12,000 alkaloids have been isolated from diverse plant species [7]. Alkaloids are primarily solids that are found in higher plants. They are found in the following botanical families: Apocynaceae, Annonaceae, Amaryllidaceae, Berberidaceae, Boraginaceae, Gnetaceae, Liliaceae, Leguminoceae, Lauraceae, Loganiaceae, Magnoliaceae, Menispermaceae, Papaveraceae, Piperaceae, Rutaceae, Rubiaceae, and Ranunculaceae [14].

2.1.1 Phytochemistry and classification of alkaloids

Alkaloids exhibit a wide range of variety, not only in their botanical and biological origins but also in structure and pharmacological function. In this regard, different categorization schemes are feasible. Alkaloids can be classified structurally based on their chemical precursor, structures, and sources, or on the biological mechanisms employed to acquire the molecule. True alkaloids, protoalkaloids, and pseudoalkaloids are the three main kinds of alkaloids. True alkaloids and protoalkaloids are generated from amino acids, but pseudoalkaloids are not.

2.1.1.1 True alkaloids

These alkaloids are produced from amino acids and share a heterocyclic ring containing nitrogen. They are biologically active and extremely reactive. They generate water-soluble salts, and many of them are crystalline, forming a salt when conjugated with acid. Except for nicotine, which is a dark liquid, almost all genuine alkaloids have a bitter taste and are solid [15]. Their presence in plants takes three forms: (a) free-state, (b) N-oxide, or (c) salts. Various amino acids like L-phenylalanine, L-tyrosine, L-ornithine, L-histidine, L-lysine, and other amino acids are the main sources of true alkaloids (**Table 1**) [16]. The most prevalent genuine alkaloids found in nature are cocaine, morphine, and quinine.

Alkaloid type	Major group of alkaloid	Chemical group of alkaloid	Amino acid precursor
Tryptophan-derived alkaloids	True alkaloid	Ergot alkaloids Pyrroloindole alkaloids Indole alkaloids Aspidosperma alkaloids Quinoline alkaloids	L-Threonine L-Proline L-Tryptophan L-Serine
	Protoalkaloids	Terpenoid indole alkaloids	---
Arginine-derived alkaloids	True alkaloid	Marine alkaloids	L-Asparagine L-Alanine L-Aspartic acid L-Arginine
Ornithine-derived alkaloids	True alkaloid	Pyrrolizidine alkaloids Tropane alkaloids Pyrrolidine alkaloids	L-Ornithine
Histidine-derived alkaloids	True alkaloid	Manzamine alkaloids Imidazole alkaloids	L-Histidine
Nicotinic acid-derived alkaloids	True alkaloid	Sesquiterpene pyridine alkaloids Pyridine alkaloids	Nicotinic acid
Lysine-derived alkaloids	True alkaloid	Indolizidine alkaloids Quinolizidine alkaloids Piperidine alkaloids	L-Lysine L-Leucine L-Isoleucine
Anthranilic acid-derived alkaloids	True alkaloid	Acridine alkaloids Quinoline alkaloids Quinazoline alkaloids	Anthranilic acid
Tryptophan-derived alkaloids	Protoalkaloids	Terpenoid indole alkaloids	L-Threonine L-Proline L-Tryptophan L-Serine
Tyrosine-derived alkaloids	Protoalkaloids	Phenylethylamine alkaloids	L-Tyrosine

Table 1.
Amino acid and their involvement in alkaloid synthesis.

Parent compounds	Precursor compound	Chemical group of alkaloids	Examples
Terpenoid	Geraniol	Terpenoid-alkaloids	Gentianine Aconitine β-Skytanthine Actinidine
Sesquiterpene	Acetate	Sesquiterpene-alkaloids	Evonoline Cassinine Evorine Celapanin
Phenyl	Ferulic acid	Aromatic alkaloids	Capsaicin
Piperidine	Acetate	Piperidine-alkaloids	Pinidine Coniceine Coniine
Purine	Adenine/guanine	Purine alkaloids	Theophylline Theobromine Caffeine

Table 2.
Involvement of parent compound in pseudoalkaloids synthesis.

2.1.1.2 Proto alkaloids

This class of alkaloids has a nitrogen atom obtained from an amino acid but does not belong to the heterocyclic ring system. The major precursors of these categories of alkaloids are L-tryptophan and L-tyrosine. This small category structurally consists primarily of simple alkaloids. The primary alkaloids in this category include yohimbine, mescaline, and hordenine. They are used to treat a variety of medical conditions, including mental illness, pain, and neuralgia [17].

2.1.1.3 Pseudo alkaloids

Pseudoalkaloids' fundamental carbon skeleton is not generated directly from amino acids. Instead, they are linked to amino acid pathways, where they are produced from forerunners or postcursors of amino acids via amination or transamination processes [16, 18]. Pseudoalkaloids can also be produced by nonamino-acid precursors. They can be generated from phenylalanine or acetate. Pseudoalkaloids are commonly found in capsaicin, caffeine, and ephedrine (**Table 2**).

2.1.2 Classification established upon the ring structure

Based on the existence of a fundamental heterocyclic nucleus in their structure, this is the most fully recognized categorization.

2.1.2.1 Tropane alkaloid

The tropane (C_4N skeleton) nucleus characterizes this class of alkaloids. They are plentiful in the Solanaceae family. They are created by combining ornithine with acetoacetate. Pyrolines are the structural precursors of these alkaloids. The majority of them are mono, di, and trihydroxytropane esters with a variety of hydroxylation configurations. Cocaine, atropine, scopolamine, and their derivatives have been

DOI: http://dx.doi.org/10.5772/intechopen.108030

extensively researched since the nineteenth century because of their significant pharmacological activities [19–21] (**Figure 1A**).

2.1.2.2 Pyrrolizidine alkaloids

The pyrrolizidine nucleus distinguishes this class of alkaloids. They are found in plants of the Asteraceae and Fabaceae families. The majority of pyrrolizidine alkaloids are found in plants as N-oxides; senecionine is the most well-known alkaloid of this kind (**Figure 1B**) [22–27].

2.1.2.3 Piperidine alkaloids

The fundamental ring system of this category of alkaloids is the piperidine nucleus. True piperidine alkaloids are distinguished by the presence of monocycle molecules with the C_5N nucleus. Piperidine alkaloids are distinguished by the presence of odor. They cause long-term neurotoxicity. Many of them evolved from plants. Lobeline is an important alkaloid in this class (**Figure 1C**) [28].

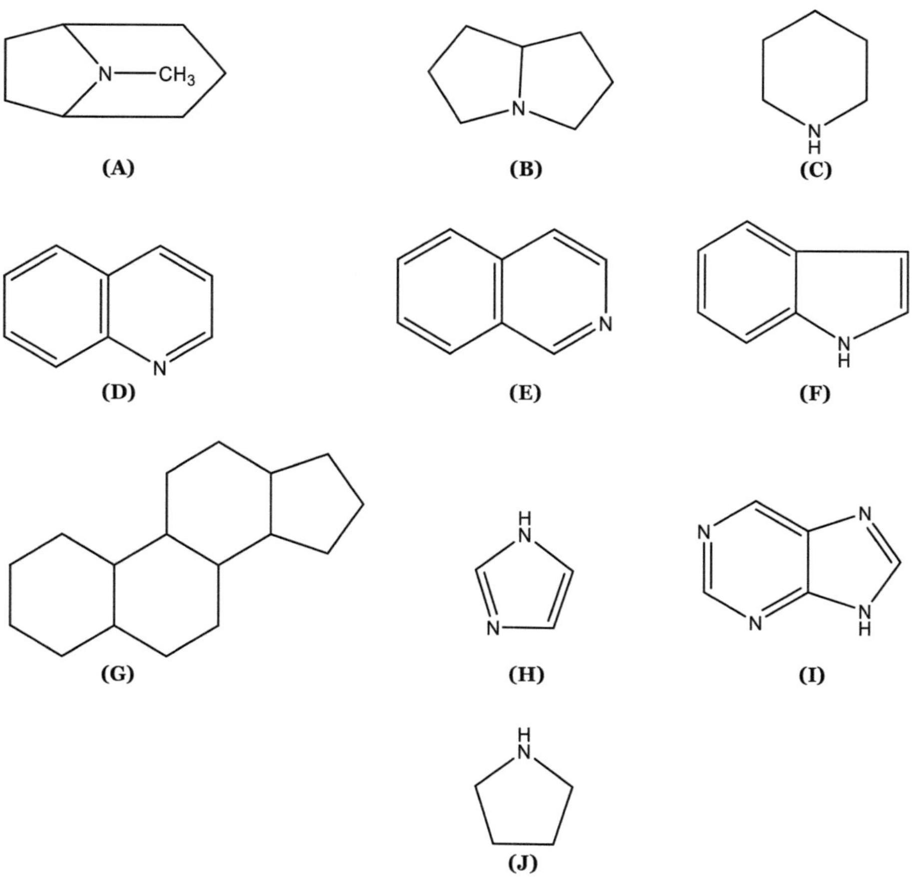

Figure 1.
(A) Basic structure of the tropane nucleus, (B) basic structure of the pyrrolizidine nucleus, (C) basic structure of the piperidine nucleus, (D) basic structure of the quinoline nucleus, (E) basic structure of the isoquinoline nucleus, (F) basic structure of the indole nucleus, (G) basic structure of the steroidal alkaloid nucleus, (H) basic structure of the imidazole nucleus, (I) basic structure of the purine nucleus, (J) basic structure of the pyrrolidine nucleus.

2.1.2.4 Quinolines alkaloids

This quinolone-nucleus-containing alkaloid can only be obtained from the bark of the Cinchona plant. However, many simple heteroaromatic quinolines have been identified from diverse marine sources (4,8-quinolinediol from cephalopod ink and 2-heptyl-4-hydroxyquinoline from a marine pseudomonad). Cinchonine, Cinchonidine, Quinine, and Quinidine are the primary alkaloids in this category (**Figure 1D**) [29, 30].

2.1.2.5 Isoquinoline alkaloids

Isoquinoline alkaloids are a diverse category of alkaloids found mostly in higher plants. However, only a few classes of isoquinolinoid marine alkaloids exist. These alkaloids offer a wide range of therapeutic effects, including antiviral, antifungal, anticancer, antioxidant, antispasmodic, and enzyme inhibitor activities. Morphine and codeine are the most well-known and researched isoquinoline alkaloids. They are made from either tyrosine or phenylalanine. They are created by combining a precursor of dopamine (3,4-dihydroxytryptamine) with a ketone or aldehyde. This group of alkaloids is further classified as follows: Simple isoquinoline alkaloids (e.g., salsoline, mimosamycin), benzyl isoquinoline alkaloids (e.g., reticuline, imbricatine), bisbenzyl isoquinoline alkaloids (e.g., fumaricine), manzamine alkaloids (e.g., manzamine a), pseudo benzyl isoquinoline alkaloids (e.g., polycarpine, ledecorine),

Seco bisbenzyl isoquinoline alkaloids (e.g., baluchistanamine), bis benzyl isoquinoline alkaloids containing one ether link (e.g., dauricine), bis benzyl isoquinoline alkaloids containing two ether links (e.g., berbamine), bis benzyl isoquinoline alkaloids containing aryl links only (e.g., pisopowetine), bis benzyl isoquinoline alkaloids containing one aromatic link and one or two ether links (e.g., rodiasine) (**Figure 1E**) [31].

2.1.2.6 Indole alkaloids

This is the most significant and intriguing alkaloid group produced from tryptophan. Simple tryptamine derivatives, carbazoles (where the ethanamine chain has been removed), a variety of alkaloids with one or more prenyl residues mixed with tryptamine, and others with the integration of typical monoterpenoid or diterpenoid units are examples of notable alkaloids from this category. Although structural diversity differs depending on the terrestrial and marine sources, traditional research investigations on alkaloids from both sources and the fungal source have been conducted. Polyhalogenation is a characteristic of these alkaloids. They are further classified as follows: simple indole alkaloids (e.g., Aplysinopsin, Gramine), bisindoles (e.g., Indirubin, 6,6′-dibromoindigotin), simple tryptamine alkaloids (e.g., tryptamine), cyclotryptamine alkaloids (e.g., Physostigmine), quinazolinocarbazole alkaloids (e.g., Rutaecarpine), β-carboline alkaloids (e.g., Harman), carbazole alkaloids (e.g., ekeberginine), indolonaphthyridine alkaloids (e.g., Canthin-6-one), ergot alkaloids (e.g., ergotamine) (**Figure 1F**) [32–38].

2.1.2.7 Steroidal alkaloids

The 1,2-Cyclopentane phenanthrene ring structure is unique to this class of alkaloids. They are mainly derived from higher plants of the Liliaceae, Solanaceae, Apocynaceae, and Buxaceae families, although some have also been isolated from amphibians. These alkaloids are further subdivided into several subtypes, the most basic of which are various forms of aminopregnanes. The others types of steroidal alkaloids are Salamandra type (e.g., cyclo neosamandione), jerveratrum type (e.g., jervine), spirosolane type (e.g., soladulcidine), solanidine type (e.g., rubijervine), cerveratrum type (e.g., 3,6-cevanediol), conanine type (e.g., didymeline), Buxus type (e.g., cyclobuxine), pregnane type (e.g., 20α-dimethylamino-3β-senecioylamino-16β-hydroxy-pregn-5-ene), cephalostatins/ritterazines (e.g., ritterazinesa), miscellaneous steroidal alkaloids (e.g., bufotoxin) (**Figure 1G**) [39–43].

2.1.2.8 Imidazole alkaloids

This class of alkaloids is distinguished by its imidazole ring structure. Because the imidazole ring of these alkaloids is already formed at the precursor stage, they are exempt from the structural transformation operation. This class of alkaloids includes several structurally distinct instances, notably among marine and microbial alkaloids. They exhibit a diverse range of biological activity as well as great medicinal promise. Pilocarpine is the most important imidazole alkaloid in medicine (**Figure 1H**) [44, 45].

2.1.2.9 Purine alkaloids

Purine is a nitrogenous nucleotide (a building unit of DNA and RNA) that consists of a purine ring, pentose sugar, and another base, pyrimidine. Purine alkaloids include caffeine, theophylline, and theobromine. They are well-known as plant alkaloids, but they may also be found in marine species as substituted purines (e.g., Phidolopin) and a variety of terpenoid-purine alkaloids, including the age lines and others (**Figure 1I**) [46, 47].

2.1.2.10 Pyrrolidine alkaloids

The fundamental nucleus of pyrrolidine alkaloids is pyrrolidine (C_4N skeleton). Plants have a large number of pyrrolidine alkaloids. Some examples of this class of alkaloids are Hygrine (biosynthesized from ornithine), Ficine (where the pyrrolidine ring is associated with a flavone nucleus), and Brevicolline (where it is coupled to a ß-carboline unit) (**Figure 1J**) [48].

2.1.3 The biological activity of alkaloids

Plant secondary metabolites are a broad group of physiologically active compounds with a variety of pharmacological activities such as antibacterial, stimulant, analgesic, anthelmintic, anticoagulant, antiacne, and antioxidant [49, 50]. For many millennia, humans from practically every culture have used plant-derived substances to predict and manage a variety of health problems.

2.1.3.1 The biological activity of indole alkaloids

The most important indole alkaloids are reserpine (an antihypertensive agent) from Rauvolfia serpentine [51] vinblastine and vincristine (an anticancer lead) from Catharanthus roseus [52]. Other indole alkaloids have important and powerful pharmacological activity such as antibacterial, antifungal, CNS stimulant, and antiviral properties. They have antiparasitic, cytotoxic, serotonin and antagonistic realms, anti-inflammatory, and antiviral properties [53]. This unique class of phytochemicals has a variety of medicinal and pharmacological properties, which will be addressed in this section.

2.1.3.1.1 Anti-cancer activity

The vinca alkaloids, vincristine, and vinblastine have mostly been employed as chemotherapeutic agents in cancer therapy. They possibly limit the development of several cancer cell lines, such as neuroblastoma cells in mice, human leukemia HL-60 cells, HeLa cells, S49 lymphoma cells from mice, and IC_{50} values for mouse leukemia L1210 cells were 33 and 15 nM, respectively. 4.1 and 5.3 nM, 1.4 and 2.6 nM, 5 and 3.5 nM, 4.4 and 4.0 nM, respectively. The cytotoxic activity of vinca alkaloids (vincristine and vinblastine) is mostly related to the disruption of mitotic spindle construction via interactions with tubulin in the microtubules that compose the mitotic spindles, resulting in metaphase arrest [54–58].

Vallesiachotamine (derived from the leaves of Palicourea rigida) exhibits substantial anticancer efficacy against human (SK-MEL-37) melanoma cells via an apoptotic mechanism [59]. Eudistomin K (derived from the Caribbean ascidian Eudistoma olivaceous) is an indole alkaloid with a new oxathiazepine ring that is an anti-tumor in L-1210, A-549, HCT-8, and P-388 cell lines [53]. Topsentin (discovered from the Caribbean deep-sea sponge Spongosorites ruetzleri) has in vitro cytotoxic effect against P-388 with IC_{50} of 3.0 and 20 μg/mL for human tumor cells, respectively (HCT-8, A-549, and T47D). At concentrations of 150 mg/kg and 37.5 mg/kg, the drug also exhibits in vivo anticancer efficacy against P-388 (T/C 137 percent) and B16 melanoma (T/C 144 percent) [53]. Dragmacidin D, a bis (indole)-derived sponge metabolite (isolated from the sponge Spongosorites sp. Dragmacidin D), has anticancer activity in vitro against P-388 and A-549, with IC_{50} values of 1.4 and 4.4 μg/mL, respectively [53]. Gelliusines A and B (derived from the deep-water New Caledonian sponge Gellius or Orina sp.) showed anticancer efficacy against KB, P-388, P-388/dox, HT-29, and NSCLCN-6 cell lines, with IC_{50} values ranging from 10 to 20 μg/mL [53, 60]. Kapakahine B, a peptide derived from the marine sponge Cribrochalina olemda, has shown promising anticancer activity against P-388 murine leukemia cells, with an IC_{50} value of 5.0 μg/mL [53]. Convolutamydine A (derived from the marine bryozoan Amathia convolute) has shown anticancer efficacy against HL-60 (human promyelocytic leukemia cells). At concentrations ranging from 0.1 to 25 μg/mL, this indole alkaloid alters culture plate adherence, produces growth arrest, and stimulates phagocytosis [53].

2.1.3.1.2 Anti-oxidant activities

The DPPH radical-scavenging test revealed that reserpine inhibits the DPPH radical by 42%. Lind et al. investigated the antioxidant activity of Barettin using two distinct biochemical tests, FRAP (Ferric-Reducing Antioxidant Power) and ORAC (Oxygen Radical Absorbance Capacity). According to their findings, Barettin has a possible antioxidant profile that is dose-dependent. Barettin showed FRAP and ORAC values of 77 and 5.5 μM Trolox equivalents (TE) at a concentration of 30 μg/mL, respectively [61].

2.1.3.1.3 Anti-hypertensive activities

Reserpine is widely used as first-line therapy in the treatment of primary hypertension. A reserpine dosage of 0.5 mg/day or higher resulted in statistically significant

SBP (systolic blood pressure) effects [62]. The fundamental mechanism of reserpine's antihypertensive activity is that it lowers the levels of catecholamines in peripheral sympathetic nerve terminals. Reserpine has a greater affinity for VMAT2 (vesicular monoamine transporter), binds to their receptors irreversibly, and inhibits VMAT2 irreversibly [63]. VMATS transports released and liberated nor-adrenaline or nor-epinephrine, dopamine, and serotonin (5-HT) from the presynaptic nerve terminal cytoplasm into storage vesicles for subsequent release into the synaptic cleft [64, 65]. Reserpine has a greater affinity for VMAT2 and binds to their receptors permanently. It is an effective antihypertensive and sedative, but long-term use promotes prolactin secretion and causes breast cancer.

2.1.3.2 The biological activity of tropane alkaloids

2.1.3.2.1 Effect on asthma

Atropine is extracted from the dried leaves and blooming tops of Datura metal, a member of the Solanaceae family. It works against Nocturnal Asthma. Atropine methyl nitrate can successfully cure nocturnal asthma, atropine sulfate [66], atropine in combination with metaproterenol [67], and albuterol Correspondingly. Atropine inhalation can enhance lung mucociliary function in humans.

2.1.3.2.2 Activity against hyperglycemia and parkinsonism

Atropine reduces hyperglycemia caused by neostigmine [68]. Atropine affects diabetes individuals' vagal tone [69]. Atropine can relieve tremors in a monkey model of parkinsonism.

2.1.3.2.3 Anti-cancer and anti-inflammatory activity

Colchicine is beneficial against chronic myelocytic leukemia and gout at toxic or almost toxic doses [70].

2.1.3.3 The biological activity of isoquinoline alkaloids

2.1.3.3.1 Anti-bacterial activity

Berberine has antibacterial action at a minimum inhibitory concentration (MIC) of 78 μg/mL by severely disrupting bacterial cell membrane structure by inhibiting cellular proteins, as proven by TEM and SDS-PAGE. This substance influenced bacterial DNA synthesis. It also inhibits methicillin-resistant S. aureus (MRSA) biofilm development in a concentration-dependent manner ranging from 1 to 64 μg/mL by reducing phenol soluble modules (PSMs) aggregation into amyloid fibrils.

2.1.3.3.2 Anti-diabetic activity

Berberine (methanolic extract) has anti-diabetic activity at a dosage of 500 mg/kg. Berberis aristata (methanolic extract) has potential effects on glucose metabolism, as well as HDL and cholesterol levels, in addition to anti-diabetic action [71].

2.1.3.3.3 Anti-osteoporosis activity

Berberine has modest laxative and hypocholesterolemic properties [72]. Berberine and its methanolic extract have strong antiosteoporosis action, which supports its ethnic usage in the treatment of postmenopausal osteoporosis [73].

2.1.4 Current and potential industrial applications of alkaloids

2.1.4.1 Pharmaceutical application

Alkaloids have led to the development of herbal remedies and their components based on the medical approach. The alkaloidal structure is changing chemically to improve therapeutic response. In general, synthetic medications perform better after modification than natural pharmaceuticals. Alkaloids, on the other hand, play an important part in phototherapy, homeopathy, and alternative medicine [15]. Indole, isoquinoline and tropane compounds are clinically important. In the pharmaceutical business, natural medications are transformed into medical goods to get a greater therapeutic response than synthetic pharmaceuticals. Physicians are interested in prescribing herbal treatments for the treatment of various ailments. Tropane derivatives such as atropine, hyoscine, and hyoscyamine are widely advocated for both recreational and therapeutic uses. Atropinol, for example, comprises the active component of atropine sulfate. Buscopan is a hyoscine derivative. Transdermal plasters include it. Another component of Bella sanol is hyoscyamine [15, 74]. Key alkaloids including boldine, codeine, narceine, and morphine have important roles in clinical care. Oxyboldine and Bold oval have morphine-like pharmacological effects. Codeine is a common ingredient in over 250 medicinal medications on the market. Codicaps and Codipront can be used for the same thing. Every single product is derived from opium. Narceine-containing drugs are related to codeine. It is mainly used for cough treatment [15, 75]. Tubocurarine derivatives such as tubarine and jexin have been used to relax muscles. Morphine-containing medicines, such as morphalgin and spasmofen, are utilized in extreme circumstances like surgical procedures and postoperative care [15]. The indole alkaloid chemical constituents such as ephedrine, ergotamine, ergometrine, and yohimbine are used in various combination formulations. Ephedrine is the primary active component of Dorex or Endrine. It is used for a variety of applications, including the treatment of nasal cold symptoms and bronchial asthma [15]. Ergotamine is the primary chemical ingredient of ergot. Because of its several uses; ergotamine is widely accessible on the market. Ergostat and Migral are commercialized ergotamine-based medications. These alkaloids are used in the treatment of migraines. Yohimbine is the primary active molecule in aphrodyne or yohimex. Based on this alkaloid, at least 20 distinct compounds have been created. These medications are used to treat male impotency. Alkaloids have a wide range of applications. Strychnine, for example, is used to treat a variety of illnesses, including eye ailments. Strychnine, which is used in clinical quantities, is the active component of Dysurgal or Pasuma [15, 76].

2.1.4.2 Agricultural application

Alkaloids are a source of worry and debate in food crops due to potential health risks and the fact that they must be eliminated from plants through breeding, particularly hybridization. As a result, alkaloid-rich (bitter) and alkaloid-poor (sweet)

DOI: http://dx.doi.org/10.5772/intechopen.108030

cultivars are created [77]. Total alkaloids cannot be eliminated by breeding. However, by employing an appropriate application, alkaloid content can be reduced. Industrial processing also removes alkaloids from raw materials [15]. Alkaloids are sometimes used as biological fertilizers in agriculture.

Alkaloids are high in nitrogen and carbon. Nitrogen and carbon, on the other hand, play an essential role in organic farming. The balance of macro and micronutrients is critical in carbon and nitrogen-based soil management methods.

2.2 Flavonoids

Flavonoids are secondary metabolites that are abundant in plants, fruits, and seeds and are responsible for color, aroma, and flavor. Flavonoids have several roles in plants, including controlling cell development, attracting pollinators and insects, and defending against biotic and abiotic stressors [78]. These chemicals have been linked to a wide range of health advantages in humans, including anti-inflammatory, anticancer, anti-aging, cardioprotective, neuroprotective, immunomodulatory, antidiabetic, antibacterial, antiparasitic, and antiviral effects [79–81]. Flavonoids have a $C_6-C_3-C_6$ flavone skeleton with two benzene rings (A and B) connected by a three-carbon pyran ring (C). The location of the catechol B-ring on the pyran C-ring, as well as the quantity and position of hydroxy groups on the catechol group of the B-ring, affect the antioxidant activity of flavonoids [82]. Flavonoids' functional hydroxy groups can donate electrons through resonance to stabilize free radicals and mediate antioxidant protection [83]. Flavonoids are categorized into six primary types based on their structure: Flavan-3-ols, Flavones, Flavonols, Flavanones, Isoflavones, and Anthocyanins [83]. Because of their remarkable antioxidant qualities, Flavonoids are used in the food, cosmetic, and pharmaceutical industries [84].

2.2.1 Flavonoids biosynthesis, structure, and classification

Flavonoids are phenolic chemicals or polyphenols that have over 6000 distinct configurations [83]. Flavonoids are generated from two biochemical processes in plants: the phenylpropanoid system, which generates the phenylpropanoid skeleton (C_6-C_3), and the polyketide pathway, which generates blocks for polymeric C_2 units [85]. Almost all flavonoids have a $C_6-C_3-C_6$ structure with two benzene rings, A and B, linked by an oxygen-containing heterocycle pyrene ring (C). Flavonoids are classified into two broad groups based on the degree of central heterocyclic ring saturation [79]. Anthocyanidins, Flavones, Flavonols, and Isoflavones, for example, have a $C_2{=}C_3$ unsaturation, whereas Flavanones, Dihydroflavonols, and Flavan-3-ols are saturated flavonoids (**Figure 2**).

2.2.1.1 Anthocyanins

Anthocyanins are responsible for the hues of flowers, which range from pink to blue, but they are also found in leaves, fruits, and roots. Anthocyanins are the anthocyanidins O-glycosides from a chemical standpoint, as previously stated. Anthocyanidins (**Figure 2g**), which are highly oxidized 2-aryl-3-hydroxychromenylium, are also colored pigments, but they are less stable, so there are fewer examples in nature. The most common derivatives are cyanidin, which is responsible for red to magenta colors, delphinidin, which is responsible for purple to blue colors and pelargonidin, which is responsible for orange to pink colors (**Figure 3**). The presence

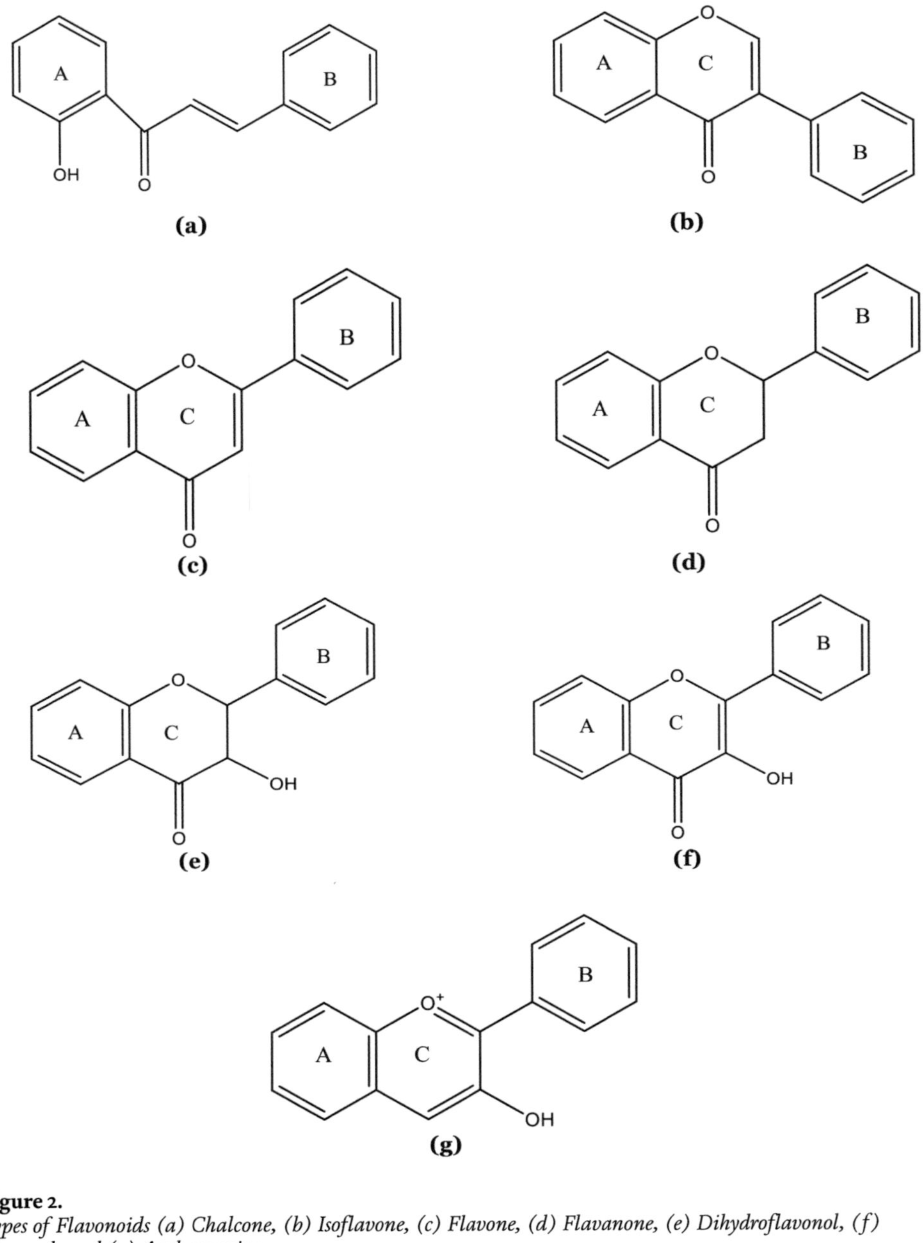

Figure 2.
Types of Flavonoids (a) Chalcone, (b) Isoflavone, (c) Flavone, (d) Flavanone, (e) Dihydroflavonol, (f) Flavonols and (g) Anthocyanins.

of a sugar moiety causes several color brightness alterations. The most frequent sugar with a β-linkage is glucose, but galactose, rhamnose, and xylose are also present [86].

2.2.1.2 Flavanones and dihydroflavonols

Flavanones, 2-arylchroman-4-ones (**Figure 2d**), are formed via ring closure isomerization of 20-hydroxychalcones, which results in a stereogenic center at carbon C_2. As a result, naturally occurring flavanones are optically active, mostly with a (2S) stereogenic structure, as in naringenin (**Figure 4**), a structure seen in natural flavanones. Many natural flavanones are also connected to sugars, mainly

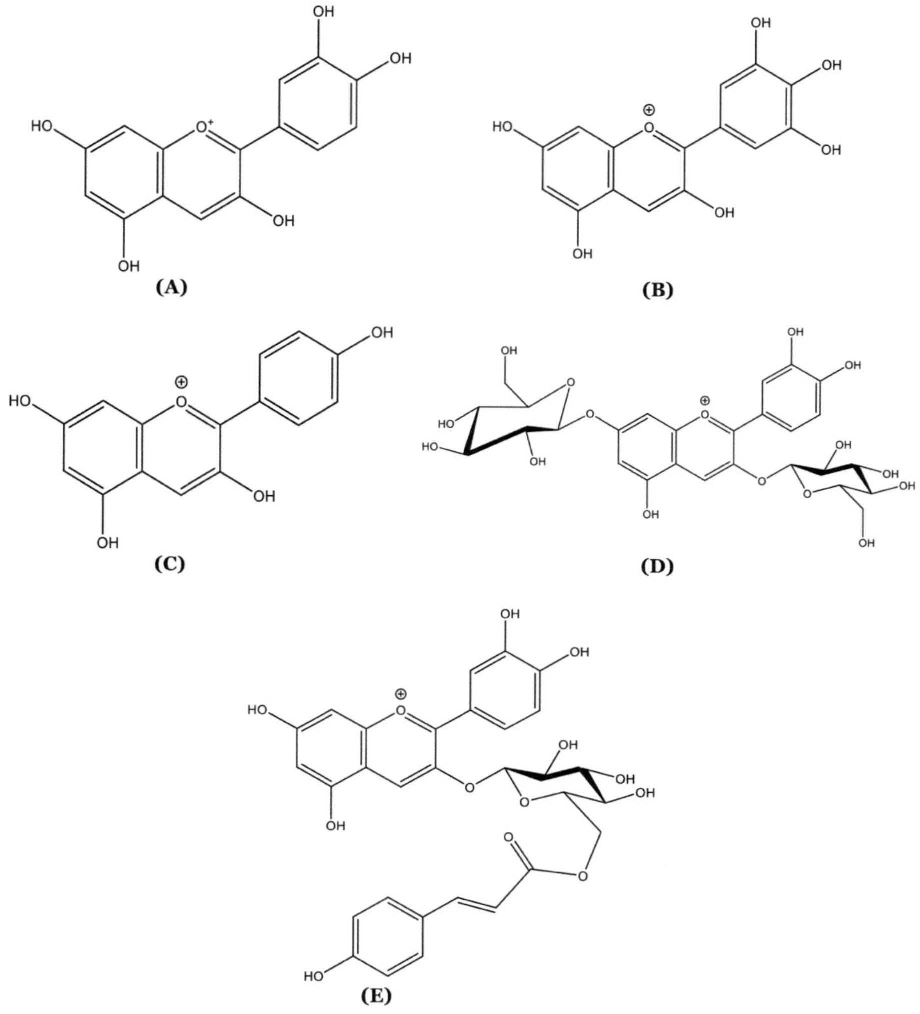

Figure 3.
Examples of representative anthocyanidins and anthocyanins. (A) Cyanidin, (B) Delphinidin, (C) Pelargonidin, (D) Seranin, (E) Hyacinthin.

as 7-O-glycosides, although others include prenyl side chains [87]. Dihydroflavonol, 2-aryl-3-hydroxychroman-4-one (**Figure 2e**), the biosynthesis of flavanones requires an oxidative hydroxy group addition at the C-3 position, which is why they are sometimes referred to as 3-hydroxyflavanones. Taxifolin is a common derivative that also serves as the principal scaffold for various other naturally occurring dihydroflavonols (**Figure 4**). These flavonoids are also discovered connected to sugars, with astilbin being an important example, as it has outstanding anti-inflammatory action [88] and is related to other groups such as prenyl and methoxy groups.

2.2.1.3 Isoflavones

Isoflavones, also known as 3-aryl-4H-chromen-4-ones (**Figure 2b**), are synthesized from flavanones by a rearrangement that favors 2,3-aryl migration followed by dehydrogenation. Although the word isoflavonoids is derived from the isolation of other

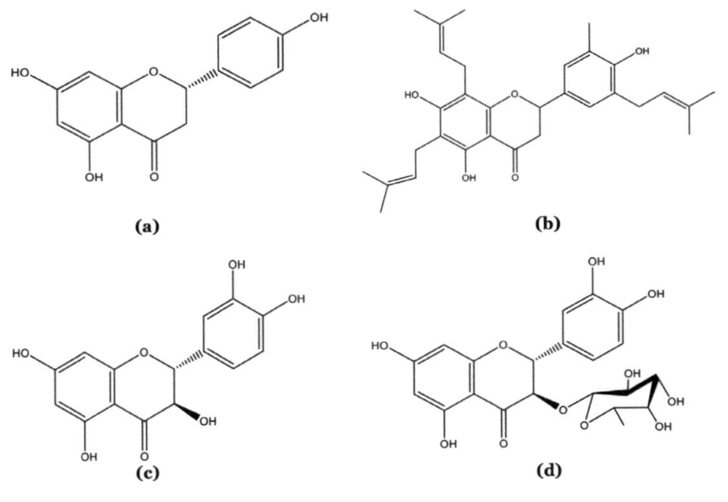

Figure 4.
Examples of representative Flavanones and Dihydroflavonols. (a) (2S)-Naringenin, (b) Amorisin, (c) (2R,3R)-Taxifolin and (d) Astilbin.

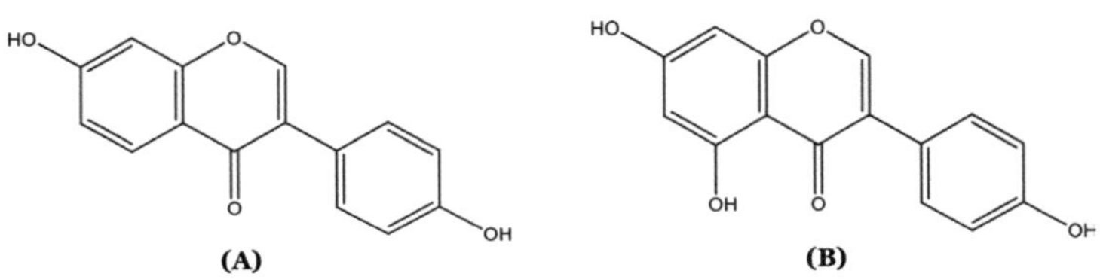

Figure 5.
Examples of representative isoflavones. (A) Daidzein (B) Genistein.

chemicals, such as isoflavanones or isoflavans, isoflavones remain the most prevalent. Isoflavones are still found only in a few subfamilies of the Leguminosae family [89]. Nonetheless, these metabolites have significant estrogenic action [90], and the anti-inflammatory benefits of several therapeutic plants are due to their isoflavone content [91]. The most prevalent scaffolds are daidzein and genistein (**Figure 5**), which are also discovered coupled to sugars however, there are just a few cases.

2.2.1.4 Flavones and flavonols

Flavones, 2-aryl-4H-chromen-4-ones (**Figure 2c**), and flavonols, 2-aryl-3-hydroxy-4H-chromen-4-ones (**Figure 2f**), are formed via dehydrogenation of flavanones and dihydroflavonols, respectively. Flavones are the most common and typical class of flavonoids, moreover if it is considered that flavonols are 3-hydroxyflavones. Flavones have piqued the curiosity of scientists due to their abundance in nature and documented biological activity [92]. Flavones are further classified based on their substitution pattern and wide dispersion, such as O-methylated, C-methylated, and isoprenylated, among others. Flavones are members of the flavonoid family that exist as both O- and C-glycosides, with the most common aglycones being apigenin and luteolin (**Figure 6**). Although various sugar moieties have been identified, glucose is the most prevalent, and the flavone-preferred O-glycosylation site is C_7. It's worth noting that many sugar units can be connected to C-glycosides, as shown in carlinoside (**Figure 6d**), the most common flavonol is quercetin (**Figure 6e**), which has

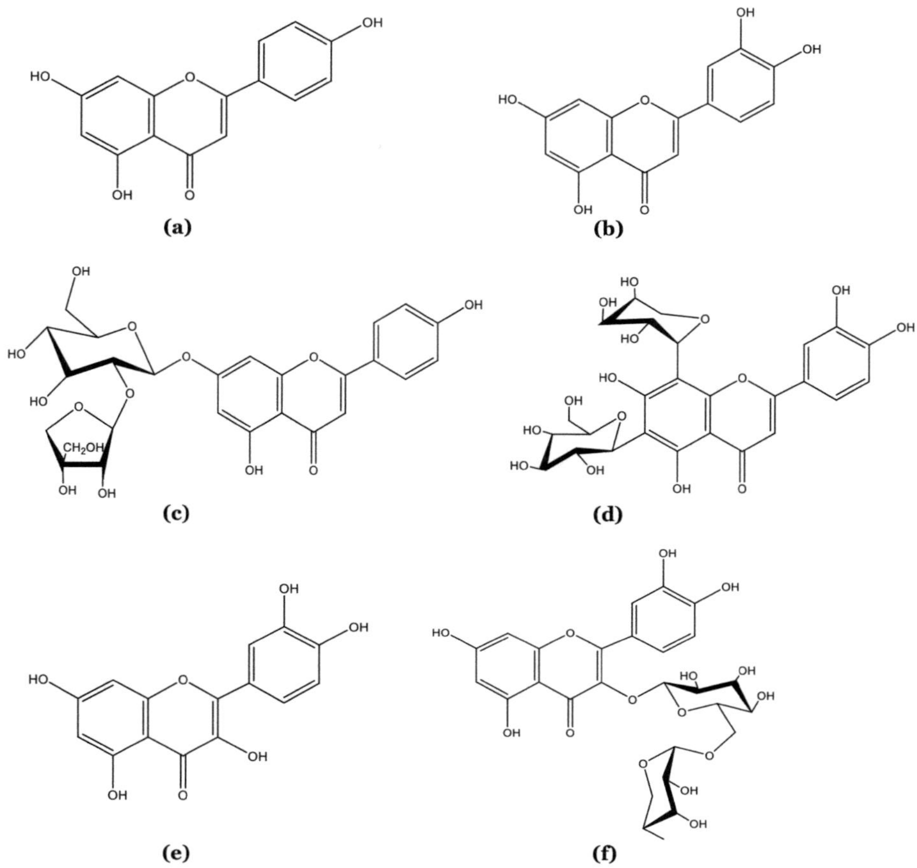

Figure 6.
Examples of representative flavones and flavonols. (a) Apigenin, (b) Luteolin, (c) Apiin, (d) Carlinoside, (e) Quercetin and (f) Rutin.

numerous biological features established [93], and which exists in both aglycone and oglycoside forms. In the case of rutin, O-glycosylation occurs at C_3 (**Figure 6f**). The most common flavonol glycoside in the plant kingdom.

2.2.2 Sources of flavonoids

Flavonoids may be found in a variety of drinks and foods, including wine, beer, and tea, but the largest concentrations of natural flavonoids can be found in fruits, vegetables, flowers, and seeds [94]. The quantity of these chemicals, however, is determined by various factors, including plant cultivar/genotype, growing environment circumstances, soil characteristics, harvest, and storage. Green leaves, fruits, and grains are high in flavonols such as quercetin, kaempferol, fisetin, isorhamnetin, and myricetin (**Table 3**) [95, 96]. Lettuce, cranberry, apple, peaches, and red pepper, for example, are high in quercetin and kaempferol [97]. Rutin, spinacetin glycosides, and patuletin glycosides are abundant in spinach leaves but kaempferol 3-O-glycosides are abundant in broccoli, kale, endive, potatoes, onions, grapes, and tomatoes [98]. Myricetin can be found in a variety of foods, including nuts, berries, tea, and red wine [98, 99]. Flavones, which include luteolin, apigenin, sinensetin, isosinensetin, nobiletin, tangeretin, galangin, and chrysin, are among the most significant flavonoids (**Table 3**) [95].

No.	Flavonoid classes	Examples	Food sources
1	Flavonols	Quercetin-Kaempferol-Fisetin-Isorhamnetin-Myricetin	Cranberry-Apple-Peaches-Grapes-Red pepper-Lettuce-Broccoli-Kale-Endive-Potatoes-Onions-Tomatoes-Nuts-Tea
2	Flavones	Luteolin-Apigenin-Sinensetin-Isosinensetin-Nobiletin-Tangeretin-Galangin-Chrysin-Baicalin	Citrus fruits-Green Tea-Red pepper-Lettuce-Broccoli-Oliveoil-Oregano-Thyme-Rosemary-Peppermint-Parsley-Cacao
3	Flavanols	Catechin-Epicatechin-Epicatechin gallate-GalloCatechin-EpigalloCatechin-EpigalloCatechin gallate	Tea-Cocoa-Raspberry-Apple-Red grape- Nectarine-Peach-Mango-Pear-Plum
4	Flavanones	Naringenin-Naringin-Hesperetin-Hesperidin-Eriodicytol	Orange-Mandarin-Lime-Lemon-Grape fruit
5	IsoFlavones	Daidzein-Genistein-Daidzin	Soyabean-Lupin-Fava beans-Chickpeas-Common beans- Kudzu roots-Peanuts
6	Anthocyanins	Pelargonidin-Cyanidin-Delphinidin-Peonidin-Petunidin-Malvidin	Cranberries-Blueberries-Raspberries-Bilberry-Strawberries-Blackberries-Red cabbage-Grapes-Cherries-Plums-Red turnip-Black beans-Purple corn

Table 3.
Flavonoid classes and examples of natural food sources

These chemicals are mostly found in leaves, flowers, and fruits as apigenin, luteolin, and diosmetin glucosides [96]. Apigenin-7-O-glycoside, for example, is plentiful in celery, while luteolin and apigenin glycosides are abundant in numerous citrus fruits, green and red peppers, lettuce, broccoli, olive oil, cocoa, oregano, thyme, rosemary, peppermint, and parsley [98]. Flavanols, also known as flavan-3-ols, are a group of compounds that include catechin, epicatechin, epicatechin gallate, gallocatechin, epigallocatechin, and epigallocatechin gallate (**Table 3**) [100]. Flavanols such as (−)-epigallocatechin gallate, (−)-epicatechin gallate, (−)-epigallocatechin, and (−)-epicatechin are abundant in Camellia sinensis, the tea plant, and tea drinking is one of the most significant sources of these flavonoids [101]. Furthermore, fruits high in (+)-catechin, (−)-epicatechin, and (−)-epigallocatechin include apples, red grapes, peaches, mangoes, pears, plums, nectarines, and raspberries. Catechins can be found in cocoa and red wine [97, 98]. Flavanones, also known as dihydroflavones, is a kind of flavonoid found in citrus fruits (**Table 3**). Flavanone glycosides such as naringin, naringenin, and naringenin 7-O-neohesperidoside may be found in grapefruits, hesperidin, hesperetin, and hesperetin 7-O-rutinoside in oranges, mandarins, limes and lemons, and eriocitrin, eriodictyol, and eriodictyol 7-O-rutinoside in lemons [96, 97]. Isoflavones have a more restricted distribution in plants, being generated mostly in legumes [102]. Soybeans are high in genistin, glycitin, and daidzin glycosides, as well as malonylated isoflavones [98] (**Table 3**). Genistin can also be found in lupin, fava beans, and kudzu roots. Isoflavones are found in small amounts in common beans, peanuts, and chickpeas [102]. Anthocyanins are flavonoids that give some flowers, foliage, and fruits their blue, purple, red, and orange colors. This family of chemicals is found in anthocyanidin glycosides such as cyanidin, pelargonidin, delphinidin, peonidin, petunidin, and malvidin [97]

(**Table 3**). Cranberries, blueberries, raspberries, bilberries, strawberries, blackberries, plums, grapes, cherries, and sweet potatoes for example contain significant levels of anthocyanins [98]. Red cabbage, red turnips, and purple sweet potatoes are high in acylated anthocyanins. Furthermore, black beans, and purple maize contain cyanidin 3-O-glucoside [96]. Some flowers are blue because of delphinidin, while others are orange because of pelargonidin. Natural flavonoids can be isolated and utilized in the food business instead of manufactured chemicals to improve food quality.

In recent years, restrictions on the use of some synthetic antioxidants, such as butylated hydroxyanisole (BHA), butylated hydroxytoluene (BHT), and propyl gallate, have increased interest in natural flavonoids, owing to their ability to slow oxidative degradation of lipids, improve food quality and nutritional value and reduce toxicity [103]. Flavonoids can be utilized as food preservatives, preventing lipid oxidation and safeguarding vitamins and enzymes, as microbial growth inhibitors in foods, as additions in human nutritional supplements and animal feed, as flavorings, and colorants and as flavorings and colorants (e.g., anthocyanins) [103]. Some flavonoids also decrease fungal spore germination and have been recommended as a fungal disease control agent in certain meals [104]. Flavonoids are extremely adaptable, with photochemical capabilities that can be employed to protect drinks against light-induced color loss [105]. Because flavonoids are natural chemicals with low toxicity, plentiful in plants, and affordable, their rising usage as food additives in place of synthetic preservatives will contribute to the sustainability of the food business.

2.2.3 Biological activity of flavonoids

Flavonoids have been demonstrated to have various health advantages in humans and a diet high in these substances can help avoid several chronic illnesses [94]. Flavonoids have numerous functions, but the capacity to scavenge free radicals and serve as antioxidants is unquestionably the most important. The antioxidant potential of flavonoids varies depending on the kind of functional group and its placement around the nuclear structure [106]. The amount and location of hydroxy groups in the catechol B-ring, as well as their position on the pyran C-ring, affect free radical scavenging capabilities [82]. Flavonoids' antioxidant activity methods include (a) direct scavenging of ROS, (b) suppression of ROS creation via trace element chelation (e.g., quercetin possesses iron-chelating and iron-stabilizing capabilities), or inhibition of enzymes involved in free radical production (e.g., glutathione S-transferase, microsomal monooxygenase, mitochondrial succinoxidase, NADH oxidase, and xanthine oxidase) and (c) antioxidant defense activation (e.g., upregulation of antioxidant enzymes with radical scavenging ability) [97, 106]. The majority of flavonoids occur as glycosides and the number and position of linkages with the sugar determine the flavonoid's antioxidant effects [107]. However, aglycone forms have a stronger antioxidant capability but are less available. In addition to antioxidant capabilities, flavonoids have been shown to have anti-inflammatory, anticancer, cardioprotective, antibacterial, and antiviral activities (**Table 4**). Inflammation develops as a result of a variety of factors, including tissue physical damage or trauma, chemical exposure, and microbial infection. In most circumstances, inflammation is brief and self-limiting, but in rare cases, continuous inflammation contributes to the development of chronic or degenerative illnesses such as cancer, diabetes, cardiovascular and neurological diseases, and obesity [108]. Flavonoids can serve as antioxidants in an inflammatory process, (a) scavenging ROS or lowering free radical buildup, (b) inhibitors of regulatory enzyme activity (e.g., protein kinases and phosphodiesterase), and

No.	Flavonoid classes	Compounds	Biological activities
1	Flavonols	Quercetin-Myricetin-Kaempferol-Isorhamnetin	Anti inflammatory-anticancer-cardioprotective-antifungal-anti bacterial-antiviral
2	Flavones	Apigenin-Luteolin-Chrysin-Baicalin-Acacetin	Anti inflammatory-anti cancer-cardioprotective-anti bacterial- antifungal-antiviral
3	Flavanols	Catechin-Epigallocatechin-Epicatechin-Epigallocatechin gallate	Anti cancer-anti bacterial-antiviral
4	Flavonones	Hesperetin-Hesperidin-Naringenin	Anti inflammatory-anti cancer-cardioprotective-antifungal
5	IsoFlavones	Genistein-Daidzein-Glabridin	Anti cancer-anti bacterial-antifungal-antiviral-cardioprotective
6	Anthocyanins	Cyanidin	Anti inflammatory-Anti Cancer

Table 4.
Flavonoid classes and some examples of their biological activities.

transcription factors involved in the regulation of mediators involved in the inflammatory process, and (c) immune cell activity modulators (e.g., suppression of cell activation, maturation, signaling transduction, and secretion processes) [108]. The inflammatory process is influenced by both hereditary and environmental factors.

Several studies have shown that a nutritious diet rich in fruits and vegetables, as well as non-processed and low-sugar meals, along with an active lifestyle, might help avoid inflammatory disorders [108]. Some flavonoids, such as flavonols (e.g., quercetin, rutin, and morin), flavanones (e.g., hesperetin and hesperidin), flavanols (e.g., catechin), isoflavones (e.g., genisten), and anthocyanins (e.g., cyanidin) have been demonstrated to exhibit anti-inflammatory functions during in vitro and in vivo experiments and clinical studies.

2.2.3.1 Cardiovascular protection

Flavonoids can protect the heart by reducing oxidative stress (preventing the oxidation of low-density lipoproteins), causing vasodilation, and regulating apoptotic processes in the endothelium [109]. Flavonoids can interact with lipid metabolism and minimize platelet aggregation, hence avoiding a variety of cardiovascular disorders [110]. Some research has shown that quercetin, naringenin, and hesperetin have vasodilator characteristics, with naringenin lowering blood pressure and relaxing vascular smooth muscles [108]. Isoflavones appear to protect against inflammatory vascular disorders and quercetin possesses cardioprotective characteristics against heart damage as well as an atheroprotective activity linked to oxidative stress reduction [108]. Baicalin has been shown to prevent apoptosis in heart tissue and alleviate cardiac dysfunction [111]. Chrysin inhibits platelet activity, while genistein has antihypertensive characteristics [109]. Anthocyanins reduce the risk of myocardial infarction in humans, enhance systolic blood pressure, and lower triglyceride total, and LDL cholesterol levels [112]. Furthermore, quercetin lowers systolic blood pressure and LDL cholesterol levels [81].

2.2.3.2 Antiviral action

Flavonoids can inhibit virus binding and penetration into cells, interfere with viral reproduction or translation and impede virus release [113]. Apigenin, for example, has been shown to inhibit viral protein synthesis in various DNA and RNA viruses, including herpes simplex virus, types 1 and 2, hepatitis C and B viruses, and the African swine fever virus [114]. Baicalein can inhibit avian influenza H_5N_1 virus multiplication in humans [115], while luteolin can inhibit HIV-1 reactivation [115]. Epigallocatechin gallate has an antiviral impact at several stages of the HIV-1 life cycle [115]. By interfering with HIV-mediated actin dynamics, genistein can prevent HIV infection of CD4 T cells and macrophages [116]. In addition, kaempferol can limit HIV replication in target cells [117] and prevent herpes simplex virus types 1 and 2 from adhering to and entering the host cell [116]. Wu et al. demonstrated the antiviral activity of quercetin, kaempferol, and epigallocatechin gallate against different influenza virus strains [118].

2.2.3.3 Antibacterial action

Flavonoids have multiple methods of action against bacteria. They can damage bacterial membranes and hinder many activities such as biofilm development, cell envelope creation, nucleic acid synthesis, electron transport chain, and ATP generation [119].

Catechin, epicatechin, and epigallocatechin gallate, as well as the flavonol quercetin, appear to cause an oxidative burst, boosting ROS generation and thereby increasing membrane permeability and damage [120]. Apigenin can disrupt membrane structure by disordering and disorienting membrane lipids, resulting in membrane leakage [119]. Flavonoids such as apigenin, chrysin, naringenin, kaempferol, quercetin, daidzein, and genistein limit biofilm development, whereas luteolin, myricetin and baicalein hinder bacterial DNA replication [119]. Epigallocatechin gallate and baicalein may limit bacterial ATP production [121].

2.2.3.4 Antifungal action

Flavonoids have several antifungal mechanisms, including disruption of the plasma membrane, activation of numerous mitochondrial dysfunctions, and suppression of cell wall production, cell division, and RNA and protein synthesis [122]. Apigenin and Baicalein can serve as antifungals by lowering lipid peroxidation and preventing membrane disruption [123]. Some isoflavones, such as glabridin, can impede the formation of fungal cell wall components such as β-glucans and chitin [124]. Quercetin can influence numerous mitochondrial activities, including the suppression of oxidative phosphorylation and the modification of ROS generation [125]. Apigenin disrupts the cell cycle, whereas myricetin, kaempferol, quercetin, luteolin, naringenin, and genistein inhibit DNA, RNA, and protein synthesis [126].

2.2.4 Conclusions

Alkaloids are of enormous medicinal and societal importance as a source of innovative leading chemicals for medication development against a variety of severe illnesses. Among them, the indole, tropane, and isoquinoline alkaloids are widely known for their medicinal potential in the treatment of hypertension, cancer, microbial infection, neurological disorders, and other conditions. They are structurally distinct bioactive compounds with potential therapeutic properties. Finally, an extensive study on their metabolic transformation, the introduction of a wide variety of scientific instruments, and the collaborative collaboration of specialists from other scientific fields will speed up research on this hotspot and give new and significant healthcare chances. Also, flavonoids as another secondary chemical have different roles in growth and development as well as stress prevention. A greater understanding of the positive effects of flavonoids on human health has led to increased consumption and interest in using flavonoids in food processing and for medicinal purposes. Flavonoids are abundant in vegetables, flowers, and seeds, and methods have been developed to extract these compounds from these natural sources for use as food additives and preservatives. The recognition of natural flavonoids as a good and safer source of antioxidants provides new avenues for further research on these chemicals, focusing on new structures, new approaches and technologies, and other new natural sources.

Acknowledgements

In this section, I'd like to thank my dear parents for all of their hard work on my behalf.

Author details

Hamed Zandavar* and Mojtaba Afshari Babazad
Malek Ashtar University of Technology, Tehran, Iran

*Address all correspondence to: zandavar_hamed@yahoo.com

References

[1] Daviss B. Growing pains for metabolomics: The newest'omic science is producing results and more data than researchers know what to do with. The Scientist. 2005;**19**(8):25-29

[2] Jordan KW et al. Metabolomic characterization of human rectal adenocarcinoma with intact tissue magnetic resonance spectroscopy. Diseases of the Colon and Rectum. 2009;**52**(3):520-525

[3] Mera IF, Falconí DE. Secondary metabolites in plants: Main classes, phytochemical analysis and pharmacological activities. Bionatura. 2019;**4**(4):1000-1009

[4] Návarová H et al. Pipecolic acid, an endogenous mediator of defense amplification and priming, is a critical regulator of inducible plant immunity. The Plant Cell. 2012;**24**(12):5123-5141

[5] Ishtiyak P et al. Traditional use of medicinal plants among tribal communities of Bangus Valley, Kashmir Himalaya. India. Studies on Ethno-Medicine. 2017;**11**(4):318-331

[6] Amirkia V, Heinrich M. Alkaloids as drug leads – A predictive structural and biodiversity-based analysis. Phytochemistry Letters. 2014;**10**:xlviii-liii

[7] Kaur RAJBIR, Arora SAROJ. Alkaloids-important therapeutic secondary metabolites of plant origin. Journal of critical reviews. 2015;**2**(3):1-8

[8] Roy A. A review on the alkaloids an important therapeutic compound from plants. IJPB. 2017;**3**(2):1-9

[9] Qiu S et al. Natural alkaloids: Basic aspects, biological roles, and future perspectives. Chinese Journal of Natural Medicines. 2014;**12**(6):401-406

[10] Manske RHF, Holmes HL, editors. The Alkaloids: Chemistry and Physiology. Elsevier; 2014

[11] McNaught AD, Wilkinson A. Compendium of Chemical Terminology. Blackwell Science Oxford; 1997

[12] Lewis RA. Lewis' Dictionary of Toxicology. CRC Press; 1998

[13] Croteau R, Kutchan TM, Lewis NG. Natural products (secondary metabolites). Biochemistry and Molecular Biology of Plants. 2000;**24**:1250-1319

[14] Boit HG. Ergebnisse der Alkaloid-Chemie bis 1960. Berlin: Akademie Verl; 1961

[15] Aniszewski T. Alkaloids-Secrets of Life:: Aklaloid Chemistry, Biological Significance, Applications and Ecological Role. Elsevier; 2007

[16] Dewick PM. Medicinal Natural Products: A Biosynthetic Approach. John Wiley & Sons; 2002

[17] Chini C et al. Protoalkaloids from Boscia angustifolia. Planta Medica. 1992;**58**(05):476-476

[18] Eagleson M. Concise Encyclopedia Chemistry. Walter de Gruyter; 1994

[19] Biastoff S et al. Chapter 2 Calystegines. In: Cordell GA, editor. The Alkaloids: Chemistry and Biology. Academic Press; 2007. pp. 49-102

[20] Gossauer A. Monopyrrolic natural compounds including tetramic acid

derivatives. In: Gossauer A et al., editors. Fortschritte der Chemie organischer Naturstoffe / Progress in the Chemistry of Organic Natural Products. Vienna: Springer Vienna; 2003. pp. 1-188

[21] Hemscheidt T. Tropane and related alkaloids. In: Leeper FJ, Vederas JC, editors. Biosynthesis: Aromatic Polyketides, Isoprenoids, Alkaloids. Berlin Heidelberg: Springer; 2000. pp. 175-206

[22] Hartmann T et al. Biosynthesis and metabolism of pyrrolizidine alkaloids in plants and specialized insect herbivores. In: Leeper FJ, Vederas JC, editors. Biosynthesis: Aromatic Polyketides, Isoprenoids, Alkaloids, Springer. Berlin Heidelberg: Berlin, Heidelberg; 2000. pp. 207-243

[23] Jemes R, Liddell JR. Pyrrolizidine alkaloids. Natural Product Reports. 2002;**19**:773-781

[24] Rizk AF. Naturally Occurring Pyrrolizidine Alkaloids. CRC Press; 1990

[25] Robins DJ. In: Daly JW et al., editors. The Pyrrolizidine Alkaloids, in Fortschritte der Chemie organischer Naturstoffe/Progress in the Chemistry of Organic Natural Products. Vienna: Springer; 1982. pp. 115-202

[26] Schardl CL et al. Loline alkaloids: Currencies of mutualism. Phytochemistry. 2007;**68**(7):980-996

[27] Wróbel JT. Chapter 7 Pyrrolizidine alkaloids. In: Brossi A, editor. The Alkaloids: Chemistry and Pharmacology. Academic Press; 1985. pp. 327-384

[28] Strunz GM, Findlay JA. Chapter 3 pyridine and piperidine alkaloids. In: Brossi A, editor. The Alkaloids: Chemistry and Pharmacology. Academic Press; 1985. pp. 89-183

[29] Michael JP. Quinoline, quinazoline and acridone alkaloids. Natural Product Reports. 2001;**18**(5):543-559

[30] Soares MS et al. Chapter 4 alkyl, aryl, alkylarylquinoline, and related alkaloids. In: Cordell GA, editor. The Alkaloids: Chemistry and Biology. Academic Press; 2007. pp. 139-214

[31] Schiff PL. Bisbenzylisoquinoline alkaloids. Journal of Natural Products. 1987;**50**(4):529-599

[32] Kam T et al. Chapter 4 bisindole alkaloids. In: Cordell GA, editor. The Alkaloids: Chemistry and Biology. Academic Press; 2006. pp. 181-337

[33] Kawasaki T, Higuchi K. Simple indole alkaloids and those with a nonrearranged monoterpenoid unit. Natural Product Reports. 2005;**22**(6):761-793

[34] Knölker H. Synthesis of biologically active carbazole alkaloids using selective transition-metal-catalyzed coupling reactions. Chemistry Letters. 2008;**38**(1):8-13

[35] Mukherjee J, Menge M. Progress and prospects of ergot alkaloid research. In: New Products and New Areas of Bioprocess Engineering. Berlin Heidelberg: Springer; 2000. pp. 1-20

[36] Schardl CL, Panaccione PTDG. Chapter 2 ergot alkaloids – Biology and molecular biology. In: Cordell GA, editor. The Alkaloids: Chemistry and Biology. Academic Press; 2006. pp. 45-86

[37] Somei M, Yamada F. Simple indole alkaloids and those with a nonrearranged monoterpenoid unit. Natural Product Reports. 2004;**21**(2):278-311

[38] Somei M et al. Recent synthetic studies on the ergot alkaloids and related compounds. In: The Alkaloids: Chemistry

and Biology. Academic Press; 2000. pp. 191-257

[39] Ata A et al. Chapter 3 Buxus steroidal alkaloids: Chemistry and biology. In: Cordell GA, editor. The Alkaloids: Chemistry and Biology. Academic Press; 2008. pp. 191-213

[40] Habermehl G. Chapter 9 The Steroid Alkaloids: The Salamandra Group**Supplementary to Volume V, page 321. In: Manske RHF, editor. The Alkaloids: Chemistry and Physiology. Academic Press; 1967. pp. 427-439

[41] Keeler RF. Teratology of steroidal alkaloids. Alkaloids: Chemical and Biological Perspectives. 1986;**4**:389-425

[42] Ripperger H. Chapter Two – Solanum steroid alkaloids – An update. In: Pelletier SW, editor. Alkaloids: Chemical and Biological Perspectives. Pergamon; 1998. pp. 103-185

[43] Zhao H et al. A novel pregnane-type alkaloid from Pachysandra terminalis inhibits methicillin-resistant staphylococcus aureus in vitro and in vivo. Phytotherapy Research. 2015;**29**(3):373-380

[44] Jin Z. Imidazole, oxazole and thiazole alkaloids. Natural Product Reports. 2006;**23**(3):464-496

[45] Maat L, Beyerman HC. Chapter 5 The imidazole alkaloids. In: Brossi A, editor. The Alkaloids: Chemistry and Pharmacology. Academic Press; 1984. pp. 281-333

[46] Ashihara H, Yokota T, Crozier A, Alkaloids P. Cytokinins, and purine-like neurotoxin alkaloids. In: Ramawat KG, Mérillon J-M, editors. Natural Products: Phytochemistry, Botany and Metabolism of Alkaloids, Phenolics and Terpenes. Berlin Heidelberg: Springer; 2013. pp. 953-975

[47] Lean MEJ, et al. Purine alkaloids: A focus on caffeine and related compounds in beverages. In: Crozier A, Ashihara H, Tomás-Barbéran F, editors. Teas, Cocoa and Coffee: Plant Secondary Metabolites and Health; 2011. pp. 25-44

[48] Cheeke PR. Toxicity and metabolism of pyrrolizidine alkaloids. Journal of Animal Science. 1988;**66**(9):2343-2350

[49] Karuna DS et al. In vitro antioxidant activities of root extract of Asparagus racemosus Linn. Journal of Traditional and Complementary Medicine. 2018;**8**(1):60-65

[50] Kundu A et al. Protective effects of Croton hookeri on streptozotocin-induced diabetic nephropathy. Food and Chemical Toxicology. 2020;**135**:110873

[51] Sagi S et al. Quantification and characterization of alkaloids from roots of Rauwolfia serpentina using ultra-high performance liquid chromatography-photo diode array-mass spectrometry. Analytical and Bioanalytical Chemistry. 2016;**408**(1):177-190

[52] El-Sayed M, Verpoorte R. Catharanthus terpenoid indole alkaloids: Biosynthesis and regulation. Phytochemistry Reviews. 2007;**6**(2):277-305

[53] Gul W et al. Indole alkaloid marine natural products: An established source of cancer drug leads with considerable promise for the control of parasitic, neurological and other diseases. Life Sciences. 2005;**78**(5):442-453

[54] Gupta DK et al. Moderate uranium disturbs the nutritional status and induces oxidative stress in *Pisum sativum* L. Journal of Plant Physiology and Pathology. 2016;**4**(1)

[55] Mohapatra S, Mittra B. Induction of glutathione, ascorbate and

associated enzymes by a low dose $CdCl_2$ pretreatment alleviate fusarium induced oxidative stress in wheat. Journal of Plant Physiolology and Pathology. 2016;**4**:1

[56] Seleim MA et al. Peroxidase and polyphenoloxidase activities as biochemical markers for biocontrol efficacy in the control of tomato bacterial wilt. Journal of Plant Physiolology and Pathology. 2014;**2**(1):2

[57] Archana US, Prasad D. Management of plant-parasitic nematodes by the use of botanicals. Journal of Plant Physiology and Pathology. 2014;**2**(1)

[58] Abduyeva-Ismayilova SM. Effect of physiological acid salts on swelling, germination and growth processes of seedlings. Journal of Plant Physiolology and Pathology. 2016;**4**:1

[59] Soares PRO et al. In vitro antiproliferative effects of the indole alkaloid vallesiachotamine on human melanoma cells. Archives of Pharmacal Research. 2012;**35**(3):565-571

[60] Bifulco G et al. (±)-Gelliusines A and B, two diastereomeric brominated tris-indole alkaloids from a deep water new caledonian Marine Sponge (Gellius or Orina sp.). Journal of Natural Products. 1994;**57**(9):1294-1299

[61] Lind KF et al. Antioxidant and anti-inflammatory activities of barettin. Marine Drugs. 2013;**11**(7)

[62] Shamon SD, Perez MI. Blood pressure-lowering efficacy of reserpine for primary hypertension. Cochrane Database of Systematic Reviews. 2016;**12**

[63] Schuldiner S, Liu Y, Edwards RH. Reserpine binding to a vesicular amine transporter expressed in Chinese hamster ovary fibroblasts. Journal of Biological Chemistry. 1993;**268**(1):29-34

[64] Blackman JG, Campion DS, Fastier FN. Mechanism of action of reserpine in producing gastric haemorrhage and erosion in the mouse. British Journal of Pharmacology and Chemotherapy. 1959;**14**(1):112-116

[65] Nammi S, Boini KM, Sreemantula SS. Reserpine-induced central effects: Pharmacological evidence for the lack of central effects of reserpine methiodide. Canadian Journal of Physiology and Pharmacology. 2005;**83**(6):509-515

[66] Owens MW et al. Nebulized atropine sulfate in the treatment of acute asthma. Chest. 1991;**99**(5):1084-1087

[67] Young GP, Freitas P. A randomized comparison of atropine and metaproterenol inhalational therapies for refractory status asthmaticus. Annals of Emergency Medicine. 1991;**20**(5):513-519

[68] Iguchi A et al. Hyperglycemia induced by hippocampal administration of neostigmine is suppressed by intrahypothalamic atropine. Neuropharmacology. 1991;**30**(10):1129-1131

[69] Julu P, Adler J, Hondo RG. Vagal Tone in Healthy-Volunteers Given Atropine and in Diabetic-Patients. New York: Cambridge University Press; 1991

[70] Wedge DE, Camper ND. Connections between agrochemicals and pharmaceuticals. In: Biologically Active Natural Products. CRC Press; 1999. pp. 13-27

[71] Saravanan G, Pari L. Effect of Cogent db, a herbal drug, on serum and tissue lipid metabolism in experimental hyperglycaemic rats. Diabetes, Obesity and Metabolism. 2003;**5**(3):156-162

[72] Chauhan NS. Medicinal and Aromatic Plants of Himachal Pradesh. Indus Publishing; 1999

[73] Potdar D, Hirwani RR, Dhulap S. Phyto-chemical and pharmacological applications of Berberis aristata. Fitoterapia. 2012;**83**(5):817-830

[74] Grynkiewicz G, Gadzikowska M. Tropane alkaloids as medicinally useful natural products and their synthetic derivatives as new drugs. Pharmacological Reports. 2008;**60**(4):439

[75] Ahmad S et al. In vitro production of alkaloids: Factors, approaches, challenges and prospects. Pharmacognosy Reviews. 2013;**7**(13):27-33

[76] Schmeller T et al. Utilization of alkaloids in modern medicine. In: Roberts MFW, editor. Alkaloids: Biochemistry, Ecology, and Medicinal Applications. Boston, MA: Springer; 1998. pp. 435-459

[77] Tadeusz A. The alkaloid-rich and alkaloid-poor Washington lupine (Lupinus polyphyllus Lindl.) as a potential industrial crop. Industrial Crops and Products. 1992;**1**(2):147-155

[78] De Luna SLR, Ramírez Garza SOSSRE. Environmentally friendly methods for flavonoid extraction from plant material: Impact of their operating conditions on yield and antioxidant properties. The Scientific World Journal. 2020;**2020**:6792069

[79] Saini N, Gahlawat SK, Lather V. Flavonoids: A nutraceutical and its role as anti-inflammatory and anticancer agent. In: Gahlawat SKS, Siwach RK, Duhan P, Singh J, Kumar SK, editors. Plant Biotechnology: Recent Advancements and Developments. Singapore: Springer; 2017. pp. 255-270

[80] Jucá MM et al. Flavonoids: Biological activities and therapeutic potential. Natural Product Research. 2020;**34**(5):692-705

[81] Fraga CG et al. The effects of polyphenols and other bioactives on human health. Food & Function. 2019;**10**(2):514-528

[82] D'Amelia V et al. The antioxidant properties of plant flavonoids: Their exploitation by molecular plant breeding. Phytochemistry Reviews. 2018;**17**(3):611-625

[83] Šamec D et al. The role of polyphenols in abiotic stress response: The influence of molecular structure. Plants. 2021;**10**(1)

[84] Kumar S, Pandey AK. Chemistry and biological activities of flavonoids: An overview. The Scientific World Journal. 2013;**2013**:162750

[85] Nabavi SM et al. Flavonoid biosynthetic pathways in plants: Versatile targets for metabolic engineering. Biotechnology Advances. 2020;**38**:107316

[86] Dias MC et al. Plant flavonoids: Chemical characteristics and biological activity. Molecules. 2021;**26**(17)

[87] Brahmachari G. Naturally occurring flavanones: An overview. Natural Product Communications. 2008;**3**(8):193

[88] Shukla R et al. Chapter 18 role of flavonoids in management of inflammatory disorders. In: Watson RR, Preedy VR, editors. Bioactive Food as Dietary Interventions for Arthritis and Related Inflammatory Diseases. Second ed. Academic Press; 2019. pp. 293-322

[89] Wong E. The isoflavonoids. In: Harborne JB, Mabry TJ, Mabry H, editors. The Flavonoids. Boston, MA: Springer; 1975. pp. 743-800

[90] Vitale DC et al. Isoflavones: Estrogenic activity, biological effect and bioavailability. European Journal of

Drug Metabolism and Pharmacokinetics. 2013;**38**(1):15-25

[91] Pinto DCGA, Simões MAM, Silva AMS. Genista tridentata L.: A Rich Source of Flavonoids with Anti-Inflammatory Activity. Medicine. 2020;**7**(6)

[92] Singh M, Kaur M, Silakari O. Flavones: An important scaffold for medicinal chemistry. European Journal of Medicinal Chemistry. 2014;**84**:206-239

[93] Batiha GE et al. The pharmacological activity, biochemical properties, and pharmacokinetics of the major natural polyphenolic flavonoid: Quercetin. Foods. 2020;**9**(3)

[94] García CR, Quesada CS, Gaforio JJ. Dietary flavonoids as cancer chemopreventive agents: An updated review of human studies. Antioxidants. 2019;**8**(5)

[95] Kozłowska A, Węgierek DS. Flavonoids – Food sources, health benefits, and mechanisms involved. In: Mérillon J-M, Ramawat KG, editors. Bioactive Molecules in Food. Cham: Springer International Publishing; 2017. pp. 1-27

[96] Terahara N. Flavonoids in foods: A review. Natural Product Communications. 2015;**10**(3):193

[97] Agrawal AD. Pharmacological activities of flavonoids: A review. International Journal of Pharmaceutical Sciences and Nanotechnology(IJPSN). 2011;**4**(2)

[98] Panche AN, Diwan AD, Chandra SR. Flavonoids: An overview. Journal of Nutritional Science. 2016;**5**:e47

[99] Basli A et al. Wine polyphenols: Potential agents in neuroprotection. Oxidative Medicine and Cellular Longevity. 2012;**2012**:805762

[100] Bae J et al. Activity of catechins and their applications. Biomedical Dermatology. 2020;**4**(1):8

[101] Dwyer JT, Peterson J. Tea and flavonoids: Where we are, where to go next. The American Journal of Clinical Nutrition. 2013;**98**(6):1611S-1618S

[102] Sharma V, Ramawat KG. Isoflavonoids. In: Ramawat KG, Mérillon J-M, editors. Natural Products: Phytochemistry, Botany and Metabolism of Alkaloids, Phenolics and Terpenes. Berlin: Springer; 2013. pp. 1849-1865

[103] Saul R. Flavonoids: Important Biocompounds in Food N2 - Flavonoids are abundant secondary metabolites found in plants and fungi that have various roles in these organisms, including pigmentation, cell signalling, plant defence and inter-organism communication. Due to their abundance in nature, flavonoids are also important components of the human diet, and the last four decades have seen an intense study focused on the structure characterization of flavonoids and on their roles in mammal metabolism. This book reviews most of the well-established activities of flavonoids, and we also present more recent research studies on the area of flavonoids, including the chemical aspects of structure characterization of flavonoids, the biosynthesis of flavonoids in model plants as well as their role in abiotic stress situations and in agriculture, the role of flavonoids in metabolism and health and their importance in foods, from consumption to their use as bioactive components. 2017: Chapter 16

[104] Redondo-Blanco S et al. Plant phytochemicals in food preservation: Antifungal bioactivity: A review. Journal of Food Protection. 2019;**83**(1):163-171

[105] Huvaere K, Skibsted LH. Flavonoids protecting food and beverages against light. Journal of the Science of Food and Agriculture. 2015;**95**(1):20-35

[106] Kaleem M, Ahmad A. Chapter 8 – Flavonoids as nutraceuticals. In: Grumezescu AM, Holban AM, editors. Therapeutic, Probiotic, and Unconventional Foods. Academic Press; 2018. pp. 137-155

[107] Sandoval V et al. Metabolic impact of flavonoids consumption in obesity: From central to peripheral. Nutrients. 2020;**12**(8)

[108] Maleki SJ, Crespo JF, Cabanillas B. Anti-inflammatory effects of flavonoids. Food Chemistry. 2019;**299**:125124

[109] Ciumărnean L et al. The effects of flavonoids in cardiovascular diseases. Molecules. 2020;**25**(18)

[110] Rolnik A et al. Quercetin and kaempferol derivatives isolated from aerial parts of Lens culinaris Medik as modulators of blood platelet functions. Industrial Crops and Products. 2020;**152**:112536

[111] Zhang Y et al. Baicalin attenuates cardiac dysfunction and myocardial remodeling in a chronic pressure-overload mice model. Cellular Physiology and Biochemistry. 2017;**41**(3):849-864

[112] Cassidy A. Berry anthocyanin intake and cardiovascular health. Molecular Aspects of Medicine. 2018;**61**:76-82

[113] Lalani S, Poh CL. Flavonoids as antiviral agents for enterovirus A71 (EV-A71). Viruses. 2020;**12**(2)

[114] Jaime MFV et al. In vitro antiviral activity of plant extracts from Asteraceae medicinal plants. Virology Journal. 2013;**10**(1):245

[115] Sithisarn P et al. Differential antiviral and anti-inflammatory mechanisms of the flavonoids biochanin A and baicalein in H5N1 influenza A virus-infected cells. Antiviral Research. 2013;**97**(1):41-48

[116] Zakaryan H et al. Flavonoids: Promising natural compounds against viral infections. Archives of Virology. 2017;**162**(9):2539-2551

[117] Behbahani M, Pourazar MSA. In vitro anti-HIV-1 activities of kaempferol and kaempferol-7-O-glucoside isolated from Securigera securidaca. Res Pharm Sci. 2014;**9**(6):463-469

[118] Wu W et al. Quercetin as an Antiviral Agent Inhibits Influenza A Virus (IAV) Entry. Viruses. 2016;**8**(1)

[119] Górniak I, Bartoszewski R, Króliczewski J. Comprehensive review of antimicrobial activities of plant flavonoids. Phytochemistry Reviews. 2019;**18**(1):241-272

[120] Fathima A, Rao JR. Selective toxicity of Catechin—a natural flavonoid towards bacteria. Applied Microbiology and Biotechnology. 2016;**100**(14):6395-6402

[121] Xu X, Wu CD. Tea catechin epigallocatechin gallate inhibits Streptococcus mutans biofilm formation by suppressing gtf genes. Archives of Oral Biology. 2012;**57**(6):678-683

[122] Al Aboody MS, Mickymaray S. Anti-fungal efficacy and mechanisms of flavonoids. Antibiotics. 2020;**9**(2)

[123] Tsang PW, Yang HP. Baicalein exhibits inhibitory effect on the energy-dependent efflux pump activity in non-albicans Candida fungi. Journal of Chemotherapy. 2015;**27**(1):61-62

[124] Lagrouh F, Dakka N, Bakri Y. The antifungal activity of Moroccan

plants and the mechanism of action of secondary metabolites from plants. Journal de Mycologie Médicale. 2017;**27**(3):303-311

[125] Oliveira MRD, Daglia M, Rastrelli L, Nabavi SM. Epigallocatechin gallate and mitochondria—A story of life and death. Pharmacological Research. 2016;**104**:70-85

[126] Cassetta A et al. Structural basis for inhibition of 17β-hydroxysteroid dehydrogenases by phytoestrogens: The case of fungal 17β-HSDcl. The Journal of Steroid Biochemistry and Molecular Biology. 2017;**171**:80-93

Chapter 6

Garlic (*Allium sativum* L.): Characterization of Bioactive Compounds and Related Health Benefits

Judita Lidiková, Natália Čeryová, Tomáš Tóth, Janette Musilová, Alena Vollmannová, Kushvara Mammadova and Eva Ivanišová

Abstract

Garlic (*Allium sativum* L.) is one of the greatest gifts of natural medicine and the oldest medicinal herbs that is cultivated all over the world. It is a widely used spice plant with well-known medicinal properties. Garlic is an important raw material of plant origin with observed and proven positive effects on the human body. *A. sativum* L. belongs to the most extensively studied medicinal herbs from genus *Allium*. In the past few decades, its biologically active compounds have been analyzed for their therapeutical properties. The most essential biologically active compound discovered in *A. sativum* is allicin, working synergistically with other phytochemicals in the prevention of many diseases. Preparation of garlic extractions can be done in liquid form and solid form. The composition and bioactivity of the extraction depend on the strain, age, method of preparation, and consumption method. When extracted and isolated, the bioactive compounds of garlic show a wide range of beneficial health effects: platelets inhibitory and antithrombic activities, hepatoprotective, antimicrobial, antihyperglycemic, antidiabetic, and antitumor. The present chapter describes botanical characterization of garlic, its chemical composition regarding bioactive compounds, and its health benefits.

Keywords: scallion, health benefits, polyphenols, antioxidant, sulfur compounds

1. Introduction

The name "*Allium sativum*" is derived from the Celtic word "all" meaning burning or pricking and the latin word "*sativum*" meaning planted or cultivated. Garlic is known by various names, such as "stinking rose", "nectar of the gods", "Russian penicillin", "natural antibiotic", "herbal viagra", "herbal talisman", "snake grass", some names are still used today [1, 2].

Garlic is known to have been used for medicinal purposes as far back as the middle ages, as evidenced by ancient writings from China, Egypt, Greece, and India [3]. Garlic has been used in various cultures for thousands of years, dating back to the time when the Egyptian pyramids and ancient Greek temples were being built. In 1720, garlic was used to save the inhabitants of Marseille from the black plague. Garlic was often used in funerals and religious ceremonies to mummify bodies. The Greeks used garlic as a remedy against aging and disease. Interestingly, Greek athletes participating in the olympic games chewed garlic to improve their stamina, strength, and endurance [4]. In Roman times, workers and soldiers chewed garlic before battle, and the Slavs claimed that it protected them from snakebites. In Africa, fishermen painted their bodies with garlic extract to ward off crocodiles. In Europe, garlic was believed to be able to ward off vampires, demons, evil spirits, and other magical properties. Even the Bible refers to its use [5]. This aromatic vegetable is mentioned in the Bible because the Israelites were tired of eating simple manna and longed for the pleasant varieties that were eaten in Egypt. Garlic has been used among several ancient civilizations around the world in addition to Egypt, Greece, Rome, India, and China to treat various ailments, including poisoning, respiratory and stomach ailments, abnormal growth, headache, insomnia, and depression [6]. The ancient Greek physician Hippocrates (ca. 460–370 BC), known today as the "father of western medicine," prescribed garlic for a wide range of ailments. Hippocrates recommended the use of garlic to treat respiratory problems, parasites, indigestion, and fatigue [7]. Garlic is an effective medicine against diseases, including viral diseases. Ingestion of fresh garlic or intravenous preparation of its extracts has also been used to treat patients with cryptococcal meningitis in China. In Asia and Europe, garlic was used to treat cold, fever, cough, asthma, and wounds. Garlic has been used in traditional African medicine (in Ethiopia and Nigeria) to treat infections, including sexually transmitted diseases, tuberculosis, respiratory tract infections, and wounds [8]. Throughout history, in the Middle East, East Asia, and Nepal, garlic has been used to treat bronchitis, hypertension (high blood pressure), tuberculosis, liver disorders, dysentery, flatulence, intestinal worms, rheumatism, diabetes, and fever [7].

Nicolas Culpeper wrote in the Complete Herbal, 1653, "...a remedy for all diseases and injuries. It induces urine and menses, helps in bites of mad dogs and other venomous creatures, kills worms in children, cuts and destroys tough phlegm, clears the head, helps lethargy, and is a good preservative and remedy for any pestilential, sore, or foul sores." Garlic was already used by the ancient Egyptians for both medicinal and food purposes. Several bulbs of garlic were found in the tomb of Tutankhamun, probably to protect the young king on his way to the afterlife [9].

During World War I, garlic was widely used as an antiseptic to prevent gangrene, and today people use garlic to prevent atherosclerosis, improve high blood pressure, and relieve coughs and bronchitis [10]. Garlic has attracted special attention in modern medicine because of the widespread belief in its effects on maintaining good health. In some western countries, sales of garlic preparations are comparable to prescription drugs [11]. The main garlic growing countries are China, India, Spain, Egypt, Argentina, Italy, and the United States [12]. Currently, China is the largest producer and exporter of garlic [6].

Multiple studies have shown the multifaceted health effects of garlic, which is why it is recommended as a dietary supplement all over the world. Because of these proven effects, its consumption has increased, especially in the culinary field [13]. Replace the entirety of this text with the introduction to your chapter. The introduction section should provide a context for your manuscript and should be numbered as first heading. When preparing the introduction, please bear in mind that some readers will not be experts in your field of research.

2. Chemical composition of garlic

Garlic is considered one of the 20 most important vegetables with various uses around the world, either as a raw vegetable for culinary purposes or as part of traditional and modern medicine [14].

Its health-promoting properties are attributed to its chemical composition. The chemical composition of garlic is significantly influenced by the variety, growing conditions, and growing practices. In particular, the fertilization regime and soil properties can have a significant impact on quality properties, such as mineral composition, dry matter, protein content, and total soluble solids content [15]. Due to the fact that garlic is commonly consumed cooked and as a dried spice, several authors have also investigated and found that heating can affect the chemical composition of garlic, including its antioxidant properties. The health benefits of garlic depend on the content of biologically active compounds that differ between varieties and geographical areas [16].

Fresh garlic contains approximately 63% water, 28% carbohydrates (fructans), 2.3% organosulfur compounds, 2% protein (allinase), 1.2% free amino acids (arginine), and 1.5% fiber [1, 17]. Other authors [18] reported approximately 65% water, 28% carbohydrates, 2.3% organosulfur compounds, 2% protein, 1.2% free amino acids, and 1.5% fiber in garlic.

Garlic contains 17 amino acids, which include lysine, histidine, arginine, threonine, aspartic acid, glutamine, proline, serine, glycine, alanine, cysteine, valine, methionine, isoleucine, leucine, tryptophan, and phenylalanine. A very effective component of garlic is polysaccharides, which are becoming more and more attractive due to their various pharmacological effects. They exhibit various biological activities, including antioxidant and hepatoprotective effects. Garlic polysaccharides consist of monosaccharides, such as fructose, glucose, and sucrose [19]. These polysaccharides have a high molecular weight, form one of the active components of garlic, and are characterized by low toxicity. In garlic, they represent approximately 26–30% of the fresh weight [20].

Study [21] reported that the main carbohydrate in kitchen garlic is sucrose, which ranged from 1.99 to 3.29 g.100 g-1 fresh mass and represented up to 97% of the total carbohydrate content in garlic. Fructose was detected in relatively low amounts, and glucose was not recorded in the monitored garlic varieties. Dried garlic heads contain mainly water (62–68%) and carbohydrates (26–30%), while proteins are detected in a relatively smaller amount (1.5–2.1%). The energy content is approximately 140 kcal.100 g-1 of fresh mass.

Garlic contains a high content of vitamins, especially vitamin C and group B vitamins. Vitamin C has beneficial effects on the immune system. Ensuring sufficient intake of vitamin C through the diet is essential for the body's resistance to infections [22].

Garlic contains relatively large amounts of vital minerals and trace elements, such as calcium, phosphorus, potassium, sodium, magnesium, aluminum, iron, copper, manganese, chromium, molybdenum, selenium, germanium, and iodine. The most represented minerals in garlic are potassium, phosphorus, and calcium [23]. Other authors [24–26] state the rich content of sodium, magnesium, potassium as well as vitamin C and group B in garlic. Potassium is one of the main blood minerals called electrolyte, it is important for cellular function; a high concentration of potassium helps to prevent hypertension [27].

The health effects of garlic depend on the level of some mineral elements, such as Se, K, Zn, and Ca [28]. Lee et al. [29] reported that potassium, phosphorus, magnesium, and calcium are the main constituents of garlic. Sulfur, selenium, and germanium are also found in kitchen garlic [30].

Turan et al. [31] reported that consumption of 100 g of garlic represents 3–5% of the recommended daily intake of Zn and Mn for adults. Mineral elements prevent various diseases, such as osteoporosis, cardiovascular disease, and aging.

The vitamins and minerals found in kitchen garlic are essential for proper functioning and health, so they must be obtained through an adequate balanced diet. They are considered micronutrients and act mainly as cofactors [32]. Garlic is an important source of nicotinic acid, thiamin, and riboflavin. It also contains citral, linalool, geraniol, α-phellandrene, valeraldehyde, and propionaldehyde [33]. A wide range of other organic compounds in garlic, such as steroid glycosides, essential oils, lectins, prostaglandins, adenosine, glycolipids, and phospholipids are reported [34].

Garlic is a source of other nonvolatile phytonutrients with significant medicinal and therapeutic properties, of which special emphasis is placed on flavonoids, saponins and sapogenins, phenolic compounds, nitrogen oxides and amides, and proteins [35].

2.1 Sulfur compounds in garlic

The specific smell and taste of garlic caused by sulfur-containing phytochemicals [36, 37]. The most characteristic volatile and odorous organosulfur compounds of garlic are released after disruption of the cell membrane. Garlic contains bioactive compounds, such as organic sulfur compounds, phenols, and saponins, which exhibit various biological activities, namely antioxidant, immunomodulatory, anti-inflammatory, anticancer, hepatoprotective, cardiovascular protective, antidiabetic, antiobesity, renal, neuroprotective, antibacterial, and antifungal activities [38–40]. The synergistic interactions between the individual components present contribute to these remarkable health effects of garlic [41].

Garlic contains at least 33 sulfur compounds. Organosulfur compounds are effective scavengers of free radicals. A unique group of plants of the genus Allium are alk(en)yl-cysteine sulfoxides, which are responsible for their typical smell and taste. These sulfoxides include S-methyl-L-cysteine sulfoxide (methine), S-allyl-L-cysteine sulfoxide (alliine), S-propyl-L-cysteine sulfoxide (propiine), S-ethyl-L-cysteine sulfoxide (ethiine), and S-butyl-L-cysteine sulfoxide (butyin) [42, 43]. Untreated fresh garlic also contains high amounts of glutamylcysteine. These compounds can be hydrolyzed and oxidized to form alliin. In fresh garlic, alliin is present in the amount of 10 mg/g, while in dried garlic its level is 30 mg/g [44].

After processing, such as cutting, crushing, chewing, or dehydration, allinase rapidly cleaves cytotoxic cysteine sulfoxides (alliin) to form cytotoxic and aromatic alkylalkane thiosulfinates, such as allicin, which is the main biologically active component of garlic extract. It represents about 70% of all thiosulfinates formed in crushed garlic [45, 46]. According to Ref. [47] uncrushed garlic contains approximately 16 organosulfur compounds, while crushed garlic contains 23 organosulfur compounds. Allicin contributes to the characteristic flavor and aroma of garlic [16]. Allicin is a thio-ester of sulfenic acid and its beneficial effect on health is attributed to its antioxidant activity as well as its interaction with thiol-containing proteins (**Figure 1**) [48].

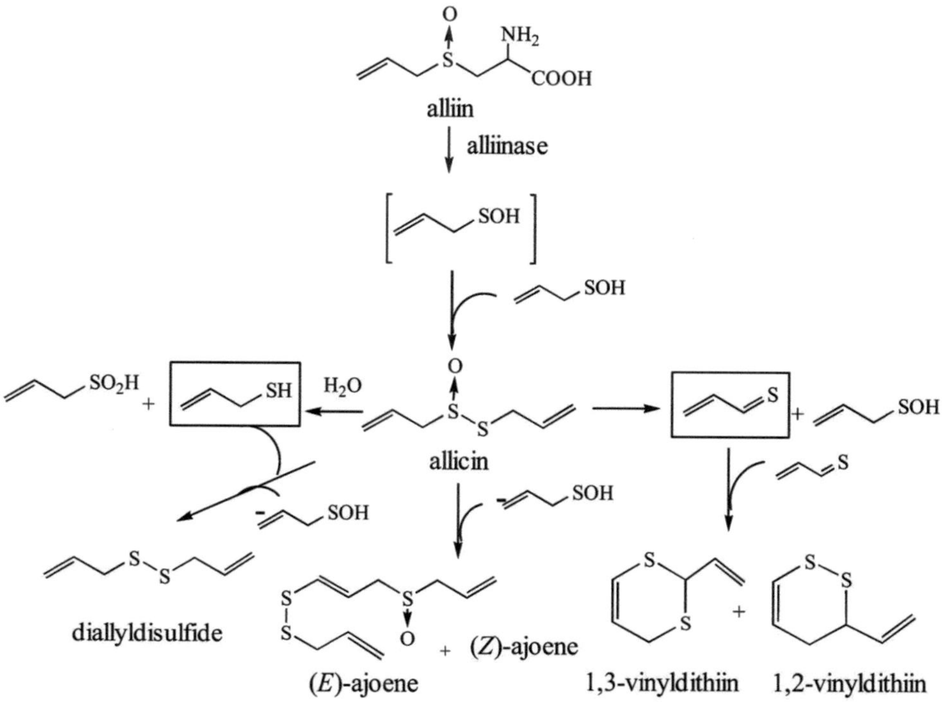

Figure 1.
Enzymatic reaction of sulfur-substituted cysteine sulfoxides. Source: [48, 49].

Garlic also contains S-propylcysteine-sulfoxide (PCSO) and S-methylcysteine-sulfoxide (MCSO). Other sulfur compounds found in garlic include diallyl sulfide, diallyl disulfide, diallyl trisulfide, S-allyl cysteine allyl mercaptan, allyl methyl disulfide, allyl methyl trisulfide and Ref. [6].

These active compounds are mainly responsible for protecting tissue from damage and various disorders [1]. Some phenolic compounds and thiosulfinates are related to the defense function of garlic, and these compounds serve as nonenzymatic antioxidants and antifungal metabolites [50]. These organosulfur compounds are very sensitive and chemically unstable; they are prone to degradation and easily undergo oxidation when exposed to light, oxygen, and high temperatures [40]. The different content of sulfur compounds in garlic varieties is determined genetically [51].

2.2 Polyphenol content and antioxidant activity of garlic

Polyphenolic compounds are a group of biologically active compounds in plant foods. Polyphenolic compounds have been identified as nutrients, plant secondary metabolites, phytonutrients, antioxidants, dietary bioactive substances, and protective factors [52].

Secondary metabolites, such as phenolics, including flavonoids and anthocyanins, have been shown to be significantly involved in plant responses to various abiotic factors, including temperature [53]. In addition to temperature, the influence of light is also considered to be one of the main influences that affect the biosynthesis of phenols in plants during growth and development. The consumption of polyphenolic compounds may play an important role in health prevention through the regulation

Phenolic acid	$mg.kg^{-1}$ FW
Pyrocatechuic acid	1.7
Caffeic acid	0.06
p-Hydroxybenzoic acid	0.05
p-Coumaric acid	2.1
Ferulic acid	4.3
FW: fresh weight.	

Table 1.
Content of phenolic acids in garlic [55, 56].

of metabolism, weight, chronic diseases, and cell proliferation. Kitchen garlic (*Allium sativum* L.) is one of the important vegetables, which is characterized by a significantly high content of polyphenolic compounds that has a positive effect on the human body. The largest share of polyphenolic compounds in garlic is represented by phenolic acids and flavonoids. Garlic is ranked second in total polyphenol content out of 23 commonly consumed vegetables [54]. Phenolic acids are among the most important antioxidants that protect the human organism against the negative effects of free radicals (**Table 1**) [55, 56].

Among the phenolic acids in garlic, caffeic acid, o-, m-, p-coumaric acid and chlorogenic acid, were identified. Of the derivatives of hydroxybenzoic acids, mainly gallic acid, protocatechuic acid, β-resorcylic acid, vanillic acid, and syringic acid. Of the other phenolic substances, mainly pyrogallol, rutin, hesperidin, resveratrol, and naringenin were identified in garlic [34]. Garlic flavonoids, such as nobiletin, tangeretin, and rutin, also significantly contribute to the pharmacological activity of garlic (**Table 2**) [57].

Beato et al. [54] mentions the presence of caffeic acid, ferulic acid, vanillic acid, p-hydroxybenzoic acid, and p-coumaric acid in garlic. Colorful varieties of garlic are rich in anthocyanins. The antioxidant properties of garlic are widely proven. Some polyphenols and sulfur-containing compounds are antioxidants and participate in protecting cells from oxidative damage. Garlic oil has been found to contain more than 30 organic sulfur-containing compounds, including diallyl trisulfide, diallyl disulfide, and diallyl sulfide with excellent antioxidant properties [58, 59]. Anwar et al. [60] attributes the antioxidant activity of garlic to organosulfur compounds that increase glutathione levels and glutathione-S-transferase activity. Garlic oil contains compounds based on sulfhydryl groups (–SH) that directly trap ROS and modulate the redox state of cells.

Flavonoid	$mg.kg^{-1}$ FW
Total flavonoid content	36.1
Quercetin	1.74
Myricetin	1.61
Kaempferol	0.26
FW: fresh weight.	

Table 2.
Content of flavonoids in garlic [56, 57].

Bozin et al. [61] describe a strong relationship between the content of polyphenolic compounds and the value of antioxidant activity in cooking garlic. The collective of authors [62] analyzed the correlation between the content of total polyphenols and antioxidant activity in 43 varieties of garlic and showed significant positive correlations. Consumption of garlic has antioxidant and antigenotoxic properties, which demonstrates a chemopreventive role against the harmful effects of hydrogen peroxide [63].

3. Health benefits of garlic

The phytochemicals found in garlic exhibit several biological effects, play a key role in maintaining health and have the potential to reduce the risk of civilization diseases. The pharmacological effects of garlic on human health are in a certain correlation with the content of bioactive compounds present in garlic. Garlic preparations, such as oils, powders, and pills, are already widely used in several cardiovascular diseases, as they effectively reduce blood lipid profiles and blood pressure [64, 65]. Antibacterial properties were first attributed to garlic by L. Pasteur. Hippocrates already observed that garlic inhibited cancer cell lines and also prevented intestinal diseases [66].

Garlic extracts are characterized by antioxidant, antidiabetic, antimicrobial, antiasthmatic, and neuroprotective effects [36, 67]. Shang et al. [68] describes the anticancer, hepatoprotective, antidiabetic, anti-obesity effects of garlic. It is known that secondary metabolites as well as organic sulfur compounds, mainly allicin and thiosulfinates, are responsible for most of the biological activities of garlic, such as antibiotic, antiviral, and antifungal properties [69, 70].

Consumption of garlic helps in the metabolism of fats, reduces the level of cholesterol and triglycerides in the blood. *In vitro* and animal studies have shown that garlic can suppress many types of cancer, such as blood, bladder, stomach, breast, oral cavity, lung cancer, colorectal cancer, skin cancer, and uterine cancer [71–73]. Epidemiological studies have shown that garlic has a role in the prevention of cardiovascular diseases due to the presence of these bioactive components [74]. Garlic consumption may protect the brain from loss of intellectual capacity and may reduce the risk of Alzheimer's disease [75].

These properties of garlic are primarily due to the beneficial content of vitamins, phenolic compounds, anthocyanins, flavonoids, and tannins in cooking garlic. Garlic has been shown to have potential anticancer properties, which is due to the content of diverse sulfur-containing compounds that have an inhibitory effect on the carcinogenic process [76]. Choi and Park [77] reported that garlic oil has an anticancer role by inducing apoptosis and inhibiting differentiation and tumor angiogenesis.

Garlic polysaccharides are characterized by antiviral as well as anti-inflammatory effects [78]. Allylsulfides have shown a hepatoprotective effect and improve liver damage. Research has confirmed that diallyl disulfide increases the activity of antioxidant enzymes and reduces lipid peroxidation [79]. Allicin has antimicrobial, anti-inflammatory, antithrombotic, and anticancer properties [46].

Diallyl sulfide suppresses the enzymatic activities of cytochrome P450-2E1, reducing the formation of reactive oxygen and nitrogen species [80]. Studies indicate that diallyl trisulfide (DATS) is responsible for the anticancer effect in garlic consumers, especially organic sulfur compounds, such as peptides of glutamylcysteine, alliin, and their degradation products, which arise when cell membranes are broken, can interact with cytochromes and P-glycoprotein, and can effectively reduce cholesterol levels [81].

Garlic extracts are also effective against *Helicobacter pylori* [82]. Consumption of garlic has been reported to have some beneficial effects in preventing changes in the lipid profile induced by the heavy metals, nickel, and chromium [83].

Ajoene present in garlic has many health benefits. It works as an antioxidant. Ajoene also has antithrombotic properties that help prevent blood clots, which reduces the risk of heart disease and stroke in humans. Ajoene exhibits potential virucidal properties against a range of viruses, including vesicular stomatitis, human rhinovirus, and herpes. Ajoene has a wide spectrum of antimicrobial (antibacterial and antifungal) properties. Ajoene reduces the tumor size of basal carcinoma cells by inducing apoptosis, it is effective in inhibiting the growth of tumor cells [84]. Regular consumption of garlic may have a chemo-preventive role against various human cancers including colon, liver, breast, stomach, and pancreatic cancer. Garlic polyphenols lower blood glucose levels in a variety of ways, such as preventing β-cell damage, reducing insulin resistance, increasing insulin sensitivity and secretion, and suppressing the activity of glucosidase enzymes. Bioactive substances found in garlic suppress lipid peroxidation, nitric oxide synthetase activity, alleviate cardiovascular complications, allergic reactions, and delay aging [66]. Garlic oil inhibits proliferation and induces apoptosis in a pancreatic cancer cell line [85].

4. Conclusions

Garlic has been considered a source of highly promising functional foods and traditional herbal medicine for millennia. Overall, garlic is an excellent natural source of bioactive sulfur-containing compounds and has promising applications in the development of functional foods and for the prevention and treatment of some diseases. Garlic (*A. sativum* L.,) is most important vegetable in agriculture, food industry, and gastronomy that has been widely utilized as flavoring, culinary, and in herbal remedies and seasoning. The consumption of traditional plants, especially garlic has progressively increased worldwide because of their great effectiveness, fewer side effects, and relatively low cost. Garlic is well known to contain various phytochemicals. These compound play key role in maintaining human health and having potential to reduce many diseases. It has distinct nutritional profile with special reference to its various bioactive components that can be used in different diet-based therapies to cure various life-style related disorders and also in developing of foods with added values.

Acknowledgements

This work was supported by the Operational Program Integrated Infrastructure within the project: Demand-driven Research for the Sustainable and Innovative Food, Drive4SIFood 313011 V336, cofinanced by the European Regional Development Fund.

Conflict of interest

The authors declare no conflict of interest.

Author details

Judita Lidiková[1], Natália Čeryová[1], Tomáš Tóth[1], Janette Musilová[1], Alena Vollmannová[1], Kushvara Mammadova[2] and Eva Ivanišová[1*]

1 Institute of Food Sciences, Faculty of Biotechnology and Food Sciences, Slovak University of Agriculture in Nitra, Nitra, Slovak Republic

2 Department of Hygiene and Food Safety, Faculty of Veterinary Medicines, Azerbaijan State Agricultural University, Ganja, Azerbaijan

*Address all correspondence to: eva.ivanisova@uniag.sk

References

[1] Divya BJ, Suman B, Kumar LL, Venkataswamy M, Eswari B, Thyagaraju K. The role of Allium sativum (garlic) in various diseases and its health benefits: A comprehensive review. International Journal of Advances Research. 2017;**5**(8):2320-2407. DOI: 10.21474/ijar01/5094

[2] Bhandari PR. Garlic (Allium sativum L.): A review of potential therapeutic applications. International Journal of Green Pharmacy. 2012;**6**:118-129. DOI: 10.4103/0973-8258.102826

[3] Cardelle-Cobas A, Soria AC, Corzo-Martine ZM, Villamiel M. A comprehensive survey of garlic functionality. In Garlic Consumption and Health. USA: Nova Science Publishers; 2009. pp. 1-60. ISBN 978-1607-41642-5

[4] Estes JW. Staple foods: Domesticated plants and animals: Onion. In: Kiple KF, Conee K, editors. The Cambridge World History of Food. Omelas: Cambridge University Press; 2000. DOI: 10.1017/chol9780521402149.010

[5] Majewski M. Allium sativum: Facts and myths regarding human health. Roczniki Państwowego Zakładu Higieny. 2014;**65**(1):1-8

[6] Myneni AA, Chang SC, Niu R, Liu L, Swanson MK, Li J, et al. Raw garlic consumption and lung cancer in a Chinese population. In Cancer Epidemiology, Biomarkers & Prevention. 2016;**25**(4):624-633. DOI: 10.1158/1055-9965.epi-15-0760

[7] Butler N. Garlic: Proven health benefits and uses. Medical News Today; 2017. Available from: https://www.medicalnewstoday.com/articles/265853

[8] Rouf R, Jamal Uddin S, Kumer SD. Antiviral potential of garlic (Allium sativum) and its organosulfur compounds: A systematic update of pre-clinical and clinical data. In Trends in Food Science & Technology. 2020;**104**:219-234. DOI: 10.1016/j.tifs.2020.08.006

[9] Aviello G, Abenavoli L, Borelli F, Capasso R, Izzo AA, Lembo F, et al. Garlic: Empiricism or science? Natural Product Communications. 2009;**4**(12):1785-1796. DOI: 10.1177/1934578X0900401231

[10] Medina JC, García HS. Garlic: Post-harvest Operations. INPhO Post-harvest Compendium. FAO; 2007. pp. 1-43

[11] Bayan L, Koulivand PH, Gorji A. Garlic: A review of potential therapeutic effects. Avicenna Journal of Phytomedicine. 2014;**4**(1):1-14

[12] Muhammad I, Shafiullah I, Muhammad I, Shah FA, Khan A, Rukh S, et al. Comparison of different garlic (Allium sativum) varieties for yield and yield components grown at agriculture Research Station. International Journal of Environmental Sciences & Natural Resources. 2018;**13**(5):555873. DOI: 10.19080/IJESNR.2018.13.555873

[13] Suleria HAR, Butt MS, Khalid N, Sultan S, Raza A, Alee M, et al. Garlic (Allium sativum): Diet based therapy of 21st century. In Asian Pacific Journal of Tropical Disease. 2015;**5**(4):271-278. DOI: 10.1016/s2222-1808(14)60782-9

[14] Lenková M, Bystrická J, Tóth T, Hrstková M. Evaluation and comparison of the content of total polyphenols and antioxidant activity of selected species of the genus Allium. Journal of Central European Agriculture. 2016;**17**(4):1119-1133. DOI: 10.5513/jcea01/17.4.1820

[15] Čeryová N, Čičová I, Lidiková J, Šnirc M, Horváthová J, Lichtnerová H, et al. The content of bioactive compounds and antioxidant activity of garlic (Allium sativum l.). Potravinarstvo Slovak Journal of Food Sciences. 2021;**15**:1104-1111. DOI: 10.5219/1694

[16] Szychowski KA, Rybczynska-Tkaczyk K, Gawel-Beben K, Swieca M, Karas MJ, A, Gminski, J. Characterization of active compounds of different garlic (Allium sativum L.) cultivars. Polish Journal of Food and Nutrition Sciences. 2018;**68**(1):73-81. DOI: 10.1515/pjfns-2017-0005

[17] Kimura S, Tung YC, Pan MH, Su NW, Lai YJ, Cheng KC. Black garlic: A critical review of its production, bioactivity, and application. Journal of Food and Drug Analysis. 2017;**25**(1):62-70. DOI: 10.1016/j.jfda.2016.11.003

[18] Oosthuizen CB, Reid AM, Lall N. Garlic (Allium sativum) and its associated molecules, as medicine. In: Medicinal Plants for Holistic Health and Well-Being. USA: Academic Press; 2018. pp. 277-295. ISBN 978-0-12-812475-8

[19] Jiang XY, Liang JY, Si-Yuan J, Pan Z, Feng T, Jia L, et al. Garlic polysaccharides: A review on their extraction, isolation, structural characteristics, and bioactivities. Carbohydrate Research. 2022;**518**:108599. DOI: 10.1016/j.carres.2022.108599

[20] Yan JK, Wang C, Yu YB, Wu LX, Chen TT, Wang ZW. Physicochemical characteristics and in vitro biological activities of polysaccharides derived from raw garlic (Allium sativum L.) bulbs via three-phase partitioning combined with gradient ethanol precipitation method. Food Chemistry. 2021;**339**:128081. DOI: 10.1016/j.foodchem.2020.128081

[21] Petropoulos SA, Fernandes Â, Ntatsi G, Petrotos K, Barros L, Ferreira IC. Nutritional value, chemical characterization and bulb morphology of Greek garlic landraces. Molecules. 2018;**23**(2):319. DOI: 10.3390/molecules23020319

[22] Carr AC, Maggini S. Vitamin C and immune function. Nutrients. 2017;**9**(11):1211. DOI: 10.3390/nu9111211

[23] Gambelli L, Marconi S, Durazzo A, Camilli E, Aguzzi A, Gabrielli P, et al. Vitamins and minerals in four traditional garlic ecotypes (Allium sativum L.) from Italy: An example of territorial biodiversity. Sustainability. 2021;**13**:7405. DOI: 10.3390/su13137405

[24] Akinwande BA, Olatunde SJ. Comparative evaluation of the mineral profile and other selected components of onion and garlic. International Food Research Journal. 2015;**22**(1):332-336

[25] Prianshu A, Singh M, Kumar M, Malik S, Sahahi U, Lodhi S. Effect of integrated nutrient management on yield and quality of garlic cv. Yamuna Safed-3: Effect of INM on garlic yield and quality. Journal of Agriculture Search. 2020;**7**(4):251-254. DOI: 10.21921/jas.v7i04.19399

[26] Evrendilek GA. In: Jaiswal A, editor. Nutritional Composition and Antioxidant Properties of Fruits and Vegetables. London, UK: Academic Press; 2020. pp. 89-105

[27] Abiola TT, Amoo IA, Ayoade GW. Evaluation of nutritional composition and antioxidants properties of onion (Allium Cepa) and garlic (Allium sativum). The International Journal of Science and Technology. 2017;**5**(10):1-6

[28] Vadalà R, Mottese A, Bua G, Salvo A, Mallamace D, Corsaro C, et al. Statistical analysis of mineral concentration for the geographic identification of garlic

samples from Sicily (Italy), Tunisia and Spain. Food. 2016;**5**(4):20. DOI: 10.3390/foods5010020

[29] Lee JH, Lee J, Whang J, Nam JS, Lee J, Kim SM, et al. Changes in nutritional components of the northern and southern types garlic by different heat treatments. Korean Journal of Food and Cookery Science. 2016;**32**(3):245-252. DOI: 10.9724/kfcs.2016.32.3.245

[30] Sohrabi M, Mehrjerdi MZ, Karimi S, Tavallali V. Using gypsum and selenium foliar application for mineral biofortification and improving the bioactive compounds of garlic ecotypes. Industrial Crops and Products. 2020;**54**:112742. DOI: 10.1016/j.indcrop.2020.112742

[31] Turan MA, Taban S, Taban N, Ersan LY. Characterization of garlic (Allium sativum L.) according the geographical origin by analysis of minerals. Fresenius Environmental Bulletin. 2017;**26**(6):4292-4298

[32] Tardy AL, Pouteau E, Marquez D, Yilmaz C, Scholey A. Vitamins and minerals for energy, fatigue and cognition: A narrative review of the biochemical and clinical evidence. Nutrients. 2020;**12**:228. DOI: 10.3390/nu12010228

[33] Lanzotti V. The analysis of onion and garlic. Journal of chromatography A. 2006;**1112**(1-2):3-22. DOI: 10.1016/j.chroma.2005.12.016

[34] Nagella P, Thiruvengadam M, Ahmad A, Yoon J, Chung I. Composition of polyphenols and antioxidant activity of garlic bulbs collected from different locations of Korea. Asian Journal of Chemistry. 2014;**26**(3):897-902. DOI: 10.14233/ajchem.2014.16143a

[35] Lanzotti V, Scala F, Bonanomi G. Compounds from Allium species with cytotoxic and antimicrobial activity. Phytochemistry Reviews. 2014;**13**:769-791. DOI: 10.1007/s11101-014-9366-0

[36] Poojary MM, Putnik P, Kovačević DB, Barba FJ, Lorenzo JM, Dias DA, et al. Stability and extraction of bioactive sulfur compounds from Allium genus processed by traditional and innovative technologies. Journal of Food Composition and Analysis. 2017;**61**:28-39. DOI: 10.1016/j.jfca.2017.04.007

[37] Kamenentsky R, Rabinowitch HD. Physiology of domesticated alliums: Onions, garlic, Leek, and minor crops. Encyclopedia of Applied Plant Sciences,2nd ed. 2017;**3**:255-261

[38] Nicastro HL, Ross SA, Milner JA. Garlic and onions: Their cancer prevention properties. Cancer Prevention Research. 2015;**8**(3):181-189. DOI: 10.1158/1940-6207

[39] Alide T, Wangila P, Kiprop A. Effect of cooking temperature and time on total phenolic content, total flavonoid content and total in vitro antioxidant activity of garlic. BMC Resesrch Notes. 2020;**13**:564. DOI: 10.1186/s13104-020-05404-8

[40] Tavares L, Santos L, Noreña CPZ. Bioactive compounds of garlic: A comprehensive review of encapsulation technologies, characterization of the encapsulated garlic compounds and their industrial applicability. Trends in Food Science & Technology. 2021;**114**:232-244. DOI: 10.1016/j.tifs.2021.05.019

[41] Durazzo A. Study approach of antioxidant properties in foods: Update and considerations. Food. 2017;**6**:17. DOI: 10.3390/foods6030017

[42] Gebreyohannes G, Gebreyohannes M. Medical values of garlic: A review. International Journal of Medicine and Medical Sciences. 2013;**5**(9):401-408

[43] Hasib A, Ourouadi S, Moumene H, Zaki N, Boulli AA, Ouatmane A. Garlic (Allium sativum): A source of multiple nutraceutical and functional components (review). Journal of Chemical, Biological and Physical Sciences. 2016;7(1):9-21

[44] Block E. The chemistry of garlic and onions. Scientific American. *1985*;*252*(3):114-121

[45] Abdel-Daim MM, Abdelkhalek NK, Hassan AM. Antagonistic activity of dietary allicin against deltamethrin-induced oxidative damage in freshwater Nile tilapia; *Oreochromis niloticus*. Ecotoxicology and Environmental Safety. 2015;**111**:146-152. DOI: 10.1016/j.ecoenv.2014.10.019

[46] Naheed Z, Cheng Z, Wu C, Wen Y, Ding H. Total polyphenols, total flavonoids, allicin and antioxidant capacities in garlic scape cultivars during controlled atmosphere storage. Postharvest Biology and Technology. 2017;**131**:39-45. DOI: 10.1016/j.postharvbio.2017.0

[47] Verma SK, Jain V, Verma D. Garlic-" the spice of life": Composition, cooking, chemistry and preparations. Journal of Herbal Medicine and Toxicology. 2008;**2**(2):2008

[48] Miron T, Rabinkov A, Mirelman D, Wilchek M, Weiner L. The mode of action of allicin: Its ready permeability through phospholipid membranes may contribute to its biological activity. Biochimica et Biophysica Acta (BBA)-Biomembranes. 2000;**1463**(1):20-30. DOI: 10.1016/S0005-2736(99)00174-1

[49] Amagase H. Clarifying the real bioactive constituents of garlic. The Journal of nutrition. 2006;**136**(3):716S-725S. DOI: 10.1093/jn/136.3.716S

[50] Okada Y, Tanaka K, Fujita I, Sato E, Okajima H. Antiodidant activity of thiosulfinates derived from garlic. Redox Report. 2005;**10**(2):96-102. DOI: 10.1179/135100005X38851

[51] Prajapati H. Evaluation of varieties/ local cultivars (races) of garlic (Allium sativum L.) for Malwa region. Annals of Plant and Soil Research. 2016;**18**(4):315-318

[52] Cory H, Passarelli S, Szeto J, Tamez M, Mattei J. The role of polyphenols in human health and food systems: A mini-review. Frontiers in Nutrition. 2018;**5**:87. DOI: 10.3389/fnut.2018.00087

[53] Herrera MD, Servín-Palestina M, Reveles-Hernández M, Zegbe JA. Garlic cloves (Allium sativum L.) conditioned at low temperatures and planting dates enhance the polyphenolic content of garlic cataphylls. Journal of Applied Research on Medicinal and Aromatic Plants. 2021;**25**:100316. DOI: 10.1016/j.jarmap.2021.100316

[54] Beato VM, Orgay F, Mansilla F, Montano A. Changes inphenolic compounds in garlic (Allium sativum L.) owing to the cultivar and location of growth. Plant Foods for Human Nutrition. 2011;**66**(3):218-223. DOI: 10.1007/s11130-011-0236-2

[55] Piazzon A, Vrhovsek U, Masuero D, Mattivi F, Mandoj F, Nardini M. Antioxidant activity of phenolic acids and their metabolites: Synthesis and antioxidant properties of the sulfate derivatives of ferulic and coffeic acids and of the acyl glucuronide of ferulic acids. Journal of Pharmacy and Pharmacology. 2012;**64**:1119-1127. DOI: 10.1021/jf304076z

[56] Drozd M, Thomas M, Nowak R. Determination of phenolic acids in raw garlic (Allium sativum L.) and onion (Allium cepa L.) bulbs. Annales

Universitatis Mariae curie-Sklodowska. Sectio DDD: Pharmacia. 2011;**24**:121-127

[57] Berginc K, Milisav I, Kristl A. Garlic flavonoids and organosulfur compounds: Impact on the hepatic pharmacokinetics of Saquinavir and Darunavir. Drug Metabolism and Pharmacokinetics. 2010;**25**(6):521-530. DOI: 10.2133/dmpk.dmpk-10-rg-053

[58] Yashin A, Yashin Y, Xia X, Nemzer B. Antioxidant activity of spices and their impact on human health: A review. Antioxidants. 2017;**6**(3):70. DOI: 10.3390/antiox6030070

[59] Ekeleme Egedigwe Chima A, Famurewa Ademola C, David Ebuka E, Eleazu Chinedum O, Egedigwe UO. Antioxidant potential of garlic oil supplementation prevents cyclophosphamide-induced oxidative testicular damage and endocrine depletion in rats. Journal of Nutrition & Intermediary Metabolism. 2019;**18**:100109. DOI: 10.1016/j.jnim.2020.100109

[60] Anwar MM, Meki ARM. Oxidative stress in streptozotocin-induced diabetic rats: Effects of garlic oil and melatonin. Comparative Biochemistry and Physiology Part A: Molecular & Integrative Physiology. 2003;**135**(4):539-547. DOI: 10.1016/S1095-6433(03)00114-4

[61] Bozin B, Mimica-Dukic N, Samojlik I, Goran A, Igic R. Phenolics as antioxidants in garlic (Allium sativum L., Alliaceae). Food Chemistry. 2008;**111**(4):925-929. DOI: 10.1016/j.foodchem.2008.04.071

[62] Chen S, Shen X, Cheng S, Li P, Du J. Evaluation of garlic cultivars for polyphenolic content and antioxidant properties. PLoS One. 2013;**8**(11):79730. DOI: 10.1371/journal.pone.0079730

[63] Park JH, Park YK, Park E. Antioxidative and Antigenotoxic effects of garlic (Allium. Sativum L.) prepared by different processing methods. Plant Foods for Human Nutrition. 2009;**64**(4):244-249. DOI: 10.1007/s11130-009-0132-1

[64] El-Saber Batiha G, Magdy Beshbishy AG, Wasef L, Elewa YHA, Al-Sagan A, Abd El-Hack ME, et al. Chemical constituents and pharmacological activities of garlic (Allium sativum L.): A review. Nutrients. 2020;**12**(3):872. DOI: 10.3390/nu12030872

[65] Chen CY, Tsai TY, Chen BH. Effects of black garlic extract and Nanoemulsion on the deoxy corticosterone acetate-salt induced hypertension and its associated mild cognitive impairment in rats. Antioxidants. 2021;**10**(10):1611. DOI: 10.3390/antiox10101611

[66] Mughal MF. Garlic polyphenols: A diet based therapy. Biomedical Journal of Scientific & Technical Research. 2019;**15**(4):11453-11458. DOI: doi; 10.26717/BJSTR.2019.15.002721

[67] Shin NR, Kwon HJ, Ko JW, Kim JS, Lee IC, Kim JC, et al. S-allyl cysteine reduces eosinophilic airway inflammation and mucus overproduction on ovalbumin-induced allergic asthma model. International Immunopharmacology. 2019;**68**:124-130. DOI: 10.1016/j.intimp.2019.01.001

[68] Shang A, Cao SY, Xu XY, Gan RY, Tang GY, Corke H, et al. Bioactive compounds and biological functions of garlic (Allium sativum L.). Food. 2019;**8**(7):246. DOI: 10.3390/foods8070246

[69] Borlinghaus J, Albrecht F, Gruhlke MC, Nwachukwu ID, Slusarenko AJ. Allicin: Chemistry and biological properties. Molecules. 2014;**19**(8):12591-12618. DOI: 10.3390/molecules190812591

[70] Cavalcanti VP, Aazza S, Bertolucci SKV, Pereira MMA, Cavalcanti PP, Buttrós VHT, et al. Plant, pathogen and biocontrol agent interaction effects on bioactive compounds and antioxidant activity in garlic. Physiological and Molecular Plant Pathology. 2020;**112**:101550. DOI: 10.1016/j.pmpp.2020.101550

[71] Karmakar S, Choudhury Subhasree R, Banik Naren L, Ray Swapan K. Molecular mechanisms of anti-cancer action of garlic compounds in neuroblastoma. Anti-Cancer Agents in Medicinal Chemistry (Formerly Current Medicinal Chemistry-Anti-Cancer Agents). 2011;**11**(4):398-407. DOI: 10.2174/187152011795677553

[72] Aggarwal B, Prasad S, Sung B, Krishnan S, Guha S. Prevention and treatment of colorectal cancer by natural agents from mother nature. Current Colorectal Cancer Reports. 2013;**9**(1):37-56. DOI: 10.1007/s11888-012-0154-1

[73] Ciric A, Krajnc B, Heath D, Ogrinc N. Response surface methodology and artificial neural network approach for the optimization of ultrasound-assisted extraction of polyphenols from garlic. Food and Chemical Toxicology. 2020;**135**:110976. DOI: 10.1016/j.fct.2019.110976

[74] Zhou L, Guo X, Bi J, Yi J, Chen Q, Wu X, et al. Drying of garlic slices (Allium sativum L.) and its effect on thiosulfinates, total phenolic compounds and antioxidant activity during infrared drying. Journal of Food Processing and Preservation. 2017;**41**(1):e12734. DOI: 10.1111/jfpp.12734

[75] Javed H, Khan MM, Khan A, Vaibhav K, Ahmad A, Khuwaja G, et al. S-allyl cysteine attenuates oxidative stress associated cognitive impairment and neurodegeneration in mouse model of streptozotocin-induced experimental dementia of Alzheimer's type. Brain Research. 2011;**1389**:133-142. DOI: 10.1016/j.brainres.2011.02.072

[76] Catanzaro E, Canistro D, Pellicioni V, Vivarelli F, Fimognari C. Anticancer potential of allicin: A review. Pharmacological Research. 2022;**117**:106118. DOI: 10.1016/j.phrs.2022.106118

[77] Choi YH, Park HS. Apoptosis induction of U937 human leukemia cells by diallyltrisulfide induces through generation of reactive oxygen species. Journal of Biomedical Science. 2012;**19**:50. DOI: 10.1186/1423-0127-19-50

[78] Shao X, Sun C, Tang X, Zhang X, Han D, Liang S, et al. Anti-inflammatory and intestinal microbiota modulation properties of Jinxiang garlic (Allium sativum L.) polysaccharides toward dextran sodium sulfate-induced colitis. Journal of Agricultural and Food Chemistry. 2020;**68**(44):12295-12309. DOI: 10.1021/acs.jafc.0c04773

[79] Chekki R, Najjaa H, Zouari N, Máthé Á, Bouzouita N. Detection of Organo-Sulphur volatiles in Allium sativum by factorial design. Natural Products Chemistry & Research. 2016;**4**:211. DOI: 10.4172/2329-6836.1000211

[80] Abdel-Daim MM, Shaheen HM, Abushouk AI, Toraih EA, Fawzy MS, Alansari WS, et al. Thymoquinone and diallyl sulfide protect against fipronil-induced oxidative injury in rats. Environmental Science and Pollution Research International. 2018;**25**: 23909-23916. DOI: 10.1007/s11356-018-2386-3

[81] Shord SS, Shah K, Lukose A. Drug-botanicals interactions: A review of the laboratory, animal and human data for 8 common botanicals. Integrative Cancer Therapies. 2009;**8**:208-227. DOI: 10.1177%2F1534735409340900

[82] Cellini L, Di Campli E, Masulli M, Di Bartolomeo S, Allocati N. Inhibition of helicobacter pylori by garlic extract (Allium sativum). FEMS Immunology and Medical Microbiology. 1996;**13**:273-277. DOI: 10.1111/j.1574-695X.1996.tb00251.x

[83] Amrita DG, Das SN, Dhundasi SA, Das KK. Effect of garlic (Allium sativum) on heavy metal (nickel II and ChromiumVI) induced alteration of serum lipid profile in male albino rats. International Journal of Environmental Research and Public Health. 2008;**5**: 147-151. DOI: 10.3390/ijerph5030147

[84] Dharshini HP, Devi A. A study on extraction of Ajoene from Allium sativum and its applications. Journal of Medicinal Plants Studies. 2017;**5**(5):111-116

[85] Lan XY, Sun HY, Liu JJ, Lin Y, Zhu ZY, Han X, et al. Effects of garlic oil on pancreatic cancer cells. Asian Pacific Journal of Cancer Prevention. 2013;**14**(10):5905-5910. DOI: 10.7314/APJCP.2013.14.10.5905

Chapter 7

Herbs and Spices' Antimicrobial Properties and Possible Use in the Food Sector

Madonna Ngwatshipane Mashabela, Peter Tshepiso Ndhlovu and Wilfred Otang Mbeng

Abstract

With increased consumer knowledge of food safety and quality, there is a strong demand for preservative (synthetic)-free food and the use of natural products as preservatives. Natural antimicrobials derived from various sources are used to keep food safe from spoilage and pathogenic microbes. Plants are the primary source of antimicrobials and include a variety of essential oils that have antimicrobial properties. Many essential oils are found in herbs and spices, such as rosemary, sage, basil, oregano, thyme, cardamom, and clove. These antimicrobial compounds are also used in conjunction with edible coatings to prevent bacteria from growing on the surface of food and food products.

Keywords: biological assays, food, medicinal plants, nutrition, essential oils

1. Introduction

Fresh foods, such as horticulture, seafood, and meat, have a short shelf life and are linked to foodborne disease outbreaks caused by pathogenic microbes. In recent years, much effort has been expended on search for natural antimicrobials that can inhibit fungal, bacterial, and viral growth in food. Simultaneously, the food industry has sought to replace/supplement traditional food preservation techniques, such as heat treatment, acidification, salting, drying, and chemical preservation with newer, less invasive methods (pulsed light, high-pressure, pulsed electric field, ultrasound, oscillating magnetic field, and UV treatments) [1, 2]. The reason for this is that some consumers chose minimally processed foods over processed meals, preferring those with less additives and/or containing natural ingredients [1].

Natural antimicrobials are defined as substances that are naturally occurring and directly derived from biological systems without alteration or modification in a laboratory setting. These can be sourced from a variety of organisms, including algae, fungi, bacteria, and plants. Plant extracts have the advantage of having been consumed by people for thousands of years. In addition to being utilized as antimicrobials, many plants are also used in traditional medicine, functional foods, dietary supplements, and the production of recombinant proteins. Their ability to prevent/

regulate the growth of bacteria, particularly pathogenic bacteria (food safety), and to manage natural spoiling processes (food preservation) gives them their function as antimicrobials [3]. The ability of plants to manufacture a number of chemical compounds with complicated structures and antibacterial activity through secondary metabolism has been linked to their potential antimicrobial qualities. These antimicrobial substances are created naturally by plants to strengthen their defense mechanisms in challenging environments [4, 5]. Plants produce phytochemicals to protect themselves from bacteria, fungi, and viruses, but they also prevent foods from going stale [6]. There has been a surge in interest in employing natural preservatives in food products. Natural preservatives boost human health by protecting against disease [1]. Approximately 1340 plants have been identified as possible sources of antioxidant and antibacterial components [7], while over 250,000 plant species contain a diverse range of bioactive components. Plant extracts are designated as "aromatic and flavoring compounds," which comprise "all natural products and corresponding synthetic products," and can be taken by any animal species with no restrictions on product dose. Due to their widespread public acceptance, these products stand to replace synthetic preservatives in future, and the quest for novel compounds is a vital area of research in the field of food additives. All of this has led to the use of natural preservative substances, which are either directly added to food products or ingested by the source species.

Herbs and spices are examples of natural chemicals that are employed as food preservatives because they contain components with strong antioxidant and antibacterial capabilities [8]. Plant extracts have been utilized for centuries to enhance the organoleptic qualities of food. In addition, Chipault [9] and Chipault, Mizuno [10] articulated plant extracts have preservation characteristics in various types of spices, and there is already a wealth of knowledge about the chemicals and mechanisms involved in lipid peroxidation inhibition. They are GRAS (generally recognized as safe), which means that consumers and regulatory authorities perceive them to be more appropriate for use in food than manufactured substances. Butylated hydroxyanisole (BHA) and butylated hydroxytoluene (BHT) are two examples of synthetic preservatives that have been employed in the food business for many years. However, there is a lot of evidence that these substances are potentially carcinogenic, so there is a lot of interest in alternative products that safeguard against oxidation but are more natural [11, 12].

Plant materials from the Labiatae family have been extensively researched for their preservation characteristics [13]. In addition to antibacterial and antioxidant action, natural extracts contain immunomodulatory, anti-inflammatory, spasmolytic, and sedative properties. Because their individual activities are substantially lower than their combined activity, natural extracts frequently owe their biological activity to the synergism between their numerous components. The toxicity of extracts is thought to be lower when all of their components are present rather than when they are purified, a process known as buffering. As previously stated, food companies are increasingly interested in incorporating natural antioxidants and antimicrobials into food in response to consumer demand for safer and more natural foods and their rejection of synthetic antioxidants, which are being reassessed for the potential toxicity and carcinogenicity of the components formed during their degradation. Several studies have been conducted over the last decade to identify natural compounds capable of suppressing lipid auto-oxidation events in meat products and precooked meats after being added during processing procedures [14, 15]. *Origanum vulgaris, Rosmarinus officinalis,* and *Thymus vulgaris* have received special attention due to their high antioxidant activity [16]. However, it is important to remember that the efficiency of plant extracts is dependent on the type of substrate on which they operate [16] as well as the provided dose. Plant-derived antioxidants, on average, exhibit prooxidant activity at low doses and antioxidant activity above a critical concentration [16]. Plants' putative antibacterial effects have been linked to their ability to create various chemical compounds with complicated structures through secondary metabolism. These antibacterial components are naturally created to help a plant's defense system during harsh situations [4, 5]. This study provides an overview of the current state of knowledge and recent advances in the use of plant-derived compounds generated from herbs and spices as antimicrobials in foods, as well as their potential and problems.

2. Classification of herbs and spices

Spices and herbs are classified into numerous categories based on their flavor and color, such as mild (paprika and coriander), strong (mustard, chilies, cayenne pepper, and black and white peppers), aromatic spices (cinnamon, cumin, nutmeg, clove, dill fennel, and mace), and aromatic herbs (basil, bay leaf, marjoram, thyme, garlic, shallot, and onion). Based on their color (turmeric) and herbaceous (rosemary and sage) or taste (bitter, sweet, sour, spicy, and sharp) (**Figure 1**) [19].

3. Active compounds in herbs and spices

Antioxidants are compounds that prevent or delay the initiation of oxidation. Because of safety concerns regarding synthetic antioxidants, natural antioxidants are becoming increasingly popular. Furthermore, people are becoming

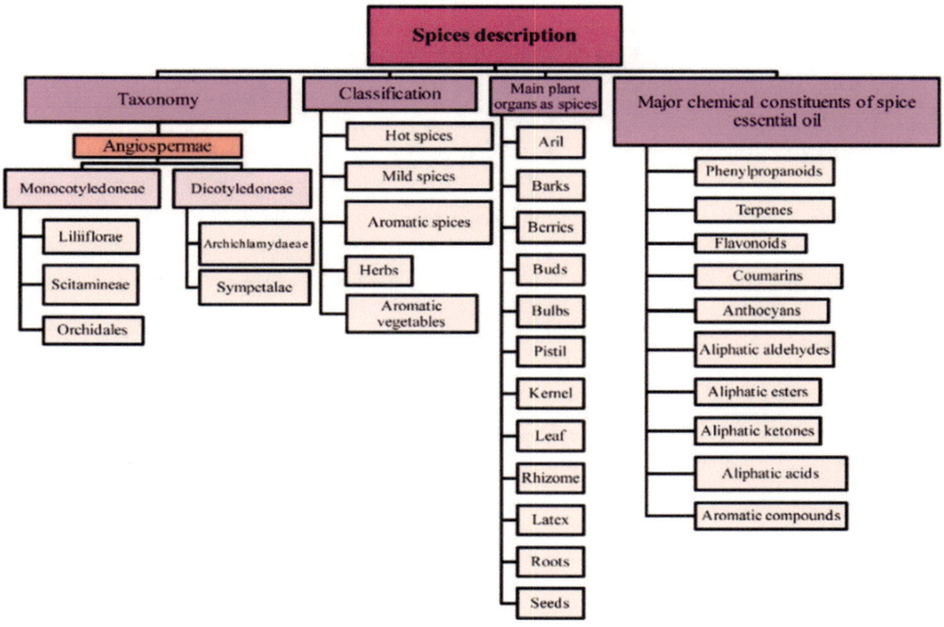

Figure 1.
Spices and herbs classification [17, 18].

more interested in natural products and less ingredients in food products [19]. Flavonoids, coumarins, carotenoids, curcumins, saponins, lignans, polyphenolics, terpenoids, sulfides, phthalides, and plant sterols are all found in herbs and spices. The most powerful antioxidants found in herbs and spices are phenolic compounds, which have at least two hydroxylic groups in the ortho or para orientations, such as caffeic acid. These compounds have been employed as antioxidants in the form of herbs, ground spices and extracts, capsules, or emulsions [19, 20]. The antioxidants contained in herbs and spices can be classed based on their chemical structure. Flavonoids, phenolic acids, catechins, volatile phenols, phenolic diterpenes, poly-alkoxybenzenes, ligans, sulfuric compounds, and ascorbic acid are the primary families of chemicals [19].

More than 6000 flavonoids have been recognized as ubiquitous in photosynthesizing cells, and they are frequently found in vegetables, fruits, nuts, stems, seeds, flowers, tea, wine, propolis, and honey [21]. Plants use phenolic compounds to defend themselves, build structures and attract pollinators and seed-dispersing animals. Plants produce these compounds to protect themselves from UV radiation and to adapt to their surroundings [19]. Flavonoids may also be beneficial in the human body, treating conditions, such as flu and colds (due to their antiviral, antibacterial, and antifungal activity), cancer (particularly lycopene and quercetin), allergies (quercetin), cardiovascular disease, and neurodegenerative disorders, including Parkinson's disease, multiple sclerosis, Alzheimer's disease, Huntington's disease, and amyotrophic lateral sclerosis. It may also function as a preventative strategy against eye diseases (cataracts and macular degeneration) (anthocyanins and lycopene), and in protecting the eye from the harmful effects of UV radiation (lutein and zeaxanthin) [22]. Some flavonoid metabolites, such as sulfates, omethylated, and glucuronides, may participate directly in plasma antioxidant activities by scavenging reactive oxygen and nitrogen species in the bloodstream [23]. Common antioxidants that occur in herbs and spices are presented in **Table 1**.

Scientific name and plant family	Spice/herb	Antioxidant compounds	Mode of action
Allium cepa L Amaryllidaceae	Onion	Kaempferol, quercetin, cyanidin glucosides, taxifolin, peonidin glucosides, allicin	Free radical scavenger
Allium sativum L Amaryllidaceae	Garlic	Vanillic, allicin, p-hydroxybenzoic, p-coumaric acids, caffeic	Metal chelator, free radical scavenger
Brassica nigra, alba, juncea Syn: *Brassica carinata A.Braun* Brassicaceae	Mustards	Glucosinolates, carotenes,	Free radical scavenger
Capsicum frutescence L Solanaceae	Chili pepper	Capsaicinol, capsaicin	Free radical scavenger
Coriandrum sativum L Apiaceae	Coriander	Beta-sitosterol, tannin, beta-carotene, camphene, caffeic acid, isoquercitrin, myricene, gamma-terpinene, protocatechuic acid, p-hydroxy-benzoic acid, myristicin, quercetin, rhamnetin, rutin, scopoletin, trans-anethole, vanillic acid, terpinen-4-ol,	Metal chelator, free radical scavenger

Scientific name and plant family	Spice/herb	Antioxidant compounds	Mode of action
Curcuma domestica Valeton Zingiberaceae	Turmeric	4-hydroxycinnamoyl methane, curcumins, p-cumaric acid, carotenes, curcumin, ascorbic acid, caffeic acid	Free radical scavenger, oxygen scavenger, free radical scavenger, metal chelator,
Cumimum cyminum L Apiaceae	Cumin	Cuminic alcohol, cuminal, linalool, pinocarveol, 1-methyl-2-(1-methylethyl) benzene, luteolin, p-cymene, γ-terpinene, β-pinene, carotol, cuminaldehyde, apigenin	Metal chelator, free radical scavenger
Eugenia caryophyllata Thunb Myrtaceae	Clove	Tannins, phenolic volatile oils (acetyl eugenol, isoeugenol, eugenol), flavonol glucosides, phenolic acids (gallic acid),	Metal chelator, free radical scavenger
Laurus nobilis L Lauraceae	Laurel or bay leaf	Ascorbic acid, beta-carotene, methyl eugenol, tocopherols, eugenol, eudesmol, kaempferol, kaempferol-3-rhamnopyranoside, kaempferol-3,7-dirhamnopyranoside, α-terpinyl acetate, cinnamtannin B1, catechin, terpinen-4-ol, 8-cineole,	Oxygen scavenger, free radical scavenger
Majorana hortensis Moench Lamiaceae	Marjoram	Phenol, ursolic acid, beta-sitosterol, linalyl-acetate plant, caffeic acid, tannin, myricene, beta-carotene, caffeic acid, carvacrol, hydroquinone, beta-carotene, trans-anethole, oleanolic acid, terpinen-4-ol, myricene, rosmarinic acid, eugenol	Free radical scavenger
Mentha x piperita L Lamiaceae	Peppermint	Glucoside, isorhoifolin, beta-carotene, eriodictyol, narirutin, eriodictyol 7-O-β- eriocitrin, , rosmarinic acid, caffeic acid, piperitoside, lithospermic acid, ascorbic acid, luteolin 7-O-β-glucoside, menthoside, diosmin, hesperidin, luteolin 7-O-rutinoside	Oxygen scavenger, free radical scavenger
Origanum vulgaris L Lamiaceae	Oregano	Linalyl-acetate, carvacrol, Camphene, protocatechuic acid, thymol, myricene, dihydrokaempferol, terpinen-4-ol, rosmarinic acid, 2-caffeoyloxy--3-[2-(4-hydroxybenzyl)-4,5-dihydroxy] phenylpropionic acid; flavonoids—apigen, eriodictyol, caffeic acid, dihydroquercetin, gamma-terpinene,	Free radical scavenger
Salvia officinali L Lamiaceae	Sage	Cirsimaritin, salvigenin, terpinen-4-ol, carnosol, gamma-terpinene, carnosic acid, hispidulin, rosmanol, ursolic acid, methyl and ethyl esters of carnosol, rosmarinic acid, beta-carotene, camphene, labiatic acid, oleanolic acid, selenium, nevadensin, cirsileol, apigenin, beta-sitosterol, ascorbic acid, rosmadial	Free radical scavenger
Rosmarinus officinalis L Lamiaceae	Rosemary	Rosmarinic acid, carnosol, rosmariquinone, carnosic acid, rosmanol, rosmadial, diterpenes (epirosmanol, rosmaridiphenol, isorosmanol)	Metal chelator, scavenge superoxide radicals, lipid antioxidant

Scientific name and plant family	Spice/herb	Antioxidant compounds	Mode of action
Thymus vulgaris L Lamiaceae	Thyme	Isochlorogenic acid, thymol, phenolic acids (caffeic acid, gallic acid, rosmarinic acid), flavonoids, labiatic acid, p-coumaric acid, rosmarinic acid, carvacrol, p-Cumene-2,3-diol, ascorbic acid, beta carotene, phenolic diterpenes	oxygen scavenger, free radical scavenger
Piper nigrum L Piperaceae	Black pepper	ubiquinone, piperine, quercetin, eugenol, beta-carotene, camphen, carvacrol, methyl eugenol, kaempferol, ascorbic acid, rhamnetin, gamma-terpinene	Free radical scavenger

Based on: [19, 20, 24].
The botanical names of the plants were verified using the World flora online (http://www.worldfloraonline.org/).

Table 1.
Antioxidants isolated from herbs and spices.

4. Herbs and spices in the food industry

Herbs and spices have long been used in cooking as functional food additives. One of their applications could be to assist reduce the fat, sugar content, and salt in food products. Instead of salt, use marjoram, bay leaves, thyme, basil, tarragon, coriander, lovage, or rosemary. Furthermore, several herbs and spices are high in vitamins, including A, B, K, E, D, C (particularly dill and parsley), B, and PP (especially in onion). Additional substances present in herbs and spices, such as micro- and macroelements, also play an essential role. These bioelements regulate osmotic pressure and are a component of or influence the action of numerous enzymes, acting directly or indirectly in a variety of biochemical activities and so performing a function [25]. Food poisoning is a significant issue that has an impact on both consumers and food producers. Spices and herbs can also be used to stop undesirable microorganisms from growing in meals. Food producers are always worried about the rise in illness outbreaks brought on by pathogenic and spoilage bacteria in food. Furthermore, antibiotic overuse has resulted in the development of antimicrobial resistance in bacteria involved with foodborne diseases. However, as public understanding of manufacturing methods grows, many consumers refuse to purchase goods containing synthetic preservatives. As a result, there is a growing concern about the creation of novel forms of effective and benign natural antibacterial substances for food preservation, such as extracts of herbs and spices [26]. Because of their antibacterial action, herbs and spices can be employed as natural agents in the food business to extend the shelf life of foods. A variety of antimicrobials derived from plants and spices are used to inhibit or eliminate harmful bacteria and improve the overall quality of food products [3]. There are over 1340 plants that have antibacterial chemicals that have been identified. Antibacterial action is notably strong in vanillin, lemongrass, sage, oregano, cloves, cinnamon, garlic, parsley, coriander, and rosemary [3]. Some herbs and spices, such as peppermint, thyme, red pepper, clove, oregano, fennel, ginger, parsley, coriander, sage, rosemary, common balm, black pepper, marjoram, summer savory, basil, nutmeg, spearmint, cumin, and cinnamon, are added to lipid-containing dishes.

Oxidative rancidity, a major cause of food deterioration, causes food to deteriorate and finally be rejected by consumers as a result of the formation of unwanted odors and off-flavors or color degradation [19]. Furthermore, herbs and spices have been used for generations not just to preserve foods and beverages, but also to keep the color, flavor, and aroma of food products [19]. Plant essential oils can also be employed as additives in biodegradable films and coatings to improve shelf life and add value to products [27, 28]. The inclusion of essential oils has a favorable effect on the polymer matrix's continuity, resulting in physical modifications based on the specific polymer-oil component interactions. The oil thus weakens the film structure while improving the water barrier characteristics and decreasing transparency. Essential oil-infused films offer antioxidant and antibacterial effects [27]. Some food products can also be preserved using alginate-based edible films containing bioactive components. They can be used as nanoemulsions because of their poor water solubility, which improves water dispersion and protects active components from degradation [29].

5. Effect of using herbs and spices in yogurt

Yogurt's health benefits are well known, and many yogurt-based products are consumed by people all over the world [30]. Behrad, Yusof [31] concluded that adding cinnamon did not alter yogurt fermentation but allowed *Lactobacillus* spp. to thrive during refrigerated storage. *In vitro*, cinnamon yogurt containing probiotic bacteria inhibited *Helicobacter pylori* development. The ability of these herbal yogurts to inhibit the growth of *H. pylori* in the stomach's, severely acidic environment requires more investigation [32]. Srivastava, Prasad [33] created herbal yogurt from buffalo, cow, and goat milk using varied ratios of beetroot and ginger extracts. They discovered that goat milk yogurt supplemented with 2% beetroot and 2% ginger extract had the highest antioxidant activity evaluated by the DPPH technique, followed by cow milk yogurt fortified with 2% ginger extract. Furthermore, Peter and Shylaja [17] discovered that fortifying milk and yogurt with 2% red ginseng extract increased oxygen radical absorption capacity and (DPPH) radical-scavenging activity. Furthermore, H_2O_2-induced DNA damage was reduced in yogurt enriched with red ginseng extract than in regular yogurt. However, no significant variations in DNA damage were identified between regular milk and milk supplemented with red ginseng extract. As a result, our study demonstrates that red ginseng fortification can effectively promote the antioxidant and antigenotoxic effects of dairy products. Kumar, Arvindakshan [34] made yogurt concentrate with crushed leaves mint in ratios of 2, 4, and 6%. They discovered that adding 2% mint level to yogurt was excellent in all sensory aspects. Furthermore, the shelf life of the yogurt spread at 5°C was 10 days. It was suggested that the mint-flavored yogurt be used in burgers, sandwiches, and other bakery items. Ghalem and Zouaoui [35] also supplemented yogurt with *Rosmarinus officinalis* oil at 0.14, 0.21, 0.29, and 0.36 g/L over 21 days. The herbal yoghurt enhanced with 0.14 g/L essential oil received the highest grade from panelists for taste, flavor, and texture. Furthermore, the inclusion of *R. officinalis* essential oil enhanced the properties. Furthermore, the use of *R. officinalis* essential oil improved the characteristics of yogurt by decreasing the pH, lactose, and dry matter values while increasing the titratable acidity, proteins, ash, and fat contents. Storage duration showed little effect on the physicochemical parameters of prepared yogurts in genera [35].

6. Effect of adding herbs and spices to butter

Najgebauer-Lejko, Grega [36] investigated the storage stability of sour cream butter with a 2% addition of dried herbs (sage or rosemary). They concluded that the addition of rosemary herb was more effective than sage in delaying lipolysis in butter, both supplemented products showed higher oxidative stability through storage than the control. TBA analysis revealed that the sage and rosemary butter had much less secondary oxidative compounds, such as malonoaldehyde and ketones, than the butter without herbs. Furthermore, Farag, Ali [37] reported that the addition of thyme and cumin essential oils to butter reduced degradation and was more effective than butylated hydroxytoluene.

7. *Cuminum cyminum* is used as a preservative

C. cyminum is a spice that has long been used as an antiseptic, and it shows powerful antibacterial action in humans against a variety of bacteria, and pathogenic and nonpathogenic fungi [38]. The basic chemical components of cumin essential oil are cuminaldehyde, b-pinene, p-cymene, and g-terpinene [39, 40]. Cuminaldehyde, the main constituent of cumin essential oil, possesses antimicrobial properties [39]. Cumin alcoholic extract has been shown to inhibit *Bacillus subtilis*, *E. coli*, and *Saccharomyces cerevisiae*, as well as have outstanding antimicrobial activity against *Agrobacterium tumefaciens*, *Pseudomonas oleovorans*, *B. subtilis*, *S. cerevisiae*, *Trichophyton rubrum*, and *Bacillus licheniformis* [41]. When the aldehyde fraction of cumin oil containing the antibacterial chemical component cuminaldehyde was examined, it inhibited *Aspergillus flavus* and *Aspergillus niger* by more than 90% [42, 43].

8. *Eugenia caryophyllata* is used as a preservative

E. caryophyllata is a familiar spice used for culinary purposes all over the world, but it also has unique qualities that make it a potential preservative. The major constituents of clove essential oil are beta-caryophyllene and eugenol, both of which have antibacterial activity against *Listeria monocytogenes, E. coli, Campylobacter jejuni, S. aureus,* and *Salmonella enterica* [44]. *E. caryophyllata* has essential oil that includes a high concentration of eugenol (about 88.58%) and has been demonstrated to have antimicrobial properties. *E. caryophyllata* oil treatment at 1–2% concentrations slowed the development of *L. monocytogenes* strains [45]. With a MIC of 39 mg/mL, clove plant leaf oil inhibits *Bacillus cereus* [46]. The sensitivity of different bacterial strains to clove essential oil was investigated, and the maximum level of sensitivity was discovered against five strains of *Staphylococcus epidermidis* with inhibition zones greater than 16 mm. *E. caryophyllata* has essential oil that includes a high concentration of eugenol (about 88.58%) and has been demonstrated to have antimicrobial properties. *E. caryophyllata* oil treatment at 1–2% concentrations slowed the development of *L. monocytogenes* strains has antifungal activity, and chemical components including carvacrol and eugenol have been proven to be antifungal against and *Trichophyton mentagrophytes* and *Candida albicans* [47]. Eugenol is the primary chemical component in clove that has antioxidant qualities. The primary antioxidant activity mechanisms are radical scavenging and metal ion chelation, and eugenol participates in photochemical reactions with strong antioxidant activity [48]. Clove essential oil has been shown to have chelating properties, resulting in the suppression of hydroxyl radicals due to eugenol in clove oil [49].

9. *Cinnamomum verum* is used as a preservative

C. verum is used as a preservative due to its antimicrobial and antibacterial qualities, which can inhibit the growth of bacteria, particularly gram-positive bacteria. Cinnamon oil contains a variety of chemicals, the most notable of which are cynammyldehyde, cynammyl alcohol, and eugenol [50]. *C. verum* was examined for antimicrobial activity against *S. aureus*, and it showed the ability to suppress *S. aureus* growth with an optimum inhibitory effort of 0.09%. This discovery is mostly connected to cynammyldehyde, a chemical component found in *C. verum* [51]. Cinnamaldehyde can be used to prevent bacterial growth by inhibiting cell wall formation, cell membrane function, protein synthesis, or nucleic acid synthesis [51].

10. *Piper nigrum* is used as a preservative

P. nigrum is an Indian spice whose volatile oil has been shown to have antibacterial properties [52]. The phenolic chemicals in black pepper are thought to be responsible for antibacterial activity by destroying bacterium membranes and preventing their development [53]. This essential oil was extracted using acetone and has been proven to be effective in preventing the mycelial growth of fungi, such as *Penicillium viridicatum* and *Fusarium graminearum* [54]. *P. nigrum* has been shown to have antibacterial activity, with reported minimum inhibitory concentrations of around 50–500 ppm inhibiting the growth of gram-positive bacteria, such as *Streptococcus faecalis*, *B. cereus,* and *S. aureus*, as well as some gram-negative bacteria, such as *Pseudomonas aeruginosa* [53].

11. *Rosmarinus officinalis* is used as a preservative

R. officinalis has been demonstrated to have preservation capabilities for usage in food, as its antioxidant activity has been studied in pork products, such as patties [55]. The antioxidant properties of rosemary have been attributed to a variety of phenolic compounds found in this spice, including carnosol, carnosic acid, rosmanol, rosmarinic acid, and tosemaridiphenol [56]. The most abundant compound in *R. officinalis* is carnosic acid, which is followed by other phenolic compounds, such as carnosol. The chemical elements of *R. officinalis* are classified into three groups: phenolic diterpenes with abietic acid structure, flavonoids, and phenolic acids [57]. Carnosic acid, which has a strong antioxidant activity, is primarily responsible for *R. officinalis* preservation advantages. This carnosic acid's antioxidant activity was compared to that of butylated hydroxytoluene (BHT), butylated hydroxyanisole (BHA), and tertiary butyl hydroquinone (TBHQ), and the results showed that this acid was more antioxidant than BHT and BHA. One of *R. officinalis* key active chemicals, carnosic acid, is generated from isopentenyl diphosphate *via* methylerythritol phosphate and is present as carnosol in chloroplasts and intracellular membranes [57]. *R. officinalis* has been compared to several chemical preservatives and antioxidant chemicals, with efficiency comparable to currently used preservatives, showing that rosemary can be used as a natural green alternative to some chemical antioxidants with comparable effects. Because it lacks the strong flavor of other spices, such as *C. verum, R. officinalis, P. nigrum, and Zingiber officinale,* it can be used as a natural antioxidant in a number of dishes. As a result, employing rosemary as an antioxidant will not have any negative effects on the organoleptic properties of foods.

12. *Zingiber officinale* is used as a preservative

Z. officinale is a well-known spice that contains polyphenolic compounds such as 6-gingerol and its derivatives. These chemical constituents make ginger a powerful antioxidant [58]. Fresh ginger is high in proteins, fiber, water, lipids, minerals, and carbohydrates, such as calcium and iron [59]. *Z. officinale* CO_2 extracts have been demonstrated to have high polyphenol content and to operate better as an antioxidant preservative early in the fat oxidation process. *Z. officinale* exhibits antioxidant activity comparable to BHT, a chemical antioxidant that suppresses peroxidation at temperatures ranging from 37 to 80% [59]. *Z. officinale* has been shown to inhibit the growth of colon bacteria as well as other pathogens, such as *Salmonella*, *E. coli*, *Staphylococci*, *Proteus sp*, and *Streptococci* [60–62]. *Z. officinale* has antifungal activity against a variety of fungi, including *Aspergillus* [63]. The phenolic compounds in ginger work as denaturing agents, preventing microbial growth by modifying cell permeability and causing bacterial cells to shatter. Most phenolic compounds are metal chelators that bind to active sites of metabolic enzymes, limiting enzyme activity as well as bacterial metabolism and reproduction [64]. Ginger extracts at 0.4 mg/mL have been proven in tests to be more effective than commercial antibiotics, such as gentamicin against *Klebsiella pneumoniae*, *Proteus vulgaris*, *Streptococcus pyogenes*, and *S. aureus* [65].

13. Curry is used as a preservative

Curry is a common spice found in cooking. It originated in India and has since gained popularity throughout the world because of its distinctive flavor and aroma [66]. Curry has been shown to have powerful antimicrobial effects. Antimicrobial tests with coumarin extracts in petroleum ether and chloroform demonstrated considerable antibacterial and antifungal action. Curry chloroform extract has shown good inhibitory efficacy against *A. niger* and *P. aeruginosa* [67]. Curry is high in carbazole alkaloids and coumarins, both of which have antimicrobial qualities. Curry compounds have been found to have minimal inhibitory values ranging from 3.13 to 100 mg/mL [68].

The antibacterial activity of curry extracts is proportional to the concentration used, and growth inhibition has been seen against *P. aeruginosa, E. coli*, and *B. subtilis*, with a lower minimum inhibitory concentration (MIC) than *S. aureus* and *Micrococcus luteus*. According to these findings, *E. coli* is the most resistant bacteria, and higher spice doses are required to halt it [67]. Curry's antifungal and antiaflatoxigenic properties have been demonstrated. The use of curry as a natural antibacterial food preservative and a detoxifying agent during the food preservation process has been studied [69]. Because of these features, curry has established itself as an important natural preservative with an enormous potential for replacing other types of non-natural preservatives. Whole spices can be used as preservatives on their own, but their essential oils can be isolated and evaluated for quality. Spice essential oils are homogeneous mixtures of organic chemical molecules belonging to the same chemical family, such as sesquiterpenes, monoterpenes, and terpenoids.

14. Conclusions and future outlook

Herbs and spices are used for a variety of purposes, including flavoring, coloring, medicinal, and preservation purposes, and their trading is a substantial economic activity globally. Certain popular spices have created a significant demand for certain popular spices all over the world, making spices a research and economic benefit niche. Several spices have been demonstrated to inhibit the growth of some of the most common bacteria in food, such as *E. coli, Salmonella,* and *L. monocytogenes*. Thus, while spices can be used as preservatives, it is necessary to demonstrate their antimicrobial effect on various foods, such as dairy products, fruit, meat, vegetables, and poultry, to ensure a preservative effect comparable to the conventional synthetic preservative effect for each food before settling on the use of spices as preservatives for industrial or commercial purposes. Although whole spices and essential oils have been shown to have good antibacterial activity, their use is still under discussion because it can be expensive to purify them without necessarily increasing the effectiveness of their antimicrobial or antioxidant activity. Because whole spices possess these properties, they can be employed as natural preservatives in the food industry. Finally, some spices' antibacterial and antioxidant properties, such as turmeric, black pepper, clove, nutmeg, turmeric, cumin, and cinnamon, have created a research field in which they can be employed as food preservatives. For example, spices used in foods, such as meats, have a high likelihood of success and potential antimicrobial activity comparable to that of currently used nitrite-based preservatives, which have been claimed to have negative health effects, allowing researchers to investigate a method to replace chemical-based preservatives with natural-based ones for food preservation.

Author details

Madonna Ngwatshipane Mashabela[1,2], Peter Tshepiso Ndhlovu[2*] and Wilfred Otang Mbeng[2]

1 Department of Soil Sciences, Soil Cultivation, Agricultural Research Council Infruitec-Nietvoorbij, Stellenbosch, South Africa

2 School of Biology and Environmental Sciences, Faculty of Agriculture and Natural Sciences, University of Mpumalanga, Mbombela, South Africa

*Address all correspondence to: tshepsio.ndhlovu@ump.ac.za

References

[1] Carocho M et al. Adding molecules to food, pros and cons: A review on synthetic and natural food additives. Comprehensive Reviews in Food Science and Food Safety. 2014;**13**:377-399

[2] Pinto VF, Patriarca A, Pose G. Plant extracts as natural antifungals: Alternative strategies for mold control in foods. In: Novel Technologies in Food Science. New York: Springer; 2012. pp. 205-218

[3] Tajkarimi M, Ibrahim SA, Cliver D. Antimicrobial herb and spice compounds in food. Food Control. 2010;**21**:1199-1218

[4] Juneja VK, Dwivedi HP, Yan X. Novel natural food antimicrobials. Annual Review of Food Science and Technology. 2012;**3**:381-403

[5] Makwana S et al. In-vitro antibacterial activity of plant based phenolic compounds for food safety and preservation. LWT-Food Science and Technology. 2015;**62**:935-939

[6] Ayodele OD, Oyegbade O, Oseni SR. Phytochemical analysis and antioxidant activities of dry and fresh leaves of Petivera alliacea and Ocimum gratissimum. International Journal of Sciences: Basic and Applied Research. 2015;**24**:1-13

[7] Gould GW. Industry perspectives on the use of natural antimicrobials and inhibitors for food applications. Journal of Food Protection. 1996;**59**:82-86

[8] Farag R et al. Antioxidant activity of some spice essential oils on linoleic acid oxidation in aqueous media. Journal of the American Oil Chemists' Society. 1989;**66**:792-799

[9] Chipault J. The antioxidant properties of spices in foods. Food Technology. 1956;**10**:209-211

[10] Chipault J, Mizuno G, Lundberg W. Antioxidant properties of spices in oil-in-water emulsions [abc]. Journal of Food Science. 1955;**20**:443-448

[11] Chen C, Pearson A, Gray J. Effects of synthetic antioxidants (BHA, BHT and PG) on the mutagenicity of IQ-like compounds. Food Chemistry. 1992;**43**:177-183

[12] Imaida K et al. Promoting activities of butylated hydroxyanisole and butylated hydroxytoluene on 2-stage urinary bladder carcinogenesis and inhibition of γ-glutamyl transpeptidase-positive foci development in the liver of rats. Carcinogenesis. 1983;**4**:895-899

[13] Botsoglou N et al. The effect of dietary oregano essential oil on lipid oxidation in raw and cooked chicken during refrigerated storage. Meat Science. 2002;**62**:259-265

[14] Wanasundara U, Shahidi F. Stabilization of seal blubber and menhaden oils with green tea catechins. Journal of the American Oil Chemists' Society. 1996;**73**:1183-1190

[15] Jung M, Yoon S, Min D. Effects of processing steps on the contents of minor compounds and oxidation of soybean oil. Journal of the American Oil Chemists' Society. 1989;**66**:118-120

[16] Nieto G. A review on applications and uses of Thymus in the food industry. Plants. 2020;**9**:961

[17] Peter K, Shylaja M. Introduction to herbs and spices: Definitions, trade and applications. In: Handbook of Herbs and Spices. Cambridge, UK: Elsevier; 2012. pp. 1-24

[18] Singhal R, Kulkarni P, Rege D. Quality indices for spice essential oils.

In: Peter K, editor. Handbook of Herbs and Spices. Cambridge, UK: Woodhead Publishing; 2001. pp. 42-54

[19] Embuscado ME. Herbs and spices as antioxidants for food preservation. In: Handbook of Antioxidants for Food Preservation. USA: Elsevier; 2015. pp. 251-283

[20] Pokorný J, Pánek J. The effect of natural antioxidants in herbs and spices on food shelf-life. In: Handbook of Herbs and Spices. Cambridge, UK: Elsevier; 2012. pp. 51-71

[21] Cushnie TT, Lamb AJ. Antimicrobial activity of flavonoids. International Journal of Antimicrobial Agents. 2005;**26**:343-356

[22] Solanki I et al. Flavonoid-based therapies in the early management of neurodegenerative diseases. Advances in Nutrition. 2015;**6**:64-72

[23] Spencer JPE et al. Contrasting influences of glucuronidation and O-methylation of epicatechin on hydrogen peroxide-induced cell death in neurons and fibroblasts. Free Radical Biology and Medicine. 2001;**31**:1139-1146

[24] Cazzola R, Cestaro B. Antioxidant spices and herbs used in diabetes. In: Diabetes: Oxidative Stress and Dietary Antioxidants. London, UK: Elsevier; 2014. pp. 89-97

[25] Lohani N, Singh MB, Bhalla PL. Biological parts for engineering abiotic stress tolerance in plants. BioDesign Research. 2022;**2022**:1-41

[26] Shan B et al. The in vitro antibacterial activity of dietary spice and medicinal herb extracts. International Journal of Food Microbiology. 2007;**117**:112-119

[27] Sharma S et al. Essential oils as additives in active food packaging. Food Chemistry. 2021;**343**:128403

[28] Llana-Ruiz-Cabello M et al. Development of PLA films containing oregano essential oil (Origanum vulgare L. virens) intended for use in food packaging. Food Additives & Contaminants: Part A. 2016;**33**:1374-1386

[29] Acevedo-Fani A et al. Edible films from essential oil-loaded nanoemulsions: Physicochemical characterization and antimicrobial properties. Food Hydrocolloids. 2015;**47**:168-177

[30] El-Shibiny S et al. The use of nano-sized eggshell powder for calcium fortification of cow? s and buffalo? s milk yogurts. Acta Scientiarum Polonorum Technologia Alimentaria. 2018;**17**:37-49

[31] Behrad S et al. Manipulation of probiotics fermentation of yogurt by cinnamon and licorice: Effects on yogurt formation and inhibition of helicobacter pylori growth in vitro. World Academy of Science, Engineering and Technology. 2009;**60**:590-594

[32] Bakrm S, Salihin B. Effects of inclusion of Allium sativum and Cinnamomumverum in milk on the growth and activity of lactic acid bacteria during yoghurt fermentation. Amer-Euras. Journal of Agriculture and Environmental Sciences. 2013;**13**:1448-1457

[33] Srivastava P et al. Analysis of antioxidant activity of herbal yoghurt prepared from different milk. The Pharma Innovation. 2015;**4**:18

[34] Kumar TS et al. Development of mint flavoured yoghurt spread. Asian Journal of Dairying & Foods Research. 2013;**32**:19-24

[35] Ghalem BR, Zouaoui B. Microbiological, physico-chemical and sensory quality aspects of yoghurt enriched with Rosmarinus officinalis

oil. African Journal of Biotechnology. 2013;**12**:192-198

[36] Najgebauer-Lejko D et al. The quality and storage stability of butter made from sour cream with addition of dried sage and rosemary. Biotechnology in Animal Husbandry. 2009;**25**:753-761

[37] Farag R, Ali M, Taha S. Use of some essential oils as natural preservatives for butter. Journal of the American Oil Chemists' Society. 1990;**67**:188-191

[38] Haloci E et al. Antibacterial and antifungal activity assesment of nigella sativa essential oils. International Journal of Pharmacological and Pharmaceutical Sciences. 2012;**6**:270-272

[39] Hernández-Ochoa L et al. Use of essential oils and extracts from spices in meat protection. Journal of Food Science and Technology. 2014;**51**:957-963

[40] Hajhashemi V, Ghannadi A, Jafarabadi H. Black cumin seed essential oil, as a potent analgesic and antiinflammatory drug. Phytotherapy Research: An International Journal Devoted to Pharmacological and Toxicological Evaluation of Natural Product Derivatives. 2004;**18**:195-199

[41] De M, De A, Mukhopadhvay R. Antimicrobial activity of Cuminum cyminum L. Ars Pharmaceutica. 2003;**44**:257-269

[42] Balacs T. Cajuput components. International Journal of Aromatherapy. 1993;**5**:35

[43] Pawar V, Thaker V. In vitro efficacy of 75 essential oils against *Aspergillus niger*. Mycoses. 2006;**49**:316-323

[44] Chaieb K et al. The chemical composition and biological activity of clove essential oil, Eugenia caryophyllata (Syzigium aromaticum L. Myrtaceae): A short review. Phytotherapy Research: An International Journal Devoted to Pharmacological and Toxicological Evaluation of Natural Product Derivatives. 2007;**21**:501-506

[45] Mytle N et al. Antimicrobial activity of clove (Syzgium aromaticum) oil in inhibiting Listeria monocytogenes on chicken frankfurters. Food Control. 2006;**17**:102-107

[46] Ogunwande I et al. Studies on the essential oils composition, antibacterial and cytotoxicity of Eugenia uniflora L. International Journal of Aromatherapy. 2005;**15**:147-152

[47] Tampieri MP et al. The inhibition of Candida albicans by selected essential oils and their major components. Mycopathologia. 2005;**159**:339-345

[48] Ogata M et al. Antioxidant activity of eugenol and related monomeric and dimeric compounds. Chemical and Pharmaceutical Bulletin. 2000;**48**:1467-1469

[49] Jirovetz L et al. Chemical composition and antioxidant properties of clove leaf essential oil. Journal of Agricultural and Food Chemistry. 2006;**54**:6303-6307

[50] Herwita I. The impact cinnamon bio-insecticide to the insect biologic aspect Epilachum varivestis, Mulsant. Journal of Akta Agrosia. 2007;**1**:99-105

[51] Winias S. Effect of cynammyldehyde from cinnamon extract as a natural preservative alternative to the growth of Staphylococcus aureus bacteria. Indonesian Journal of Tropical and Infectious Disease. 2011;**2**:38-41

[52] Dorman HD, Surai P, Deans SG. In vitro antioxidant activity of a

number of plant essential oils and phytoconstituents. Journal of Essential Oil Research. 2000;**12**:241-248

[53] Karsha PV, Lakshmi OB. Antibacterial activity of black pepper (*Piper nigrum* Linn.) with special reference to its mode of action on bacteria. Indian Journal of Natural Products and Resources. 2010;**1**:213-215

[54] Singh G et al. Chemical, antioxidant and antifungal activities of volatile oil of black pepper and its acetone extract. Journal of the Science of Food and Agriculture. 2004;**84**:1878-1884

[55] Chen X et al. Lipid oxidation, volatiles and color changes of irradiated pork patties affected by antioxidants. Journal of Food Science. 1999;**64**:16-19

[56] Shahidi F, Naczk M. Phenolics in Food and Nutraceuticals, Ed. n. ed. Boca Raton: CRC Press; 2003

[57] Almela L et al. Liquid chromatograpic–mass spectrometric analysis of phenolics and free radical scavenging activity of rosemary extract from different raw material. Journal of Chromatography A. 2006;**1120**:221-229

[58] Stoilova I et al. Antioxidant activity of a ginger extract (Zingiber officinale). Food Chemistry. 2007;**102**:764-770

[59] Govindarajan V, Connell D. Ginger-chemistry, technology, and quality evaluation: Part 1. Critical Reviews in Food Science & Nutrition. 1983;**17**:1-96

[60] Gupta S, Ravishankar S. A comparison of the antimicrobial activity of garlic, ginger, carrot, and turmeric pastes against Escherichia coli O157: H7 in laboratory buffer and ground beef. Foodbourne Pathogens & Disease. 2005;**2**:330-340

[61] Ernst E, Pittler M. Efficacy of ginger for nausea and vomiting: A systematic review of randomized clinical trials. British Journal of Anaesthesia. 2000;**84**:367-371

[62] White B. Ginger: An overview. American Family Physician. 2007;**75**:1689-1691

[63] Nanir S, Kadu B. Effect of some medicinal plants extract on some fungi. Acta Botanica Indica. 1987;**2**:170-175

[64] Huang M-T, Lee CY, Ho C-T. Phenolic compounds in food and their effects on health. In: ACS Symposium Series (USA). New York: American Chemical Society; 1992

[65] Ahmed SA. Study the antibacterial activity of Zingiber officinale roots against some of pathogenic bacteria. Al-Mustansiriyah Journal of Science. 2012;**23**:63-70

[66] Sathaye S et al. Hepatoprotective effects of aqueous leaf extract and crude isolates of Murraya koenigii against in vitro ethanol-induced hepatotoxicity model. Experimental and Toxicologic Pathology. 2011;**63**:587-591

[67] Vats M, Singh H, Sardana S. Phytochemical screening and antimicrobial activity of roots of Murraya koenigii (Linn.) Spreng.(Rutaceae). Brazilian Journal of Microbiology. 2011;**42**:1569-1573

[68] Rahman MM, Gray AI. A benzoisofuranone derivative and carbazole alkaloids from Murraya koenigii and their antimicrobial activity. Phytochemistry. 2005;**66**:1601-1606

[69] Murugan K, Anandaraj K, Al-Sohaibani S. Antiaflatoxigenic food additive potential of Murraya koenigii: An in vitro and molecular interaction study. Food Research International. 2013;**52**:8-16

Chapter 8

Ethnoveterinary Practices for Indigenous Poultry Health Management by Smallholder Farmers

Wiseman Ndlovu, Nyambeni Ronald Mudimeli, Marizvikuru Mwale, Tshianeo Mellda Ndou, Ola Segun Obadire and Joseph Francis

Abstract

Most resource-constrained smallholder farmers rely on ethnoveterinary medicine to treat village chicken diseases. An in-depth literature review and empirical study was conducted to establish ethnoveterinary practices used in indigenous chicken health management. The study showed that most village chicken farmers were female (70%). Most farmers kept chickens for socio-economic purposes; food, status and income. Common birds' ailments treated and controlled using EVPs include Fowl Cholera; Pullorum; Diarrhea; Gumboro; Avian Influenza; Ngorok & Snot (Infectious Coryza); Bloody & watery diarrhea (Coccidiosis). Variety of materials were used to treat and control chicken diseases either as purely indigenous methods or in combination with conventional medicines. Among the practices, medicinal plants like *Aloe vera* emerged as the most commonly used botanical plant. More so, both literature and the empirical study, showed that farmers prepared and applied *A. vera* uniquely depending on the region and type of *A. vera*. Majority of remedies are used to treat more than one ailment. It is recommended that these practices be preserved and considered for new drug advancement and commercialization to promote cheaper and environmentally friendly options for poultry health management.

Keywords: chicken diseases, ethnoveterinary medicine, medicinal plants, village chickens, smallholder farmers

1. Introduction

The use of traditional medicinal practices in animal health management also referred to as Ethnoveterinary Practices (EVPs) dates back to the time in memorial [1, 2]. Since the onset of industrial revolution, the use of EVPS like medicinal plants and herbs began to decline as the preferred alternative to conventional medicine. Recently, their use is gaining attention and importance in modern day

IntechOpen

practices that pursue organic solutions to health problems emanating from the use of the populous conventional medicine [3]. This shift is prompted by sustainability, comprehensiveness, cost effectiveness, availability and environmental friendliness of medicinal plants, traditional practices and herbs [4]. Resultantly, this necessitated a revisit to traditional grassroots medicines and paradigm shift to modern day animal health practices. This chapter critically reviews literature and empirical documents on medicinal plants or herbs and other traditional practices and approaches used in the control and treatment of indigenous village chicken diseases. Village chickens are domestic fowls of either indigenous type or any genetic stock, improved or unimproved [5, 6]. Almost every household in rural sector owns a chicken. The chickens play a significant role towards rural household income, food security and rural development [7]. Despite their substantial importance, they are significantly affected by diseases and parasites infections and infestations. Specifically, an inventory of common indigenous chicken disease types as well as medicinal plants or herbs resources used, their availability, parts used, harvesting methods, preparation and their therapeutic value are investigated and documented. This is key to promote awareness and avoid extinction of valuable information.

2. History and background of ethnoveterinary practices

Herbs and medicinal plants along with other traditional practices play a crucial role in human and animal health management [8]. Herbs and medicinal plants are a source of drug compounds, emerging modern medicines and play a critical role in the conventional medicine revolution [1]. Thus, herbs form an important foundation in the development of medicines and are a natural blueprint in advancement of new drugs or phyto-medicine in controlling and treating livestock diseases such as indigenous chickens. Ethnoveterinary practices in general consist of local based indigenous knowledge and methods used to care for, heal and manage livestock health. These were developed over a long time through trial-and-error method [8–10]. They are a viable and valuable alternative to and complement conventional synthetic veterinary medicines in the management of chicken's health characterized by rising costs [11]. Although, EVPs such as herbs or plants are recognized for their medicinal and pesticidal value, there is consensus among farmers and science that these be documented and preserved as alternatives for and advancement of animal health management [12]. Fears are that this valuable knowledge might be lost due to rapid socio-economic, environmental and technological changes.

The EVPs are commonly used among rural communities and smallholder farmers. Evidently, they are also used in commercial breeds such as broilers [13]. The resource constrained production systems used by smallholder farmers is characterized by free ranging behavior and scavenging nature in indigenous chicken management. Birds produced under these conditions, have a high mortality, that is why indigenous chickens have low productivity as a result of accidents, predation and diseases [14]. High prevalence of diseases is one of the principal limitations to these production systems [15]. Smallholder farmers and those in peri-urban areas are resource constrained, finance included, have limited access to veterinary services, information about the prevention and treatment of animal diseases, as well as prophylactic and therapeutic veterinary medicines [16]. This forms the basis as to why farmers utilize a combination of EVPs for their indigenous chicken health management, and in most cases are inclined more to EVPs. Most of these commercial drugs are expensive and are not easily accessible and affordable to the resource-poor smallholder farmers [17]. Natural options, especially plant-based products or herbs that are locally available and easily accessible as the medicines of choice for most resource poor smallholder farmers, especially women. The knowledge of EVPs appears to be mostly in the custodian of older people, both men and women. They systematically pass it to younger generations by word of mouth. This form of communication is still the most widespread means of communication in local villages in Africa.

It is observed that a fraction of EVPs knowledge is accessible to all indigenous chicken producers, and another portion is a protectively guarded family secret [18]. In rapidly changing world driven by commercialization, EVPs are increasingly shunned upon, and viewed as backward and old fashioned. Despite, these contestations, the continued use of conventional medicines is linked to environmental damage, rising costs and adverse effects to human health [19]. There are also increasing concerns for drug resistant disease-causing microorganisms due to over and improper use of conventional medicines [20]. It is why recently, there is a paradigm shift to focus on and increased demand for organic agricultural practices globally for animal health management. Herbs and medicinal plants offer a practicable choice due to the fact that they are broader in spectrum of action. Ethnoveterinary Practices are relatively more accessible, easy to prepare and administer at a little to no cost on the farmer. Moreover, most traditional herbs have a long record of safety. Their documentation offers more new options in the advancement of science and new insights or inroads to cheaper and healthier alternatives to animal health management. This makes them an attractive and viable option for use in indigenous chickens by both commercial and resource constrained rural farmers [21, 22]. Clearly, EVPs have once again become an important component of agriculture and are set to play a crucial role in the future of animal health management [17]. This chapter, therefore, comprehensively reviews literature on EVPs and uses empirical data from Vhembe district in Limpopo province of South Africa to document herbs, medicinal plants and other traditional practices used to treat and control indigenous village chicken diseases.

3. Chapter objectives

The objectives of this chapter are to:

1. Document common ailments and diseases that afflict indigenous village chickens,

2. Produce a comprehensive inventory of traditional practices, medicinal plant resources, plants parts used, harvesting techniques, preparation, and therapeutic value associated chicken health management, and

3. Assess the sustainability of the EVPs in indigenous chicken health management.

Where applicable and necessary illustrative sketches are given. Also, socioeconomic aspects of EVPs are scrutinized with the view to understand the system of knowledge transfer and gender roles.

4. Methods used

4.1 Study design

The study used an explorative descriptive design to gather, unpack and document the medicinal plants used to cure, heal, treat and control indigenous village chicken diseases in rural communities. Systematic literature search and empirical evidence from Vhembe district of Limpopo province, South Africa provided data for the study. Pragmatic approach review of literature was followed in this study. Pragmatic approach goes beyond identifying and understanding chickens' ailments to proposing possible actionable treatment interventions that enhance effective use of EVPs [23]. This approach is considered appropriate in this work for its methodological rigor and objectivity in review and analysis of information [24]. It is used in this chapter to offer tools that describe, explain, predict, interpret and understand the usage, application and sustainability of medicinal plants/herbs and other traditional methods used in the control and treatment of indigenous village chicken ailments [23].

4.2 Data collection

Data was sourced empirical and from literature. Literature was reviewed in multiple-levels through searching for related publication in database sources (Web of Science, Ebscohost and Science Direct) and search engines (Google Search, Google Scholar). Literature published between the year 1990 to 2022 on the EVPs and medicinal plants used to treat and control indigenous village chicken ailments was used. Ethnoveterinary Practices, Ethnoveterinary Medicine (EVM), medicinal plants/herbs, indigenous chickens, village chickens, and rural poultry production were the key search words/phrases for randomly selected articles in published literature. Through snowballing by reviewing the citations in each of the identified relevant articles, more relevant literature was sourced.

A semi-structured interview guide was used to collect data from indigenous chicken farmers in Thulamela local Municipality of Vhembe district in South Africa. Postgraduate students pursuing various degree programmes at the University of Venda were recruited and trained to serve as research assistants. The study was piloted to test the data collection tool prior to the actual full-scale collection of data. Participants with similar characteristics to the study participants were used for the pilot test. The purpose was to check the usability and applicability as well as to enhance the validity and reliability of the data collection tool. Minor errors observed during the pilot study, were noted and the data collection instrument was revised. Face to-face interviews were then conducted with the smallholder farmers owning chickens. The interviews were administered to the smallholder farmers via reading the questions, recording answers, and explaining to the respondents in the local language, viz. *Tshivenda*. Demographic data, prevalent chicken diseases, medicinal plants/herbs and traditional methods used to treat and control the chickens' ailments were gathered. Moreover, data on techniques of medicinal plants/herbs harvesting, parts used, preparation method and administration were collected. Data was triangulated through consultations with key informants in the form of extension officers and traditional leaders. Similarly, the results of the empirical study were presented at conferences (Society for Medicinal Plants and Economic Development Conference). The conference had representatives from the Limpopo Province Department of Agriculture Executive Managers, extension officers, advisors and researchers in the field.

4.3 Analysis procedure

Figure 1 illustrates the analysis procedure followed in this chapter. In both cases of data collection, data was analyzed thematical by first identifying the indigenous chicken disease ailments, and EVPs used. This process was aided by Atlas-ti (Version 8) a sophisticated qualitative data analysis software. The software is recommended for large texts such as in document review and it has a network diagrams capability that joins family of codes for easier analysis and drawing conclusions. Sources and harvesting methods of medicinal plants/herbs, parts used, preparation techniques and medicine administration are also observed. The chapter also unpacked the sustainability of the herbs and different EVPs used in the control and treatment of chickens' ailments based on availability, regeneration, and harvesting techniques.

4.4 Demographic information

A total of 103 articles related to EVPs in the production of indigenous chickens were found in the literature search conducted. Only 21 were considered relevant according to the search criteria and hence used in the study [3, 6, 8–12, 15, 17, 18, 21, 25–33]. Pertaining the empirical study, **Table 1** shows the demographic information of the household heads responsible and directly involved in taking care of the birds in the empirical study are presented. It is also worth noting that the responsibility of taking care of chickens is also shared with the rest of the family members. This depends on one's availability and for skills and knowledge transfer purposes. Females accounted for 70% (42) of the farmers and slightly above half (51.7%) of all the farmers were above the age of 50 years. Thus, fewer youth and children participated in day-to-day chicken farming activities. However, they are an integral part of the process. Their least representation was influenced by the time and days of the data collection process in which majority will be at school or working elsewhere.

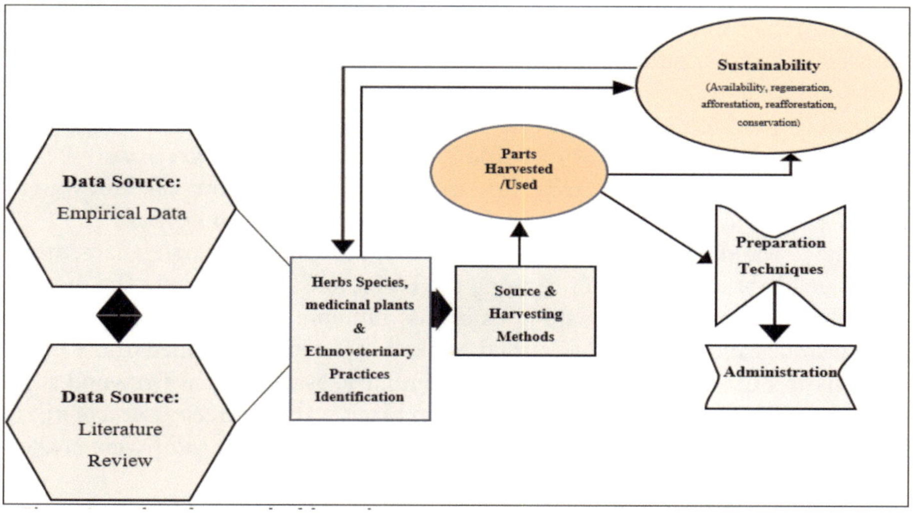

Figure 1.
Analysis framework of the study.

Variable	Category	Frequency	Proportion (%)
Gender	Male	18	30
	Female	42	70
Age group	30 years and below	5	8.3
	31 to 40	11	18.3
	41 to 50	13	21.7
	50 years and above	31	51.7

Table 1.
Demographic information of indigenous village chicken farmers (n=60).

5. Common indigenous village chickens ailments

The study identified several village chicken ailments both in literature and the empirical study. Diarrhea [*Kwingi*], Newcastle, and a disease described as a "walking duck" are the three common ailments identified that afflict indigenous village chickens in Vhembe district of Limpopo province, South Africa. In the review of literature, Fowl Cholera; Pullorum; Diarrhea; Gumboro; Avian Influenza; Ngorok & Snot (*Infectious coryza*); Bloody & watery diarrhea (Coccidiosis), Ectoparasite; Open wound; Newcastle (Fengile), kofis; Swelling of the body; depression; and swelling of head were revealed as the common diseases.

6. Ethnoveterinary practices and indigenous chicken disease management

6.1 Ethnoveterinary practices used

Smallholder farmers use several EVPs in indigenous village chickens' health management. The EVPs products used are mainly based on plants, herbs, combination of modern products with plants and other traditional practices. **Table 2** and **Figure 2** display different EVPs products used in the treatment of indigenous village chicken diseases from both literature and the empirical data. It the empirical study, farmers in Vhembe district used mainly natural occurring EVPs as one or in combination with other modern products or conventional medicines to treat and control indigenous village chicken diseases. As show in **Table 2**, these include *Capsicum frutescens* [Chilies or Peri -Peri]; *Aloe vera*; [*Mushikili*]; [Musero]; Sunflower cooking oil; Hot water; Ashes (*Mopani Musese)* - African black wattle, [*Muunga*] *Acacia nigriscen* & [*Munanaga*] - Monkey thorn); Magazine (paper); Potassium permanganate, and locally available washing powder. Among the EVPs, Aloe species were the most utilized medicinal plants in managing chickens' ailments. Most commonly, plants or herbs like chilies and Aloes were crushed, soaked in water and applied orally i.e. given to chickens as a drink or in drinking water. Similarly, ashes used as firewood at home composed of *Mopani, Acacia mearnsii* [African black wattle; *Musese*], *Acacia nigriscen* [*Muunga*] & *Acacia galpinii* [Monkey thorn, *Munanaga or Tshikwalo*] were soaked in water and given to chickens as a drink or in drinking water.

The reviewed literature showed similar results to the findings of the empirical study. From literature, the EVPs comprised of botanical or herb families like Mimosaceae (*Parkia sp.*), Caesalpiniaceae [*Cassia sp.*]; Euphorbiaceae [*Euphorbia sp.*],

No	Ethnoveterinary Practice product	Source & Harvesting Technique	Parts used	Preparation & Application methods	Therapeutic Value/ Ailment
STUDY 1: EMPIRICAL DATA					
1	Aloe [*Aloe Vera*]	In the bushes. Harvested by plucking out the whole or half	Leaves	• Dried, Crushed, fluid squeezed, mixed with salt and soaked in water for chickens to drink • Crush fruit, mix with donkey feaeces in drinking water • Crushed leaves mixed with pepper (fresh) and ashes • Crushed mixed with grinded fresh garlic and neem leaves	Diarrhea, Newcastle and Duck disease.
2	Chilies [Peri -Peri]	Grown at home. The whole fruit is plucked out and used	Whole Fruit	Crushed and mixed with water for chickens to drink	Diarrhea [*Kwingi*], Newcastle
3	[Mushikili]	Found in the bushes. Leaves are collected and used	Leaves	Soaked in water for chickens to drink	Preventative
4	[Musero]	Grown at home and found in the bushes. Wholesome leaves are collected and used	Leaves	Soaked in water for chickens to drink	Diarrhea [Kwingi]
5	Sunflower cooking oil	Bought from the shops	N/A	Put oil in the palm or deep the finger in the oil and directly apply onto the location of disease-causing parasite	Parasites
6	Hot water	Normal tape or river water.	N/A	Pour water in the chicken house to kill lice [Thatha] and Mice [Vhulive] (diseases causing parasites)	Parasites
7	Ashes	Firewood from various trees such as Mopani	Stems/ trunk	Mix it with water apply on the area infested with parasites	Diarrhea [Kwingi], Newcastle and Duck disease
8	Magazine (paper)	N/A	N/A	Burnt and the ash mixed with water for chickens to drink	

No	Ethnoveterinary Practice product	Source & Harvesting Technique	Parts used	Preparation & Application methods	Therapeutic Value/ Ailment
9	Moringa	Grown at home or found in the bushes. Leaves are pruned from small branches.	Leaves	• Leaves soaked in water and given to chickens to drink • Sun dried moringa ground into powder and mixed with chopped fresh aloe leaves add in drinking water	Diarrhea [*Kwingi*], Newcastle and Duck disease
10	Washing powder	N/A		Burn and use ashes with water for chickens to drink	

STUDY 2: LITERATURE REVIEW

No	Ethnoveterinary Practice product	Parts used	Preparation & Application methods	Therapeutic Value/ Ailment
1	Aloe [*Aloe spicata*; *Aloe ferox; Aloe Saponaria; Aloe chabaudii; Aloe excels; Aloe Vera*]	Leaves	Soaked and administered orally	Newcastle, Sleeping disease, Depression, Fowl Cholera
2	Chillies [*Capsicum annum*]	Fruit	Crushed and administered orally	Newcastle, Diarrhea, depression
3	*Albizia adianthifolia* (Mutowa)	Roots	Crushed and pasted onto the wound	
4	Lannea Stullmanni (Musosoti)	Bark	Crushed, soaked in water and administered orally	
5	Cactus [*Opuntia vulgaris*], lemon [*Citrus limon*] and red pepper [*Capsicum frutescens*]		Crushed, fluids mixed together and inoculated	Newcastle
6	Paw Paw (*Carica papaya*)	Leaves	Soaked in water mixed with feed and orally administered	Parasite worms, respiratory diseases, anti-inflammatory
7	Ginger [*Zingiber officinale*]	Rhizome	Soaked in water mixed with feed and orally administered	Respiratory diseases (prevention and cure), immunity booster.
8	Turmeric [*Curcuma sp.*]	Rhizome	Soaked in water mixed with feed and orally administered	Respiratory diseases, parasite worms, wounds and immunity booster
9	Onion [*Allium cepa*]	Bulb	Mixed with either aromatic ginger, brown sugar, vegetable oil, or garlic and given with feed to chickens	Respiratory diseases, antibiotic, immunity booster, antipyretic

No	Ethnoveterinary Practice product	Source & Harvesting Technique	Parts used	Preparation & Application methods	Therapeutic Value/ Ailment
10	Garlic [*Allium sativum*]		Bulbs	Mixed with either aromatic ginger, brown sugar, or garlic and given with feed to chickens	Respiratory diseases, antibiotic, immunity booster
No	**Ethnoveterinary Practice product**		**Parts used**	**Preparation & Application methods**	**Therapeutic Value/ Ailment**
11	Aromatic ginger		Rhizome	Soaked in water mixed with feed and orally administered	Respiratory diseases, antibiotic, immunity booster, increasing palatability, prevention of parasitic worms
12	Anacardiaceae [*Schinus mole*]				Bloody diarrhea & Ectoparasite
13	Brassicaceae [*Lepidiumstavium*]		Seeds	Grind the seeds, mix with butter and apply locally.	Open wounds
14	Euphorabiaceae [*Croton mscrostachyus*]		Leaves	Collecting juice extract and apply locally	Open wound
15	Aloceae Ret		Whole part	Squeezing and collecting juice, flower and mixing with salt and given to birds to drink	Newcastle (Fengile), Coccodios (kofis)
16	Bisana [*Euphorabiaceae*]		Leaves	Collecting juice extract and apply locally	Open wound
17	[*Allium astavium*] Allicaceae		Bulbs	Crushing it and mix with katical	Bloody diarrhea
18	Astraceae [*Verinonia amygdalin del*]		Leaves	Crushing leaves and mix with *injera* (a sour fermented pancake-like flatbread with a slightly spongy texture, traditionally made of teff flour) and fed to chickens	Watery diarrhea
19	Rutacceae [*Rutachalepensis*]		Whole	Crushing it add mixing with *injera* (a sour fermented pancake-like flatbread with a slightly spongy texture, traditionally made of teff flour) and fed to chickens	Swelling
20	*Citrus sinesis*		Fruits	Squeezing and collecting juice	Prevention and control

No	Ethnoveterinary Practice product	Source & Harvesting Technique	Parts used	Preparation & Application methods	Therapeutic Value/ Ailment
21	*Citrus ourantifoli*		Fruits	Squeeze, collect juice and mix with water for birds to drink	Diarrhea and ectoparasite
22	*Catha edulis*		Leaves	Crush leaves, mix with salt and water for birds to drink	Prevention
23	Oleaceae [*Oleaeuropaea capenesis*]		Leaves	Burn leaves and fumigate the house of chicken	Depression
24	[*Phytolaccadodecandra*] Phytolaccaceae		Whole	Crush leaves, mix with salt and water for birds to drink	Diarrhea
25	Zingibiberaceae *Zingibarofficinale*]		Rhizome	Crush a rhizome and mix it with water for birds to drink	Newcastle diseases (fengile)
No Ethnoveterinary Practice product		**Parts used**		**Preparation & Application methods**	**Therapeutic Value/ Ailment**
26	Moringaceae [*Moringa stenopetalia*]		Leaves	Crushing leaves and mix with water for birds to drink	Diseases prevention
27	Rhamnaceae [*Rhamnusprinoides*]		Leaves	Crush leaves and mix it with water for birds to drink	Depression
28	Cucurbitaceae [*Zehneriascabra*]		Leaves	Crush leaves and mix them with water for birds to drink	Swelling of head
29	Brassicaceae [*Brassica carinata*]		Seeds	Grind seeds, mix with salt and water for birds to drink	Depression
30	*Pauzzoziamixta*		Leaves	Leaves crushed and water added; animal made to Swallow the mixture	Bloat

Table 2.
Literature review.

Solanaceae [*Capsicum sp*], Cucurbitaceae [*Lagenaria sp.*]; [*Meliaceae*] (*Khaya sp.*); Anacardiaceae [*Mangifera sp.*]; *Liliaceae* (Aloe sp.); and Agavaceae [*Agave sp.*]. Herbs and plants used could be categorized into bulbs, rhizomes, fruit, leafy and ash based on medical plants like Onion (*Allium cepa*); Turmeric [*Curcuma* sp.]; Chillies [*Capsicum annum*]; Paw-paw or Papaya [*Carica papaya*]; and *Mopani*, respectively. Herbs such as [*Rutachalepensis*] Rutacceae and [*Phytolaccadodecandra*] Phytolaccaceae were used as a whole plant. The reviewed and empirical researched list of herbs and other EVPs is not exhaustive.

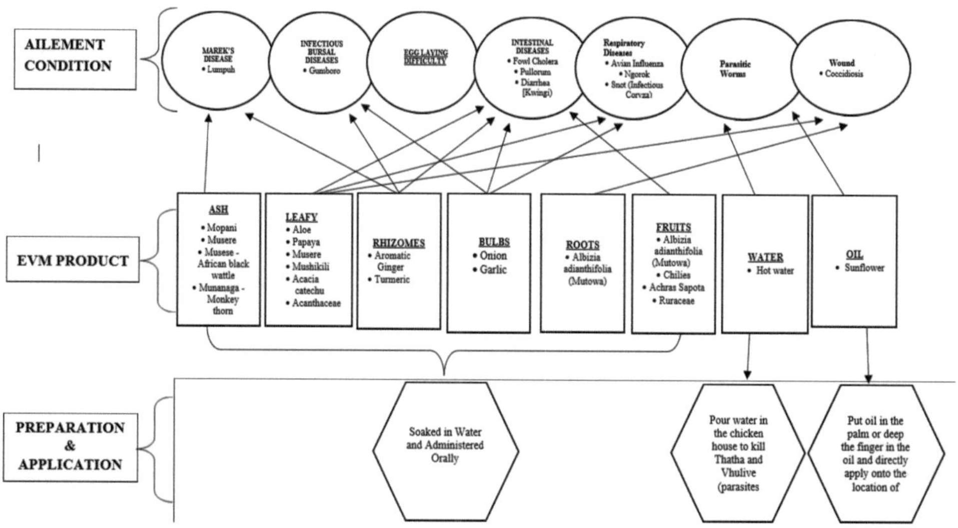

Figure 2.
Ethnoveterinary practices used to control and treat indigenous village chickens' ailments.

6.2 Preparation

Farmers prepared EVMs variedly depending on the nature and type of the EVP. Identified EVMs were mainly soaked in water and given to chickens to drink. Moreover, some herbs were combined with a number of elements and thereafter soaked in water for chickens to drink. For example, in some instances Aloe was crushed, and mixed salt, donkey feaeces, fresh pepper, neem leaves, ashes or garlic and then soaked in water for chickens to drink. In the empirical study, farmers mixed Aloe with potassium permanganate and gave to chickens as part of the drinking water. Also, onion and garlic are mixed with either aromatic ginger, brown sugar, vegetable oil, or garlic and given with feed to chickens.

6.3 Therapeutic value

Majority of EVPs were used as a preventative measure, immune boosting and for healing purposes in multiple chicken ailments. This was observed in both the empirical data and the reviewed literature. For example, Aloe was used to prevent and cure ailments such as diarrhea, Newcastle, depression, and duck disease. Similarly, Onion [*A. cepa*], Garlic [*Allium sativum*]; and Turmeric [*Curcuma sp.*] treat multiple respiratory diseases such as avian Influenza, and snot [*Infectious Coryza*]. Equally, Chillies [*Capsicum annum*], Oleaceae [*Oleaeuropaea capenesis*] and Rhamnaceae [*Rhamnusprinoides*] all treat depression.

6.4 Herbs and medicinal plants sustainability

The two studies conducted also reviewed issues of sustainability in relation to the EVPs. In relation to the herbs and medicinal plants, harvesting techniques, availability, parts used/harvested, regeneration, afforestation, reafforestation, and conservation were observed in both literature and the empirical studies. Herbs used were either found and harvested from the bushes or they were grown at home. Herbs like *Aloe*, and *Mopani* were generally harvested in the bushes. Moringa is harvested in the bushes and also grown at home for medicinal purposes for both animals and humans. In many cases, fewer tree leaves are harvested used to treat and control diseases. Aloe as the most used medicinal plant was harvests by either removing the entire leaf or by cutting the required size. The number of chickens a farmer has determines the size of the leaf to be harvested and this was also done for conservation purposes. Some plants especially fruity ones like chilies are used in whole (**Table 2**). Other EVPs are by products. For instance, sunflower oil and donkey feaeces are mixed with Aloe and used.

The sustainability of these elements depends on the primary industry like farming (sunflower & donkeys). Furthermore, firewood ashes used are products of old and drying trees. Thus, the sustainability of ashes depends on the continued adherence to traditional practices of vegetation conservation. The reviewed literature does not show how each herb or EVP is sourced. However, evidence from literature shows that while most plants are harvested in the bushes, preservation and their conservation is emphasized in practice through community ostracism, secrecy and restrictions. For example, only certain members of the community or family are permitted to harvest these herbs. Also, some herbs are a family secret while others are harvested in the night. The scarce the herb is, the higher level of protection with measures such as secrecy. Surprisingly, there is no evidence both in literature and the empirical study of attempts to preserve these plants or herbs by engaging in mass production. Privacy and secrecy are rather preferred as a preservation measure. It is also evident that most herbs used are scarce and need to be protected, cultivated and/or conserved for their future sustainability.

7. Dosage and contraindications

Literature revealed that there is no specific dosage and contraindications for different methods used in indigenous chicken health management. For instance, in the empirical study farmers indicated that depending on the number of chickens at home, different *Aloe* leaf sizes are cut, crushed and put in water for birds to drink. In some instances, the entire leaf is used. The dosage accuracy is further made difficult by the fact that most EVP practices are administered to the entire flock once the disease is suspected or when controlling diseases without systematical measured dose. This was also the case, with other herbs like *Moringa oleifera*, *C. papaya* (Papaya), *C. frutescens* (chillies) and other EVPs. Moreover, some medicine is secretly used or hidden from the general population due to cultural reasons, hence the dosages remain unknown. This is as well linked to maintaining the intellectual property rights of the community or knowledge holders. Farmers also claim that their EVPs are risk free and have no negative side effects to the health of animals. These results present an opportunity for further investigations on the actual recommended dosage ideal for a treating a particular ailment, mechanism of action, risks or contraindications associated with different herbs and other traditional medical practices.

8. Weakness and strengths of *ethnoveterinary practices*

The results show that majority of farmers relied on EVPs to manage poultry ailments. For example, an earlier study in the same area. A study reported that most farmers use herbs, plants and other traditional practices as EVMs for poultry in the area [14]. Also, in Zimbabwe it was found that over 95% of communal farmers do not use veterinary services but preferred indigenous knowledge systems in controlling or treating poultry ailments [30]. The high cost of drugs and services was cited as prohibitive by farmers. There are farmers who believe that veterinary health services aim to destroy livestock in the event of disease outbreaks. It is why, farmers do not seek assistance from extension services. Ethnoveterinary Practices perform well to a reasonable spectrum of common symptoms and conditions such as septicemia, diarrhea, wounds, colds, worms, and reproductive disorders. Evidently, EVPs cure several bacterial diseases like coccidiosis, mycobacteriosis, plague and a wide spectrum of coliform diseases.

The practice of EVP is popular in rural farmers and it lags in its development, commercialization and knowledge transfer. Another reason for this was secrecy of the practice and absence of information in the gray literature. The weakness of EVPs is they fail to treat and control epidemic or endemic infectious diseases. For instance, foot and mouth disease, rinderpest, anthrax, and acute life-threatening bacterial diseases. Their popularization creates diversity of habitat shocks in semi-arid woodland and savanna habitats. This chapter presents an evidence-based EVPs practices especially medicinal plants. The inventory also opens opportunities for herbs and traditional practices commercialization and opening further inroads into new poultry drugs development in managing birds' ailments. Intellectual property rights of the knowledge holders needs to be respected for them to benefit. Cultivation of species most at risk is an agri-business opportunity and a chance to know, conserve, manage and protect endangered herbs. Research on right soils and conditions for growing these important poultry herbs is needed to optimize their collection and sustainable use. It is also worth noting that EVPs are not universally recognized as a valid method for disease treatment and control. Variations occur from region to region as well as within communities. Additionally, the decision for the ailment is based on trial and error and deliberate experimentation. The results show that while there are similarities, EVPs are less systematic and formalized. There are also new opportunities for researchers to further validate, document and acknowledge EVM in South Africa and other tropical countries.

9. Conclusions

Herbs, medicinal plants and traditional practices identified control a wide spectrum of poultry diseases such as diarrhea, wounds, coccidiosis, respiratory diseases and reproductive disorders. The chapter revealed that there are a variety of herb species and other traditional practices used by farmers in indigenous village chicken disease management. It is evident that several medicinal plants are reliably and safely used to treat poultry ailments. However, the same are less effective in epidemic or endemic infectious diseases like foot and mouth disease, rinderpest, as well as anthrax. In most countries including South Africa legal registration of these botanical products is not yet a major hurdle or requirement for their promotion. Farmers, thus have incentives to commercialize or trade the knowledge on poultry health management without many challenges. The observed herbs and traditional medicines, offer viable alternative health care options that are environmentally friendly, safe and affordable for farmers. Also, these herbs could be used to produce alternative less harmful conventional medicine if further investigations such as laboratory tests are conducted.

There are still major gaps in the EVPs practices such as standardization of the practices. For example, there is no specific dosage for most ailments, chickens are treated collectively, and harmful effects or risks involved in the use of EVPs are yet to be scientifically studied. Lastly, medicinal plants are also not grown at large scale to support their sustainability rather farmers rely on their natural occurrence in the environment. Moreover, the knowledge is hidden to the few members of the community mainly household heads and knowledge holders. This means EVPs are at risk of extinction. Hence, to preserve EVPs with their beneficial health alternatives to chicken health management, their sustainability should be prioritized. This forms part of efforts of the fight against climate change and negative effects of conventional medicines to the environment and human health. Nonetheless, IP rights must be observed for communities and knowledge holders to benefit from the commercialization of the plants, as custodians of the indigenous knowledge.

Acknowledgements

Acknowledgements are given to the University of Venda Research and Publication Committee (Project Number SARDF/15/IRD/10/0502) for the financial support, smallholder farmers in Vhembe district, Department of Agriculture and Rural Development, village coordinators, and research assistants.

Conflict of interest

The authors declare no conflict of interest.

Author details

Wiseman Ndlovu[1], Nyambeni Ronald Mudimeli[1], Marizvikuru Mwale[1*],
Tshianeo Mellda Ndou[3], Ola Segun Obadire[2] and Joseph Francis[1]

1 Institute for Rural Development, University of Venda, Thohoyandou, South Africa

2 Directorate of International Relations and Partnerships, University of Venda, Thohoyandou, South Africa

3 Department of Environment Sciences, University of Venda, Thohoyandou, South Africa

*Address all correspondence to: marizvikuru.manjoro@univen.ac.za

References

[1] Alves R, Alves HN. The faunal drugstore: Animal-based remedies used in traditional medicines in Latin America. Journal of Ethnobiology and Ethnomedicine. 2011;**7**(1):1-43

[2] Mafimisebi TE, Oguntade AE, Fajemisin AN, Aiyelari OP. Local knowledge and socio-economic determinants of traditional medicines' utilization in livestock health management in Southwest Nigeria. Journal of Ethnobiology and Ethnomedicine. 2012;**8**(1):1-9

[3] Anand U, Jacobo-Herrera N, Altemimi A, Lakhssassi N. A comprehensive review on medicinal plants as antimicrobial therapeutics: Potential avenues of biocompatible drug discovery. Metabolites. 2019;**9**(11):258

[4] Japheth PK, Kumaresan A. Usage of herbs and spices in ethno-veterinary practice. Journal of Indian Veterinary Association, Kerala (JIVA). 2020;**18**(1): 18-34

[5] Sonaiya EB. Towards Sustainable Poultry Production in Africa. Strategies for Sustainable Animal Agriculture in Developing Countries. In: Proceedings of the FAO Expert Consultation. Rome, Italy: Food and Agriculture Organisation of the United Nations; 1990

[6] Spradbrow PB. Newcastle disease in village chickens. Poultry Science Review. 1993;**5**:57-96

[7] Mack S, Hoffmann D, Otte J. The contribution of poultry to rural development. World's Poultry Science Journal. 2005;**61**:7-14

[8] Muhammad N, Ali N, Uddin N. Ethno-veterinary practices used for treatment of various ailments in hilly areas of Melagah valley district swat KPK, Pakistan. International Journal of Botany Studies. 2019;**4**(3):171-179

[9] Mathias-Mundy E, McCorkle CM. Ethno-veterinary medicine and development: A review of the literature. In: Warren DM, Slikkerveer LJ, Brokensha D, editors. The Cultural Dimension of Development: Indigenous Knowledge Systems. London, UK: Intermediate Technology Publications. pp. 488-498

[10] McCorkle CM, Mathias-Mundy E. Ethno-veterinary medicine in Africa. Journal of the International African Institute (London). 1992;**62**(1):59-93

[11] Bakare AG, Shah S, Bautista-Jimenez V, Bhat JA, Dayal SR, Madzimure J. Potential of ethno-veterinary medicine in animal health care practices in the South Pacific Island countries: A review. Tropical Animal Health and Production. 2020;**52**(5):2193-2203

[12] Rafique Khan SM, Akhter T, Hussain M. Ethno-veterinary practice for the treatment of animal diseases in Neelum Valley, Kashmir Himalaya, Pakistan. PLoS one. 2021;**16**(4): e0250114

[13] Christy CC. Interlinks of Local Knowledge and Community in Challenging Poultry Health in Rwanda. Master Thesis. State College, PA, United States: The Pennsylvania State University, The Graduate School, College of Agricultural Sciences; 2018

[14] Ndlovu W, Mwale M, Iwara IO, Kabiti HM, Obadire OS, Francis J. Profiling village chickens predators, parasites and medicinal plants used to control the parasites. Brazilian Journal of Poultry Science. 2021;**23**:1-9

[15] Daodu OB, Jegede HO, Aiyedun JO, Oludairo OO, Olorunshola ID, Daodu OC, et al. Surveillance for avian influenza virus in captive wild birds and indigenous chickens in Nigeria. Tropical Animal Health and Production. 2020; **52**(5):2387-2393

[16] Nkonki-Mandleni B, Ogunkoya FT, Omotayo AO. Socioeconomic factors influencing livestock production among smallholder farmers in the free state province of south Africa. International Journal of Entrepreneurship. 2019;**23**(1): 1-17

[17] Mushi EZ, Binta MG, Chabo RG, Ndebele RT, Ramathodi T. Diseases and management of indigenous chickens in Oodi, Kgatleng, Botswana. World's Poultry Science Journal. 2000;**56**(2): 153-157

[18] Güler O, Polat R, Karaköse M, Çakılcıoğlu U, Akbulut S. An ethnoveterinary study on plants used for the treatment of livestock diseases in the province of Giresun (Turkey). South African Journal of Botany. 2021;**142**: 53-62

[19] Rates SMK. Plants as source of drugs. Toxicon. 2001;**39**(5):603-613

[20] Chah KF, Gómez-Sanz E, Nwanta JA, Asadu B, Agbo IC, Lozano C, et al. Methicillin-resistant coagulase-negative staphylococci from healthy dogs in Nsukka, Nigeria. Brazilian Journal of Microbiology. 2014;**45**: 215-220

[21] Matzigkeit U. Natural veterinary medicine: Ectoparasites in the tropics and subtropics. Tropical Agroecology (Germany, F.R.). 1990;**6**(6):183

[22] Shen S, Qian J, Ren J. Ethnoveterinary plant remedies used by Nu people in NW Yunnan of China. Journal of Ethnobiology and Ethnomedicine. 2010;**6**(1):1-10

[23] Braa K, Vidgen R. Interpretation, intervention, and reduction in the organizational laboratory: A framework for in-context information system research. Accounting, Management and Information Technologies. 1999;**9**(1): 25-47

[24] Stock PG, Mukhtar R, Ghersin H, Stover Fiscalini A, Esserman L. Pragmatic trials and approaches to transforming care. In: Clinical Trials. Cham, Switzerland: Springer; 2020. pp. 59-76

[25] Asmara IY, Garnida D, Sulisytati M, Tejaningsih S, Partasasmita R. Ethnoveterinary medicine and health management of Pelung Chicken in West Java, Indonesia. Biodiversitas Journal of Biological Diversity. 2018;**19**(4): 1502-1508

[26] Bizimana N. Traditional veterinary practice in Africa. In: Schriftreihe der GTZ, No 243. Eschborn, Germany; 1994

[27] Gumbochuma G, Hamandishe VR, Nyahangare ET, Imbayarwo-Chikosi VE, Ncube S. Ethno veterinary practices for poultry and cattle in Zimbabwe: A case study of Takavarasha village. Scientific Journal of Animal Science. 2013;**12**: 355-359

[28] Hassen A, Muche M, Muasya AM, Tsegay BA. Exploration of traditional plant-based medicines used for livestock ailments in northeastern Ethiopia. South African Journal of Botany. 2022;**146**: 230-242

[29] Marandure T. Concepts and key issues of ethnoveterinary medicine in Africa: A review of its application in Zimbabwe. African Journal of

Agricultural Research. 2016;**11**(20): 1836-1841

[30] Matekaire T, Bwakura TM. Ethnoveterinary medicine: A potential alternative to orthodox animal health delivery in Zimbabwe. International Journal of Applied Research in Veterinary Medicine. 2004;**2**(4):269-273

[31] Sunder J, Sujatha T, Kundu A, Kundu MS. Medicinal plant and ethnoveterinary practices used in South and North Andaman. Journal of the Andaman Science Association. 2014; **19**(1):105-115

[32] Waihenya RK, Mtambo MMA, Nkwengulila G. Evaluation of the efficacy of the crude extract of the crude extract of Aloe secundiflora in chickens experimentally infected with Newcastle disease virus Authors. Journal of Ethnopharmacology. 2002;**79**(3): 299-304

[33] Wodegebriel YW, Abebe BF, Tamir A. Medicinal plants used by farmers for treatment of major diseases of chicken in South Wollo zone, Amhara region, Ethiopia. International Journal of Advanced Research in Biological Sciences. 2018;**5**:45-58. Available at: https://github.com/citation-style-language/styles/blob/master/vancouver-brackets.csl

Chapter 9

Medicinal Plants Used by the Tay Ethnic Group, Thai Nguyen Province, Vietnam

Le Thi Thanh Huong, Nguyen Phu Hung, Hosakatte Niranjana Murthy, Do Van Hai and Nguyen Trung Thanh

Abstract

An ethnobotanical study of medicinal plants used by the Tay ethnic group in Thai Nguyen province, Vietnam has been carried out in the present study, especially in the region of Định Hoá, Phú Lương, and Võ Nhai districts. The ethnobotanical survey was conducted between 2018 and 2021 and a catalog of the medicinal plant used by the Tay ethnic group is prepared. The results of the current survey revealed that the plants used by Tay ethnic group consist of 321 species belonging to 253 genera and 103 botanical families. Majority of the plants belonging the family Euphorbiaceae (20 species), Asteraceae (19 species), Acanthaceae and Rutaceae (13 species each), Fabaceae (12 species), and Poaceae (11 species). Leaves were the most frequently used plant part (48.0%) in the preparation of medicines. The most frequent preparation method was decoction (47.7%), followed by crushing (29.9%), sauna (18.0), pickle wine (11.8%), and raw (5.6%). The major plant used by Tay ethnic people were *Schefflera heptaphylla* (L.) Frodin and *Plantago major* L., (2); *Elephantopus scaber* L. and *Achyranthes aspera* L.; *Streblus asper* Lour. We also carried out screening of some of the medicinal plant extracts for their biological activities especially the inhibition of cancer cell lines.

Keywords: medicinal plants, Tay ethnic group, traditional knowledge, biological activities, conservation, Thai Nguyen

1. Introduction

Plant resources have a long history of being used as medicinal materials. It is often cited that 80% of the world's population still relies on traditional medicines to meet their primary health care needs [1] and nearly 25% of modern medicines are derived from nature, many of which were derived from traditional uses [2]. The use of traditional medicines is generally affected by accessibility, availability, and acceptability of health care services. Especially, in remote areas of developing countries, medicinal plants may form the only available source of health care.

Vietnam possesses a vast wealth of historical, cultural, and natural richness that includes big deltas, huge limestone towers, beautiful dunes, lush green forests, and grasslands. The richness can also be seen in the diversity of flora, which is evident with an estimated number of 13,747 vascular plant species [3]. To preserve the rich biodiversity of Vietnam and their sustainable development, the government has demarcated 164 special use forest areas including 30 National Parks, 58 Natural Reserves, 11 Species Conservation Areas, 45 Forest Landscape Protection and 20 Experimental Forests of Scientific Research [3].

The use of traditional medicine in Vietnam has a vibrant history spanning thousands of years. Today, around 75% of Vietnamese people use traditional medicine as their primary source of treatment to meet their health care needs. These users mostly include inhabitants of rural or mountainous areas, which have less accessibility to hospitals or community health care centers [4].

The Tay ethnic people are one of the 54 officially recognized ethnic minorities of Vietnam, whose population is around 150,404 people, accounting for 11.69% of the Thai Nguyen province's population. They are residing mainly in areas such as districts (Định Hoá, Phú Lương, Võ Nhai) (**Figure 1**, [5]). The people belonging to the Tay ethnic group are dependent on forest resources such as wood and non-timber forest products. Their major livelihood activities include the collection of forest products such as wild honey, bamboo shoots, animals, and mushrooms for consumption [6].

Contrary to the growing demand for medicinal plants all over the world, traditional knowledge is declining rapidly, especially in developing countries. Considering the vast floristic wealth of the nature reserve and the rich knowledge of the local community, an urgent need was felt to take over this work, which could help the researchers, forest officials as well as the future generation people involved in ethnobotany research. It is worth mentioning that the knowledge of Tay ethnic people about medicinal plants is vast but poorly documented. Therefore, we were interested in

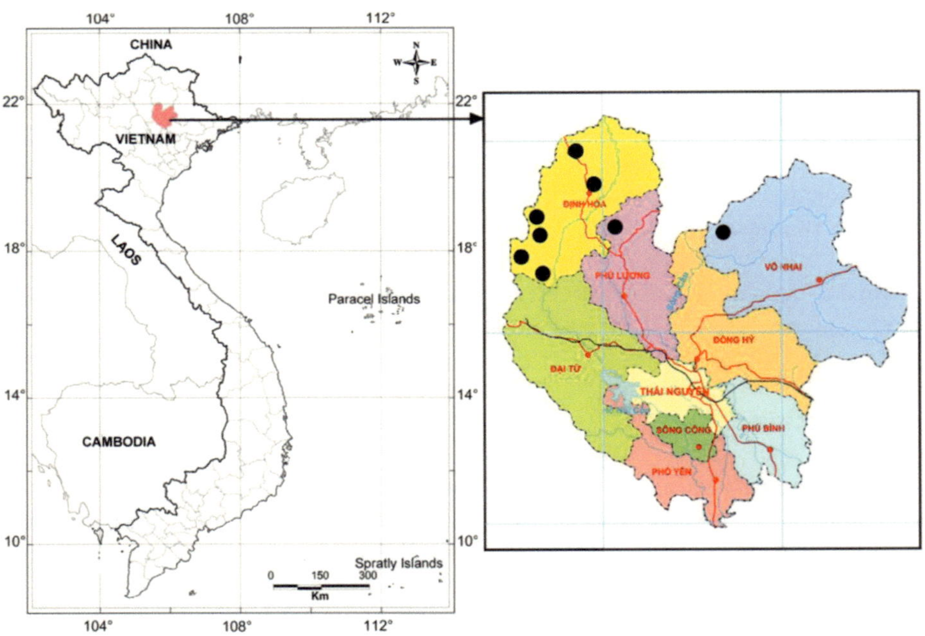

Figure 1.
Studying locations (●).

introducing medicinal plants, medicinal uses, and the experience of recognizing and collecting medicinal plants of the Tay people. Besides, also mentioned some experimental results proving the anti-cancer ability of some herbal species that have been used by the Tay people to treat diseases. Finally, conservation measures to preserve the medicinal plant resources of the Tay people in Thai Nguyen province.

2. General data on medicinal species

In this study, all investigated species were as the scientific names, Vietnamese name, name of Tay ethnic group, parts used, tree-forms, and disease treated (List of medicinal plants of Tay ethnic group in Thai Nguyen province do not show).

During (2018–2021), the result of research on medicinal plants of the Tay ethnic group in Thai Nguyen province obtained 321 species of medicinal plants belonging to 253 genera and 103 families of 3 divisions of vascular plants in Vietnam (**Table 1**, [6]).

Among these, the most diverse families (over 10 species) that the Tay people in Thai Nguyen province use as medicine are the as below: 20 species belonging to Euphorbiaceae, 19 species to Asteraceae, 13 species to Acanthaceae and Rutaceae respectively, 12 species to Fabaceae and 11 species to Poaceae (**Figure 2**). These families have been widely used in the Indo-Burma region for their medicinal properties [7–13].

3. Indigenous knowledge capital in the use of medicinal plants of the Tay ethnic group in Thai Nguyen province

Knowledge of medicinal plants depends upon ecological diversity along with differences in languages and cultures of ethnic communities. The knowledge of the use of plants varies within each ethnic group and between ethnic groups. It is of great significance to learn and research knowledge of using traditional medicinal plants to provide a database for science. Knowledge of using medicinal plants is very diverse, the same species has many different uses. Knowledge of using medicinal plants is often supplemented through experiences from medical practice, as well as from failures in the process of using medicinal plants. The knowledge used is associated with the culture, beliefs, and customs of each ethnic group and each locality.

3.1 Experience in identifying and collecting medicinal plants

Traditional knowledge of plant names and uses depends on the experience of local people. The folk names of plants are the source of the diversity of traditional

Division	**Family**		**Genus**		**Species**	
	Total	**%**	**Total**	**%**	**Total**	**%**
Polypodiophyta	9	8,8	10	3,9	11	3,5
Pinophyta	1	0,9	1	0,4	2	0,6
Magnoliophyta	93	90,3	242	95,7	308	95,9
Total	**103**	**100**	**253**	**100**	**321**	**100**

Table 1.
Total of medicinal plants used by Tay ethnic group in Thai Nguyen province.

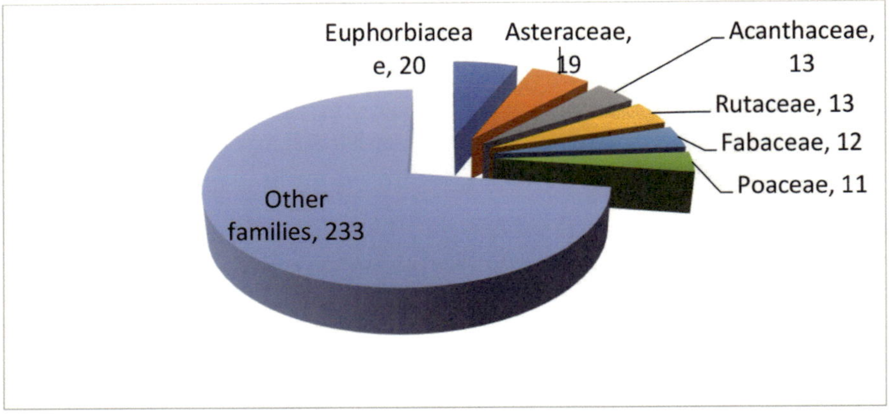

Figure 2.
Number of plant species by most representative family used for medicinal purposes in the study area.

knowledge. In addition, the system of folk names and ways of recognizing plants is passed down from generation to generation in the community.

Through research and interviews with people who have experience in using medicinal plants, it was found that the Tay people in Thai Nguyen province know how to use many types of medicinal plants. Most of the families in the Tay ethnic community know some medicine to cure some common diseases such as fever, headache, and stomachache, and are famous for treating stomach ailments, nervous breakdowns, and fractures. Depending on the type of disease, one tree or several trees can be used. The Tay people have many simple but effective remedies. In general, the use of plants to make medicine is very diverse and depends on each remedy as well as the treatment experience of the physician.

The Tay people have a unique way of naming medicinal plants, the names of medicinal plants are often based on the shape and characteristics of parts of the plant such as leaves, stems, roots, flowers, and fruits, which have similar characteristics to the shape, characteristics of a certain subspecies to name. Or the Tay people have many different ways of recognizing medicinal plants, which can be based on the plant's life form, such as "thẩu" is used to indicate the life form of climb; "nhả" refers to a life form that is mainly herbaceous, "khẩu" refers to the habitat of medicinal plants in the forest. In addition, based on the color of the parts of the tree to name them: "khảo" means "white"; "đăm" means "black"; "lưởng" means "gold"; "đẻng" means "red". This is a very interesting explanation for the naming of medicinal plants of the Tay people, helping the Tay people remember medicinal plants more easily, avoid confusion and pass it on to the next generation more effectively.

3.2 Plants parts used

Research on the used parts of medicinal plants not only shows the richness and diversity in the healing power of those parts but also has great conservation significance, at the same time, the study of medicinal plant parts partly assesses the sustainability of the exploitation and use of medicinal plant resources in ethnic minority communities. The results of the parts used as medicine according to the experience of the Tay ethnic group in Thai Nguyen province are shown in **Figure 3**, [6].

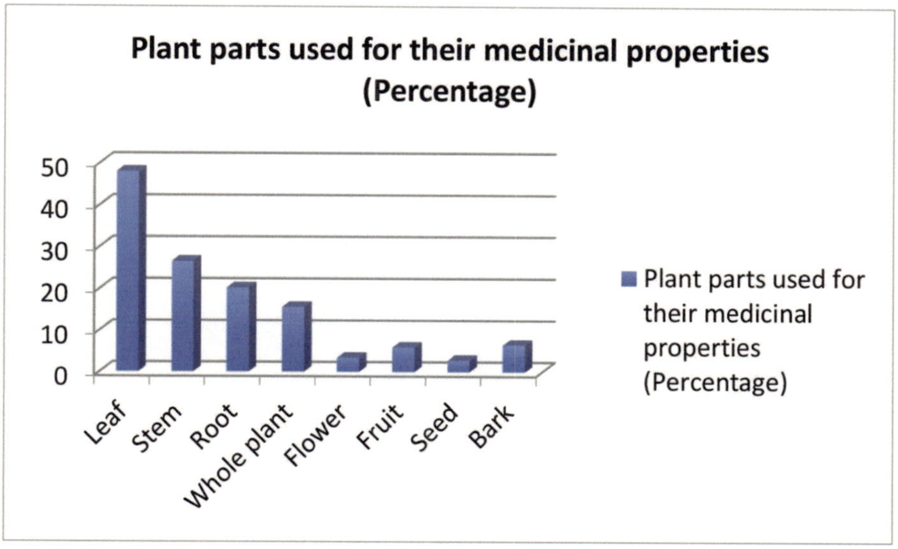

Figure 3.
Plant parts used for their medicinal properties (Percentage).

The research results on the frequency of using plant parts for healing show that leaves and stems are two parts that are used more than other parts such as flowers, fruits, seeds, roots, bark, and sap. The leaf represents the most used plant part (48.0%), followed by stem (26.5%), root (20.2%), whole plant (15.6%), flower (3.4%), fruit (5.9%), seed (2.8%), and bark (6.5%). This can be due to easy accessibility and availability of leaves among other plant parts. The use of leaves for medicinal purposes is preferred by most ethnobotanical studies because it is less likely to affect the survival of the plant as compared to roots [14–16]. Similar results were also shown in the study on medicinal plants of the Co Tu ethnic group in the buffer zone of Bach Ma National Park [17]. Many studies conducted around the world also show that leaves are used more than other parts of the plant [18–20]. The use of medicinal leaves reduces the level of threat to medicinal plants or helps in the sustainable harvesting of medicinal plants. Further, it has been reported that roots and bark are not sustainable for the development of traditional medicine [21].

Five different modes of medicine preparation were documented. Decoction (47.7%) was the most frequently quoted mode of preparation (**Figure 4**, [6]), followed by crushing (29.9%), sauna (18.0), pickle wine (11.8%), and raw (5.6%). It was also found that for some plants, different modes of preparation were used to treat different diseases. For example, leaves of *Glycosmis parviflora* (Sims) Little were prepared as a decoction for treatment of rheumatism and bone pain cure which may also be prepared as a sauna for treatment of edema.

3.3 Combination of medicinal plants

Medicinal plants make important contributions to the health care system of local communities. The collected ethnobotanical data is a valuable source for the development of new drugs in the future. The purpose of research on the conservation of ethnic medicinal plants is not only towards the conservation of medicinal plant genetic resources but also to preserve and promote the experience and knowledge of ethnic groups in the use and development of medicines.

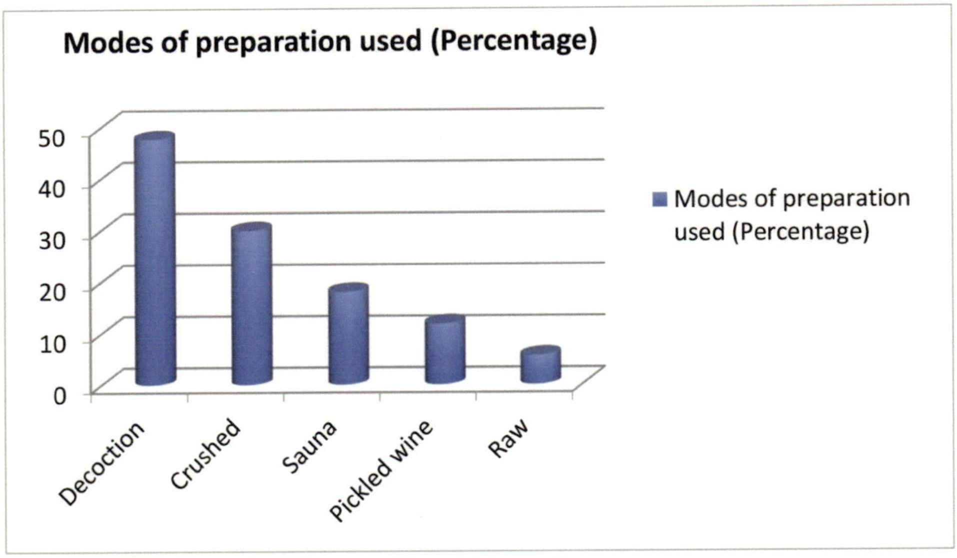

Figure 4.
Modes of preparation used (Percentage).

The Tay ethnic people in Thai Nguyen province combined some species to treat a few diseases (**Table 2**, [6]). For example, a decoction of *Abutilon indicum* (L.) Sweet (leaf), *Trevesia palmata* (Roxb. ex Lindl.) Visan. (stem), *Pandanus tonkinensis* Martelli ex. Stone (fruit), *Eclipta prostrata* L. (stem, leaf), *Schefflera heptaphylla* (L.) Frodin (root), is used to treat kidney disease. Similarly, a decoction of *Schefflera heptaphylla* (L.) Frodin (root), *Argyreia acuta* Lour. (stem and leaf), *Sigesbeckia orientalis* L. (whole plant) and *Schefflera venulosa* (Wight & Arn.) Harms in Engl. & Prantl (root) is used to treat neurological, and cerebrovascular stroke. The plants which were used more than once by Tay ethnic people to treat several diseases are *Schefflera heptaphylla* (L.) Frodin, *Plantago major* L., (2); *Elephantopus scaber* L., *Achyranthes aspera* L., (3); *Streblus asper* Lour. (4).

R = root; S = stems; W = whole plant; L = leaf; F = fruit; B = bark; RF = rind of fruit.

3.4 Rare plants conservation

Out of 321 plant species studied from this region, three plant species have been listed in the IUCN Red list [22], *Cycas balansae* Warb. as Near Threatened (NT), *Cycas bifida* (Thiselton - Dyer) K. D. Hill as Vulnerable (VU) and *Aquilaria crassna* Pierre ex Lecomte as Critically Endangered (CR). That species also is listed by the Vietnam Red book as *C. balansae* Warb. as Vulnerable (VU), *C. bifida* (Thiselton - Dyer) K. D. Hill as Vulnerable (VU), and *A. crassna* Pierre ex Lecomte as Endangered (EN) [22] and another species were listed by the Vietnam Red book and the Decree 06/2019/ND-CP of the Government of Vietnam [23, 24] (**Table 3**, [6, 22–24]).

C. balansae Warb. was distributed in Vietnam and Lao, south of China, and north of Thailand [25]. Plants grow under the forest canopy, on limestone mountains, at an altitude of about 100–500 m. Beautiful tree planted as an ornamental [26]. The studies suggest small population sizes of cycads brought about by fragmentation of their habitats, over-exploitation, and the increasing number of inbred individuals within populations [27].

Scientific name (parts used)	Preparation method	Medicinal use
Clerodendrum japonicum (Thunb.) Sweet (R, S) + *Clerodendrum chinense* (Osbeck) Mabb. (R, S) + *Psidium guajava* L. (L, B) + *Elephantopus scaber* L. (R) + *Achyranthes aspera* L. (R) + *Curcuma longa* L. (S)	Decoction/oral	Intestinal diseases
Ardisia gigantifolia Stapf. (L) + *Croton tonkinensis* Gagnep. (S, L) + *Ficus tinctoria* ssp. *gibbosa* (L) + *Hedyotis capitellata* Wall. ex G. Don (S)	Decoction/oral	Epigastric disease
Abutilon indicum (L.) Sweet (L) + *Trevesia palmata* (Roxb. ex Lindl.) Visan. (S) + *Pandanus tonkinensis* Martelli ex. Stone (F) + *Eclipta prostrata* L. (S, L) + *Schefflera heptaphylla* (L.) Frodin (R)	Decoction/oral	Kidney disease
Streblus asper Lour. (L) + *Costus speciosus* (Koenig) Smith (S, L) + *Plantago major* L. (W) + *A. aspera* L. (S, L) + *Imperata cylindrica* (L.) Beauv. (R)	Decoction/oral	Urinary tract infections
Glycosmis parviflora (Sims) Little (R) + *Sauropus androgynus* (L.) Merr. (L) + *Streblus asper* Lour. (R) + *Melastoma sanguineum* Sims (R) + *Chrysopogon aciculatus* (Retz.) Trin. (R)	Decoction/oral	White discharge in women
Oroxylum indicum (L.) Kurz (B) + *Averrhoa carambola* L. (L) + *Pistia stratiotes* L. (W)	Boil/bath	Skin rash and itching
Schefflera heptaphylla (L.) Frodin (R) + *Argyreia acuta* Lour. (L, S) + *Sigesbeckia orientalis* L. (W) + *Schefflera venulosa* (Wight & Arn.) Harms in Engl.&Prantl (R)	Decoction/oral	Neurological - cerebrovascular stroke
Streptocaulon juventas (Lour.) Merr. (S) + *Tinospora sinensis* (Lour.) Merr. (L, S) + *Piper lolot* C. DC. (S) + *Mimosa pudica* L. (R)	Decoction/oral	Joint pain
Heliciopsis lobata (Merr.) Sleum. (R) + *Glochidion eriocarpum* Champ. (R) + *Streblus asper* Lour. (R) + *E. scaber* L. (R)	Decoction/oral	Growth retardation in children
E. scaber L. (R) + *Scoparia dulcis* L. (W) + *P. major* L. (R) + *Cuscuta australis* R. Br. (S) + *Adenosma caeruleum* R. Br. (S, L)	Decoction/oral	Hepatitis
Aglaia duperreana Pierre (F) + *Raphanus sativus* L. (S) + *Polyscias fruticosa* (L.) Harms (R, L) + *Citrus nobilis* Lour. (RF)	Decoction/oral	Bronchitis
Citrus medica L. (R) + *Streblus asper* Lour. (R) + *A. aspera* L. (R) + *Clausena dimidiata* Tanaka (R)	Boil/ suck	Gingivitis
Morus alba L. (R, B) + *Ageratum conyzoides* L. (L) + *Acorus gramineus* Soland. (R)	Boil/sauna	Sinusitis

Table 2.
List of medicinal plant combinations used by Tay ethnic people.

C. bifida (Thiselton - Dyer) K. D. Hill is distributed in Vietnam, China (southern Guangxi and eastern Yunnan provinces), Southeast Asia, and Australia. The number of mature individuals ranges from 10.000 to 12.000 and the altitude range is 100 to 300 meters above sea level. The sap of cycad treats ulcers, but the megasporophyll of cycad is known to treat pain relief [28]. The Tay people use the leaf of this species to treat bone marrow disease.

Scientific name (Vietnamese name)	Family	Situation		
		IUCN Red List	VNRB	De/06/2019
Cycas balansae Warb. (Tuê ba lăng sa)	Cycadaceae	NT	VU	IIA
Cycas bifida (Thiselton - Dyer) K. D. Hill (Tuê xẻ đôi)	Cycadaceae	VU	VU	IIA
Aquilaria crassna Pierre ex Lecomte (Trâm)	Thymelaeaceae	CR	EN	
Canarium tramdenum Dai ex Yakovl. (Trám đen)	Burseraceae		VU	
Disporopsis longifolia Craib (Hoàng tinh hoa trăng)	Convallariaceae		VU	IIA
Stephania kwangsiensis H. S. Lo (Bình vôi quảng tây)	Menispermaceae			IIA
Fibraurea tinctoria Lour. (Hoàng đăng)	Menispermaceae			IIA
Melientha suavis Pierre (Rau săng)	Opiliaceae		VU	
Anoectochilus setaceus Blume (Kim tuyên tơ)	Orchidaceae		EN	IA
Paris hainanensis Merr. (Trọng lâu hải nam)	Trilliaceae			IIA

Table 3.
List of rare medicinal plants for conservation.

A. crassna Pierre ex Lecomte is endemic to the Indochina region and is known to be used in diverse Southeast Asian traditional medicine systems to treat infectious and inflammatory diseases, arthritis, and cardiac disorders [29]. The Tay people use the leaf of this species to treat cure colds and abdominal pain. According to the Dictionary of Vietnamese Medicinal Plants, *A. crassna* Pierre ex Lecomte has a beneficial effect on digestive diseases, anti-diarrhea, anti-emetic and antipyretic [27]. In the research Ethnobotanical study on medicinal plants used by local Van Kieu ethnic people of Bac Huong Hoa nature reserve, Vietnam reported the Van Kieu people use the root of this species to treat fever and abdominal pain [30]. Studies on *A. crassna* Pierre ex Lecomte revealed that the extracts from leaves and stems possess antioxidant, antimicrobial, cytotoxic, antipyretic, analgesic, antiischemic, laxative, and digestive properties [31–35].

4. Screening of medicinal plants for biological activities

From the collected data on the use of medicinal plants according to the traditional experience of the Tay ethnic people in Thai Nguyen province, the study on extracts of some herbal species *Ardisia gigantifolia* Stapf., *Excoecaria cochinchinensis* Lour., and *Heliciopsis lobata* (Merr.) Sleum. was conducted ability to inhibit cancer cells.

MTT assay (3-(4,5-dimethylthiazol-2-yl)-2,5-diphenyltetrazolium bromide) was used to check the viability of certain cancer cell lines using the above-listed plant extract. It was shown that the ethanol extract from the leaves of *Ardisia gigantifolia* Stapf. was able to effectively inhibit the proliferation of all three AGS, MKN45, and MKN74 gastric cancer cell lines with IC50 values ranging from 50 to 140 μg/mL. Meanwhile, ethanol extract of *Excoecaria cochinchinensis* Lour. was also shown to inhibit the

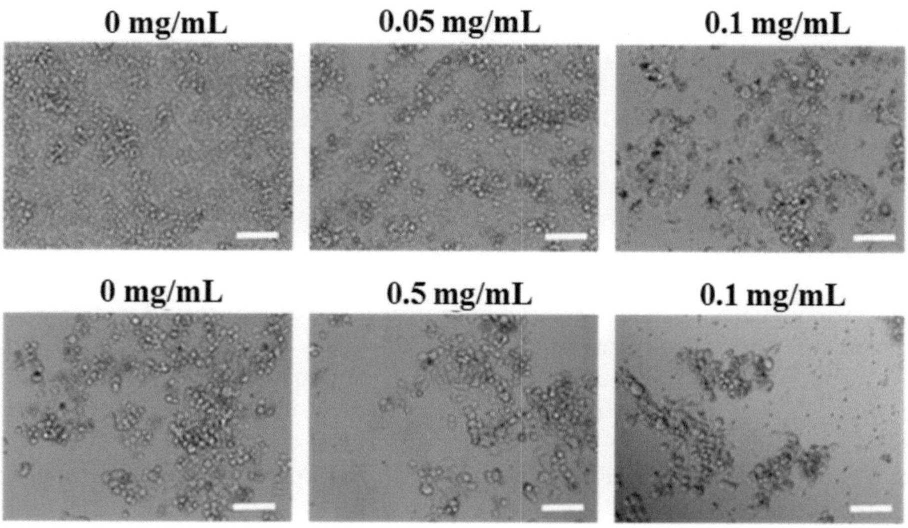

Figure 5.
Effect of Excoecaria cochinchinensis Lour. extracts on MKN45 cell proliferation. Cells were treated with extracts at different concentrations from 0.05 to 1 mg/mL. The control is extract - untreated cells (0 mg/mL): Cell image taken under an inverted microscope, 200X magnification. Scale: 50 µm.

proliferation of gastric cancer cell line MKN45 with IC50 = 70 µg/mL (**Figure 5**, [36]). Also, by MTT screening on HepG2 liver cancer cells, it was shown that the methanol extract of *Heliciopsis lobata* (Merr.) Sleum. plant effectively inhibited cell proliferation after 48 h of treatment with the extract, with IC50 value = 84 µg/mL [37].

Research on the toxicological test of new triterpenoid saponins of *Ardisia gigantifolia* Stapf., results showed that the compound triterpenoid saponin from *Ardisia gigantifolia* Stapf. was able to inhibit the growth of liver cancer cell lines and Hela cells with IC50 values determined ranging from 1.9 to 4.8 µM [38]. A later study, also showed that triterpenoid saponin AG8, an analyzed compound from *Ardisia gigantifolia* Stapf., is capable of the growth mode of various cancer cell lines such as MDA-MB-231, BT-549, and MDA-MB-157 depending on the concentration in the culture medium [39].

The extract from *Excoecaria cochinchinensis* Lour. was determined to inhibit the growth of lung cancer cell lines A549, colorectal cancer cell line Col2, gastric cancer cell line SNU638 with IC50 in the range of 0.25–0.46 µg/mL [40]. The results of the study show that the ethanol extract from *Excoecaria agallocha* L. - a species of the same genus as *Excoecaria cochinchinensis* Lour. can inhibit the growth of breast cancer cell line MCF-7 with IC50 value is 56.5 µg/mL [41].

Invasion is the initiating form of cancer cells during metastasis. Cancer cells have a stronger ability to migrate than normal cells, giving them the ability to invade surrounding tissues and metastasize distantly in the body. Cell migration is indicated by the ability to modify the cell membrane, giving the cell the ability to shift positions. Currently developed anti-cancer drugs are mostly able to attack the ability of cells to migrate to minimize the possibility of spreading to surrounding tissues. One of the effects of herbs on cancer cells of particular interest is their ability to inhibit the spread of several different types of cancer. By analysis of cell migration, it was shown that ethanol extracts of some herbal species significantly reduced the invasion of cancer cells.

This study determined that the extract from the leaves of *Excoecaria cochinchinensis* Lour. was able to inhibit the translocation or migration activity of MKN45 gastric cancer cells (**Figure 6**, [36]). MKN45 cells were treated with the extract for 48 h at concentrations of 0.05 mg/mL; 0.2 mg/mL and 1 mg/mL for 48 h to evaluate its effect on cell migration. The analysis results (**Figure 6**) showed that the extract had a clear effect on cell migration. The ability of cells to migrate into the boundary region was reduced immediately after treatment with low concentrations (0.05 mg/mL), at this concentration, the migration level of cells was determined to be only 81.5 ± 5.3% compared to the control (100%). At higher concentrations (0.2 mg/mL), migration was only approximately 50% of the control (0 mg/mL). The cells observed were mostly dead and completely lost their ability to migrate.

Extracts from *Excoecaria cochinchinensis* Lour. contain many tepotinib compounds. Tepotinib has been shown to inhibit the migration of various gastric cancer cell lines (MKN45, Hs746T, SNU638) [42]. For the first time in this study, we have demonstrated that the extract from *Excoecaria cochinchinensis* Lour. can inhibit the migration of gastric cancer cell line MKN45.

Apoptosis is programmed cell death, and plays an important role in the regulation of the cell life cycle, the balance between living and dead cells, and the prevention of cancer development. Apoptosis offers an important implication in the development of anticancer therapies. The analysis of cell nucleus morphology by nuclear staining method with DAPI (4′,6-diamidino-2-phenylindole) dye showed that herbal extracts increased the number of cells with apoptosis karyotype. The percentage of apoptotic cells was also determined by Flow cytometry. This has shown a potential to kill cancer cells of extracts from some herbal species.

The results of karyotype analysis (**Figure 7A**, [37]) showed that the leaf extract of *Heliciopsis lobata* (Merr.) Sleum. enhanced the appearance of cells with a typical karyotype of apoptosis. The cells after treatment with the extract were analyzed by Flow cytometry to determine the percentage of cells with apoptosis (**Figure 7B**, [37]). At low concentrations (0.1 mg/mL), the extract produced no significant difference in the rate of apoptosis compared with the control in either HepG2 cell line. However, at concentrations of 0.5 mg/mL or more, the increase in the percentage of apoptosis

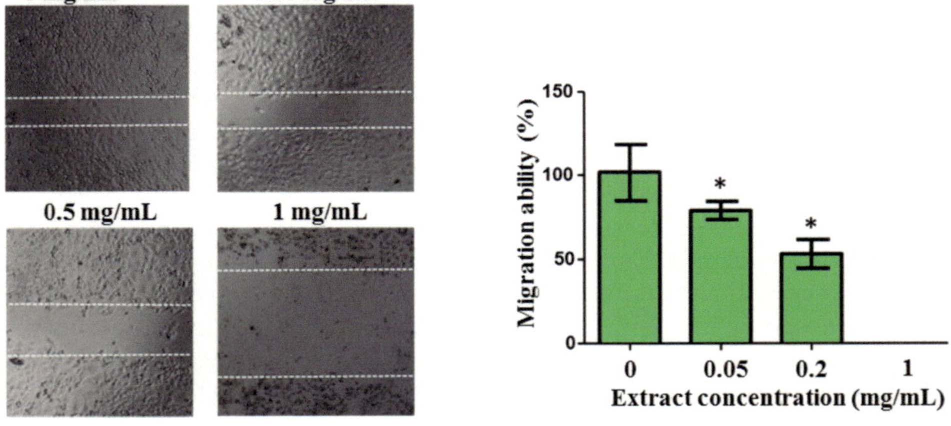

Figure 6.
Effect of Excoecaria cochinchinensis Lour. extracts on MKN45 cell migration. Cells were treated with extracts at different concentrations from 0.05 to 1 mg/mL. The control was cells that were not treated with the extract (0 mg/mL). The image was taken under an inverted microscope, at a magnification of 200X.

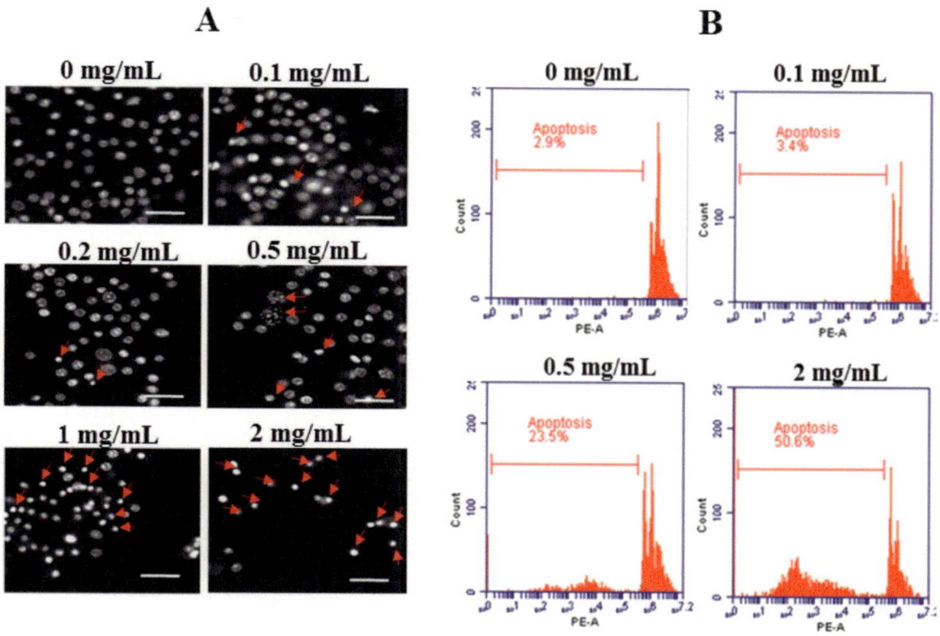

Figure 7.
Effect of Heliciopsis lobata (Merr.) Sleum. extracts on karyotype (A) and apoptosis (B) of HepG2 liver cancer cells. (A) Cells were treated with extracts at different concentrations for 48 h, followed by cell nuclei stained with DAPI dye, observed at 200X magnification, scale: 50 µm. (B) Cells after treatment with the extract were analyzed by Flow cytometry to determine the percentage of apoptosis cells.

cells was different from that of the control. In the HepG2 cell line, the rate of apoptosis induced when treated with the extract at a concentration of 0.5 mg/mL was 22.7 ± 2.7%, compared with the control was 2.5 ± 1.8%. Notably, at a high concentration (2 mg/mL), the methanol extract from the leaves of the *Heliciopsis lobata* (Merr.) Sleum. plant markedly induced apoptosis in the HepG2 cell line (50.5 ± 3.1%).

The composition of *Heliciopsis lobata* (Merr.) Sleum. has been identified to include many compounds, including myricetin, which has a significant ability to inhibit the growth of many different cancer cell lines, including cancer liver through its potentiating effect of apoptosis [43]. The research determined the inhibitory effect on HepG2 liver cancer cell proliferation of extracts from *Heliciopsis lobata* (Merr.) Sleum. through enhanced apoptosis [44]. Another study determined that an ethanol extract from *Excoecaria agallocha* L. was able to inhibit the growth of the breast cancer cell line MCF-7 by promoting the cancer cells to enter the apoptosis pathway [41].

Regulation of the cell division cycle is the way cells ensure division and maintenance of growth and development in the body, and it is strictly controlled by a series of different genes. In cancer cells, changes in genes caused by mutations can lead to changes in the cell cycle and are strongly associated with excessive proliferation compared to normal cells. Therefore, stopping the cell cycle is the anti-cancer approach of many current chemotherapy therapies. Typically, paclitaxel is an anti-cancer drug used in the treatment of cancer that currently inhibits cell division, stopping the cell cycle in the division phase (G2/M) through the mechanism of action on the control point of the mitotic cycle. Stopping the division cycle at this phase will prevent centromeric division between sister chromatids and lead to inhibition of the splitting of the mother cell into two daughter cells.

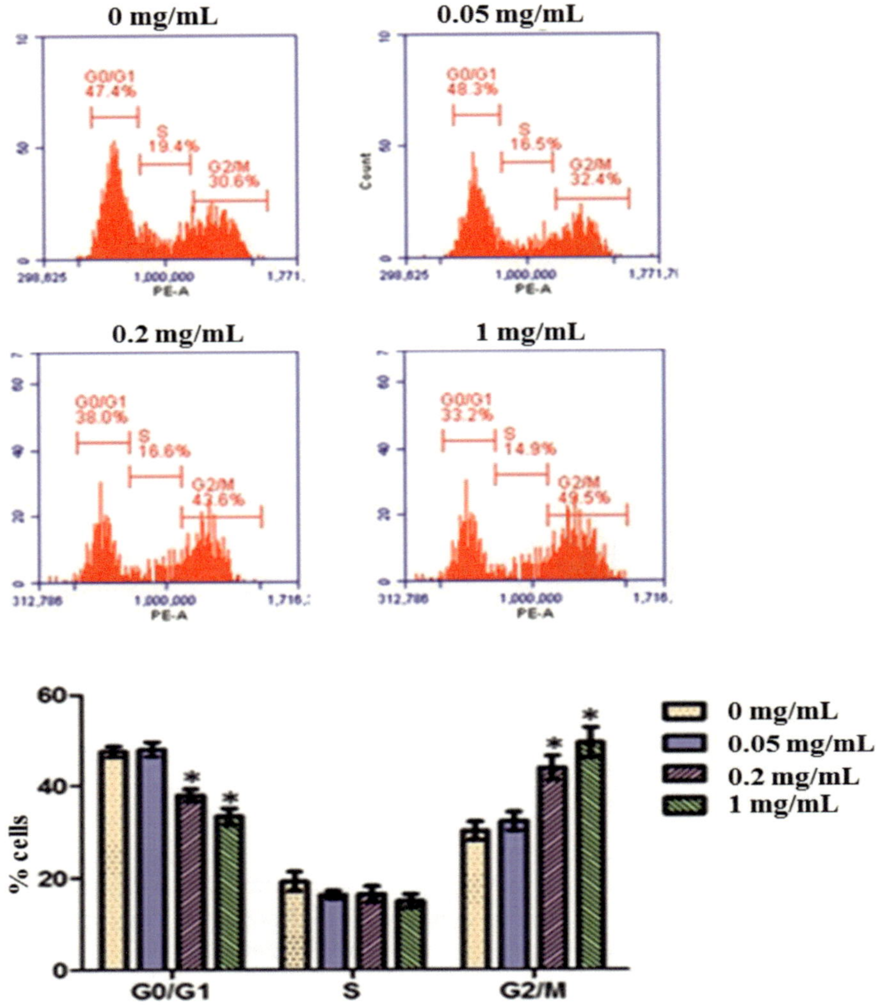

Figure 8.
*Extract of leaves of Excoecaria cochinchinensis Lour. affects the division cycle of gastric cancer cells MKN45. Cells were treated with extracts at different concentrations. The control was cells that were not treated with the extract (0 mg/mL); * $p < 0.05$; $n = 3$.*

Cell cycle arrest at the G2/M division phase is closely related to genes encoding the CDK1-cyclin B1, CDC25 and CHEK1 proteins, and PLK1, which control the phase transition during the mitotic cycle. Analysis of the effect of the extract of *Excoecaria cochinchinensis* Lour. on the division cycle of gastric cancer MKN45 cells (**Figure 8**, [36]) showed that at concentrations of 0.2 mg/mL and 1 mg/mL affected the mitotic phases of gastric cancer MKN45 cells, stopping the cell division cycle at the G2/M phase. Specifically, the percentage of cells in the G2/M phase increased to 43%–49%, compared with 33% of the control. Meanwhile, the percentage of cells in the G0/G1 phase in the treated sample was reduced to 33%–38% compared to 47% in the control.

Similar results were also shown in breast cancer cell line MCF-7 when subjected to ethanol extract from *Excoecaria agallocha* L., according to which, there was a significant increase in the proportion of cancer cells at the stage G2/M after being treated with the extract [41]. The inhibitory effect on cancer cell growth through the cessation of the cell division cycle in the G2/M phase has also been reported in various plant species. The extract of *Tamarix aucheriana* (Decne. ex Walp.) B.R. Baum inhibits the growth of colon cancer cells by stopping the cell cycle in the G2/M phase, thereby causing the cells to switch to apoptosis [45]. Another study showed the extract of *Calotropis procera* (Aiton) R. Br. enhanced apoptosis in skin melanoma cells through cyclization in the G2/M phase [46].

Experimental results have contributed to showing that the indigenous experiences of the Tay ethnic group in Thai Nguyen province are consistent with the scientific basis for the ability to inhibit some cell lines of stomach cancer and liver cancer. Explaining the scientific basis of indigenous experiences in the use of medicinal plants by experiments will strengthen and promote the conservation of folk knowledge as well as the conservation of ethnobotanical plants.

5. Some solutions for the conservation and sustainable development of medicinal plants and indigenous knowledge capital of the Tay ethnic group in Thai Nguyen province

The preservation of medicinal plants in ethnic communities is closely related to the knowledge of ethnic minorities to use, if the knowledge element is lost, medicinal plants will become wild and ineffective plants. This knowledge exists and is passed on from generation to generation, mostly by word of mouth in each family, clan, and ethnic minority community. Therefore, the conservation of medicinal plants needs to be associated with the preservation of indigenous knowledge of the Tay ethnic group in Thai Nguyen province, there should be a management mechanism and conservation methods suitable to its characteristics of local.

5.1 Conservation of endangered medicinal plants, coupled with the development of complementary planting

5.1.1. Preservation of medicinal plants

For 10 species of medicinal plants in the conservation area of Vietnam found in Thai Nguyen province (IUCN Red list, Vietnam Red Book - Part II Plants (2007), Decree No. 06/2019/ND-CP of the Government of Vietnam). Suggested solutions include:

i. *In situ conservation:* Currently in Thai Nguyen province, there are Than Sa and Võ Nhai Nature Reserves and the buffer zone of Tam Dao National Park at Quan Chu commune, Đại Từ' district, Thai Nguyen province. These are special-use forests with the function of preserving the original genetic resources of existing forest plants and animals, including medicinal plants.

Coordinate with forestry officials to plan in situ conservation of threatened medicinal plant species, specifically as follows:

- Than Sa Nature Reserve: *Stephania* ssp., *Fibraurea tinctoria* Lour.
- The buffer zone of Tam Dao National Park: *Paris hainanensis* Merr., *Disporopsis longifolia* Craib.

2. *Ex situ conservation:* Combined in the construction of the herbal garden of the old men and the mother and the garden of medicinal plants to serve the teaching requirements of professional schools in the province such as the University of Science, University of Medicine and Pharmacy, University of Agriculture and Forestry in Thai Nguyen province; Medical College of Thai Nguyen. Carrying out planting some rare and precious medicinal plants in danger of extinction for conservation and ex-situ. Based on biological characteristics, it is possible to grow most of the species in the list of 10 threatened species mentioned above.

According to ex situ conservation regulations, species need to be planted with a sufficient number of individuals, cared for, and accompanied by a regular monitoring record, to ensure the long-term survival of these species, in favorable human conditions grown, outside their inherent natural ecological environment.

5.1.2 Development of medicinal plants.

i. In-situ planting of some rare and precious medicinal plants: In parallel with the above two conservation methods, it is necessary to promote research and introduce on-site planting of some rare and precious medicinal plants that are currently in demand and have high economic value as:

- *Paris hainanensis* Merr.: Growing by seeds and cuttings. Intercropped under the canopy of moist open forest or in family gardens, in all districts in Thai Nguyen province.

- *Disporopsis longifolia* Craib: Growing by seeds and cuttings. Intercropped under the canopy of a moist forest or in family gardens, in all communes and districts in Thai Nguyen province.

ii. Developing and planting some medicinal plants that are in high demand: Besides the above rare and precious medicinal plants, in Thai Nguyen, it is possible to grow *Amomum longiligulare* T.L. Wu on forestry land for export. *Polyscias fruticosa* (L.) Harms and *Curcuma longa* L. are also medicinal plants with a large market and are perfectly suitable for production in many localities in Thai Nguyen province. The development of growing indigenous medicinal plants and other medicinal plants with high economic value is the right direction, contributing to creating more jobs and increasing incomes for people in the local ethnic communities.

5.2 Reasonable exploitation, pay attention to regeneration protection

Subjects are medicinal plants distributed in Thai Nguyen province, not in the conservation area in Vietnam. Some specific solutions are proposed as follows:

i. Develop a reasonable mining process

According to the regulations on the exploitation of medicinal plants that grow naturally in Vietnam, the sustainability of resources must be ensured. To fulfill this requirement, each medicinal plant species needs to have a technical extraction process to ensure its ability to regenerate naturally, and at the same time, it does not cause large changes to the population. The content of the mining process includes some notable points as follows:

- The name of the medicinal plant/attach the exact scientific name of the species.
- Parts used as medicine.
- Time of exploitation: In the period when medicinal plants have the highest quality, avoid the fruit season, and at the same time are most beneficial for the ability to regenerate naturally.
- How to exploit: How to collect used parts of medicinal plants to ensure natural regeneration and not affect other plants around.
- Expected volume to be harvested and rate of seed retention in the population. Note that the male/female ratio is kept, suitable for medicinal plants with different flowers.
- Exploitation cycle.

The extraction procedure needs to be compiled separately for each medicinal plant species, printed into documents, distributed to the people, and at the same time organized training to guide these processes specifically for those who harvest.

ii. *Guide the harvesting process to the community:* Depending on the target and the harvesting area, it is necessary to organize training sessions in the community, so that the technical staff can provide specific instructions on harvesting techniques for some medicinal plants for the citizen. Besides theoretical instruction, it is possible to organize direct instruction for 1-2 certain medicinal plants directly in the field. The purpose of this work is to make people more aware of the need to collect medicinal plants reasonably, to ensure natural regeneration, for the next harvest.

5.3 Preserving the indigenous knowledge capital of the community, inheriting and promoting

It is necessary to have a separate plan/program on investigating indigenous knowledge capital of ethnic groups, fully recording, and selectively publishing: Plan/chapter separate program on investigating the indigenous knowledge capital of the ethnic groups to fully record, selectively publish and promote the indigenous knowledge in the treatment of diseases with plants of the Tay ethnic group in the province. Thai Nguyen in two languages (Vietnamese and Tay ethnic language); makes practical contributions to the conservation of folk remedies and the effects of medicinal plants, which have been summed up in experiences and passed down from generation to generation in the community's development.

Select, research, and evaluate several unique remedies of the Tay ethnic group in Thai Nguyen province for wide application in the community.

5.4 Propaganda to raise public awareness

Propaganda to raise public awareness on medicinal plant conservation, indigenous knowledge conservation, sustainable exploitation, and the need to grow more medicinal plants. Integrate into communication programs on the protection of natural resources and the environment, to organize training courses on medicinal plants for the community. The contents of those training courses include:

- Disseminate guidelines and legal documents on the conservation of forest plant resources, including medicinal plants. The importance of preserving and sustainably exploiting locally available natural medicinal plants.

- Guide people to identify medicinal plants that need to be conserved in the locality, absolutely do not exploit and invade, do not collect varieties of preserved medicinal plants, and sell them to traders for illegal export across the border. Gender.

- Encourage the elderly to pass it on to young people, first of all, family members, etc. Educate the younger generation on the awareness and understanding of how to use herbs as medicine, through which the younger generation is proud of the tradition. of their forefathers and learned how to use medicinal plants found around the village.

- Incorporating the subject "Conservation of medicinal plants" into the curriculum of each grade level, to improve the understanding of medicinal plants for generations of students.

Protecting locally available medicinal plant resources needs to be associated with indigenous knowledge, which has even become a source of life for a part of the local community for many generations. If the medicinal plants here are not protected and lost, then their descendants will no longer have those medicinal plants to use. The protection of medicinal plants today also carries meaning and moral responsibility for future generations.

6. Conclusions

The research found 321 plant species belonging to 103 families and 253 genera that were used in the traditional medicine of the Tay ethnic group in Thai Nguyen province. In general, people preferred preparing medicine by boiling them in water for oral ingestion. The most used parts of plants were leaves and stems. The Tay ethnic people rely on herbal remedies for their basic health care, thus indigenous medicinal plant knowledge plays a vital role in solving local health care problems. Most of them had high use values, suggesting that they may produce bioactive compounds with strong physiological effects. That will provide basic data for further research as well as conservation of important medicinal plant including the endangered species in the study area.

Acknowledgements

The authors would like to thank the National Foundation for Science and Technology Development (Nafosted) for the financial support of project 106.03-2020.28.

Conflict of interest

The authors declare no conflicts of interest regarding the publication of this book chapter.

Abbreviations

De/06/2019	Decree 06/2019/ND-CP of the Government of Vietnam
IC50	Half-maximal inhibitory concentration
IUCN	The International Union for Conservation of Nature Red List of Threatened Species
MTT	3-(4,5-dimethylthiazol-2-yl)-2,5 diphenyltetrazolium bromide
VNRB	Vietnam Red Data Book - list of rare and endangered species
WHO	World Health Organization

Author details

Le Thi Thanh Huong[1], Nguyen Phu Hung[1], Hosakatte Niranjana Murthy[2,3], Do Van Hai[4] and Nguyen Trung Thanh[5]*

1 Faculty of Biotechnology, TNU University of Sciences, Thai Nguyen City, Vietnam

2 Department of Botany, Karnatak University, Dharwad, India

3 Department of Horticulture Science, Chungbuk National University, Cheongju, Republic of Korea

4 Institute of Ecology and Biological Resources, Vietnam Academy of Science and Technology, Hanoi, Vietnam

5 Faculty of Biology, VNU University of Science, Hanoi, Vietnam

*Address all correspondence to: thanh_nt@hus.edu.vn

References

[1] WHO. Traditional medicine. Fact Sheet No 134.2008. The Interne. 2017:EB134/24. Available from: http://www.who.int/mediacentre/factsheets/2003/fs134/en

[2] Luca VD, Salim V, Atsumi SM, Yu F. Mining the biodiversity of plants: A revolution in the making. Science. 2012;**336**:1658-1661. DOI: 10.1126/science.1217410

[3] MONRE (Ministry of Natural Resources and Environment). Vietnam National Biodiversity Strategy to 2020, vision to 2030. Vietnam. 2014;**1**:176

[4] Van-Sam H, Baas P, Kessler PJA. Traditional medicinal plants in Ben En National Park. Vietnam. Blumea. 2008;**53**:569-601. DOI: 10.3767/000651908X607521

[5] Administrative map of Vietnam with 63 provinces, 2020. The Interne. 2022. Vol. 1. Available from: https://narenca.com.vn/products/tap-ban-do-hanh-chinh-viet-nam-63-tinh-thanh-pho

[6] Trung-Thanh N, Thanh-Huong LT. Medicinal Plant Sources in Ethnic Minority Communities in Thai Nguyen Province. Hanoi: Vietnam National University Press; 2022. p. 426

[7] Thanh-Huong LT, Thi-Phuong N, Trung-Thanh N, Nghia-Thin N. Investigation of medicinal plants and experiences of using medicinal plants of San Chi ethnic at Phu Luong district, Thai Nguyen province. Journal of Medicinal Materials. 2012;**17**(1):3-8

[8] Khuankaew S, Srithi K, Tiansawat P, Jampeetong A, Inta A, Wangpakapat P. Ethnobotanical study of medicinal plants used by Tai Yai in northern Thailand. Journal of Ethnopharmacology. 2014;**151**(2):829-838. DOI: 10.1016/j.jep.2013.11.033

[9] Thanh-Huong LL, Duc-Phuong N, Hoang TT, The-An D, Trung-Thanh N, Nghia-Thin N. Investigation of medicinal plants and value of using medicinal plants of Sán Dìu Ethnic in Thai Nguyen province. VNU Journal of Science. 2014;**30**(3):14-23

[10] Kichu M, Malewska T, Akter K, Imchen I, Harrington D, Kohen J, et al. An ethnobotanical study of medicinal plants of Chungtia village, Nagaland, India. Journal of Ethnopharmacology. 2015;**166**:5-17. DOI: 10.1016/j.jep.2015.02.053

[11] Thanh-Huong LL, Van-Quan H, Van-Ve D, Trung-Thanh N. Investigation of medicinal plants and experiences of using medicinal plants of Tày ethnic at Van An commune, Van Quan district, Lang Son province. Journal of Science VNU Vietnam. 2015;**31**(4):45-55

[12] Thanh-Huong LL, Trung-Thanh N. The knowledge and experience of the medicinal plants used by minorities ethnic in Thai Nguyen province for conservation and sustainable development. VNU Journal of Science. 2016;**32**(1):55-64

[13] Phumthum M, Srithi K, Inta A, Junsongduang A, Tangjitman K, Pongamornkul W, et al. Ethnomedicinal plant diversity in Thailand. Journal of Ethnopharmacology. 2018;**214**:90-98. DOI: 10.1016/j.jep.2017.12.003

[14] Mesfin K, Tekle G, Tesfay T. Ethnobotanical study of traditional medicinal recourses and outcome measurements from a user's perspective in Ghana. Health Policy Plan. 2013;**27**:625-637

[15] Chekole G, Asfaw Z, Kelbessa E. Ethnobotanical study of medicinal plants in the environs of Tara-gedam and Amba remnant forests of Libo Kemkem district, northwest Ethiopia. Journal of Ethnobiology and Ethnomedicine. 2015;**11**:4

[16] Kefalew A, Asfaw Z, Kelbessa E. Ethnobotany of medicinal plants in Ada'a district, East Shewa Zone of Oromia regional state, Ethiopia. Journal of Ethnobiology and Ethnomedicine. 2015;**11**:25

[17] Khac-Ban N, Huong-Giang V, My-Linh T, Quynh-Lien L, Quoc-Binh N, Thien-An T, et al. Proceedings of Conference on Ecology and Biological Resources. Hanoi, Vietnam: The 5th National Scientific Conference; 2013. pp. 950-956

[18] Chevallier A. The Encyclopedia of Medicinal Plants. 1st American ed. New York: Boston: DK Pub.; Distributed by Houghton Mifflin; 1996

[19] Zaher A, Boufellous M, Jaber H, El-Hartiti H, Barrahi M, Ouhssine M, et al. Ethnobotanical Study of Medicinal Plants Used in the Province of Sidi Slimane (Morocco). Journal of Biosciences and Medicines. 2018;**6**:25-35. DOI: 10.4236/jbm.2018.69003

[20] Hu R, Lin C, Xu W, Liu Y, Long C. Ethnobotanical study on medicinal plants used by Mulam people in Guangxi, China. Journal of Ethnobiology and Ethnomedicine. 2020;**16**(40):1-50. DOI: 10.1186/s13002-020-00387-z

[21] Heinrich M, Jäger AK. Ethnopharmacology. UK: John Wiley and sons, Ltd.; 2015

[22] The IUCN. Red List of Threatened Species. Version 2022-1. 2022. Available from: https://www.iucnredlist.org

[23] Ministry of Science and Technology. Vietnamese Academy of Science and Technology. Vietnam Red Book - Part II Plants. Publisher of Science and Technology; 2007. p. 407

[24] Decree 06/2019/ND-CP. Decree No. 06 of the Government of Vietnam on the management of endangered, precious, and rare forest plants and animals and implementation of the Convention on International Trade in Endangered Species of Wild Fauna and Flora. 2019

[25] Ke-Loc P. Phylum Pinophyta. In: Vietnamese National University, Hanoi. Hanoi: List of Vietnamese plants. Publisher of Agriculture; 2001. pp. 1151-1155

[26] Chi VV. Dictionary of Vietnamese Plants. Vol. 1. Hanoi: Publisher of Science and Technology; 2003. p. 1249

[27] Minh-Tam N, Phuong-Trang NT, Ha-Giang VT. Effects of habitat fragmentation on genetic diversity in *Cycas balansae* (Cycadaceae). The ASEAN Journal on Science & Technology for Development. 2006;**23**(3):193-205. DOI: 10.29037/ajstd.104

[28] Chi VV. Dictionary of Vietnamese Medicinal Plants. Vol. 1. Vietnam: Medical Publishing House; 2012. p. 1541

[29] Loi DT. Medicinal Plants and Herbal Remedies of Vietnam. Hanoi: Publisher of Science and Technique; 1991

[30] Changyoung L, Soo-Yong K, Sangmi E, Jin-Hyub P, The-Bach T, Ashwini-Darshetkar M, et al. Ethnobotanical study on medicinal plants used by local Van Kieu ethnic people of Bac Huong Hoa nature reserve, Vietnam. Journal of Ethnopharmacology. 2019;**231**:283-294. DOI: 10.1016/j.jep.2018.11.006

[31] Dahham SS, Tabana YM, Iqbal MA, Ahamed MBK, Ezzat MO, Majid ASM, et al. The anticancer, antioxidant, and antimicrobial properties of the sesquiterpene β-caryophyllene from the essential oil of *Aquilaria crassna*. Molecules. 2015;**20**(7):11808-11829. DOI: 10.3390/molecules200711808

[32] Mamoru K, Tsuyoshi S, Hitomi K, Shigemi T, Hiroe M, Kazuhiro T, et al. Agarwood (*Aquilaria crassna*) extracts decrease high-protein high-fat diet-induced intestinal putrefaction toxins in mice. Pharmaceutica Analytica Acta. 2012;**3**:1-7. DOI: 10.4172/2153-2435.1000152

[33] Jermsri P, Jiraviriyakul A, Unajak S, Kumphune S. Effect of *Aquilaria crassna* crude extract on simulated ischemia-induced cardiac cell death. International Journal of Pharmaceutics and Biological Sciences. 2012;**3**:604-613

[34] Sattayasai J, Bantadkit J, Aromdee C, Lattmann E, Airarat W. Antipyretic, analgesic and anti-oxidative activities of *Aquilaria crassna* leaves extract in rodents. Journal of Ayurveda and Integrative Medicine. 2012;**3**:175-179. DOI: 10.4103/0975-9476.104427

[35] Kamonwannasit S, Nantapong N, Kumkrai P, Luecha P, Kupittayanant S, Chudapongse N. Antibacterial activity of *Aquilaria crassna* leaf extract against *Staphylococcus epidermidis* by disruption of the cell wall. Annals of Clinical Microbiology and Antimicrobials. 2013;**12**:20. DOI: 10.1186/1476-0711-12-20

[36] Hung NP, Huong LTT. The ethanol extract of *Excoecaria cochinchinensis* Lour. leaves inhibit cell migration and arrests cell cycle in gastric cancer cell MKN45. Vietnam Journal of Biotechnology. 2021;**19**(1):147-154. DOI: 10.15625/1811-4989/15291

[37] Nguyen PH, Pham TQ, Nguyen HH, Vu TND, Ngo TH, Nguyen TH, et al. Inhibition of cell proliferation and enhancement of apoptosis of liver and breast cancer cells by methanol extract of *Heliciopsis lobata* leaves. Hue University Journal of Science: Natural Science. 2021;**130**(1A):51-59. DOI: 10.26459/hueunijns.v130i1A.5924

[38] Li-Hua M, Ning-Yan W, Ping L. Cytotoxic triterpenoid saponins from *Ardisia gigantifolia*. Planta Medica. 2012;**78**(6):617-621. DOI: 10.1055/s-0031-1298254

[39] Li-Hua M, Li-Hua W, Teng-Fei Y, Yu-Ning W, Hong Y, Ping L, et al. Triterpenoid saponin AG8 from *Ardisia gigantifolia* Stapf. induces triple-negative breast cancer cells apoptosis through the oxidative stress pathway. Oxidative Medicine and Cellular Longevity. 2020:1-11. DOI: 10.1155/2020/7963212

[40] Park G, Lee EJ, Min HY, Choi HY, Han AR, Lee SK, et al. Evaluation of the cytotoxic potential of Indonesian medicinal plants in cultured human cancer cells. Natural Product Sciences. 2002;**8**(4):165-169

[41] Kumar-Reddy PR, Priya D, Palaniyandi T, Rajeswary H. Effect of ethanolic extract of *Excoecaria agallocha* leaves on the cytotoxic activity and cell cycle arrest of human breast cancer cell lines-MCF-7. Pharmacognosy Magazine. 2019;**15**(64):346-351. DOI: 10.4103/pm.pm_237_19

[42] Sung-Hwa S, Hee-Jung S, Bum-Jun K, Dae-Young Z. Responses to the tepotinib in gastric cancers with MET amplification or MET exon 14 skipping mutations and high expression of both PD-L1 and CD44. Cancers. 2022;**14**(14):3444. DOI: 10.3390/cancers14143444

[43] Xiao-Hong Z, Shi-Yong C, Lin T, Ying-Zhuo S, Lin L, Chen-Wei X, et al. Myricetin induces apoptosis in HepG2 cells through Akt/p70S6K/bad signaling and mitochondrial apoptotic pathway. Anti-Cancer Agents in Medicinal Chemistry. 2013;**13**(10):1575-1581. DOI: 10.2174/1871520613666131125123059

[44] Li Z, Ling H, Qiang L, Shaoyi K, Qiaoqin X, Xianjing Q, et al. N-butanol fraction of *Entada phaseoloides* ethanol extract inhibits hepatocellular carcinoma HepG2 cell proliferation by inducing apoptosis. The Balkan Union of Oncology. 2014;**19**(2):406-411

[45] Mohamed-Salah A, Al-Attiyah R, Radhika B, Ghaneim A, Mathew K, Mohammad A. Syringic acid from *Tamarix aucheriana* possesses antimitogenic and chemo-sensitizing activities in human colorectal cancer cells. Pharmaceutical Biology. 2013;**51**(9):1110-1124. DOI: 10.3109/13880209.2013.781194

[46] Aparna LJ, Pratiksha HR, Rooth M, Mahadev J, Kavitha K, Amol K, et al. *Calotropis procera* extract induces apoptosis and cell cycle arrest at G2/M phase in human skin melanoma (SK-MEL-2) cells. Natural Product Research. 2015;**29**(23):2261-2264. DOI: 10.1080/14786419.2014.1001386

Chapter 10

South African Herbs Used for Cancer Therapy in Rural Areas

Pakiso Moses Makhoahle

Abstract

South Africa is a rich country in topography and herbs used by traditional healers for the treatment of many infections. Many African ethnic groups use different herbs that are used based on their forebears' cultures and customs. Most of these plants grow none domestically and are harvested by these traditional healers and treat their patients according to their spiritual revelations and indigenous knowledge. In this chapter herbs will be grouped and comprehensibly discussed on how each tribe uses it according to their diverse cultures, customs, and beliefs. The chapter will also tap into the scientific discovery to document their toxicity for safety. Then a conclusion will be drawn combining the indigenous knowledge, culture, and scientific discovery to guide reader for potential plants.

Keywords: South Africa, medicinal herbs, diseases rural areas, traditional healers

1. Introduction

Over the past decades, herbs have become the global topic owing to recurring, (re)emerging pandemics and epidemics. In the past 2 years (2020 and 2021) medicinal plants have gained too much interest because of COVID-19 and most South African relied on concoctions for survival due to majority not affording western medication and all restricted measures of movement. Other countries also showed overwhelming trust in medicinal plants and herbs to aid in circumventing pandemic. It would have been the biggest mistake if the focus was only on the pandemic and forgetting treatment of other deadly diseases like Human Immunodeficiency Virus (HIV), tuberculosis (TB), diabetes and cancer to mention a few.

Cancer remains one of the leading causes of death globally and in sub-Saharan countries including South Africa. In the middle of the pandemic traditional healers continued to use ancestral calling guidance, culture, customs, and indigenous knowledge in the treatment of cancer and cancer related signs and symptoms. This chapter will bring most of the plants used by diverse Africans living in rural areas, highlight the scientific discoveries in relation to toxicity and impart a consolidated guidance on which plants to select hereof to avoid exposing their patients to possible toxic mixtures or concoctions.

2. Richness of south African diverse population in herbs using for cancer

South Africa have nine provinces (**Figure 1**) with a population of almost 60million, 11 spoken official languages (**Figure 2**) across with English and Afrikaans spoken by many, high unemployment rate that was escalated by the global pandemic, that encouraged traditional people to even rely on and practice the use of medicinal plants [1, 2]. Indigenous knowledge played a major role for many decades for alleviation of the diseases [3]; however, less was known to the effect that some of this herb's extracts does to the human body as most patients where happy to see the reduction to clearing of infections and the clinical symptoms possible linked to the disease at that time. This chapter will bring the documented herbs and report on the different studies done in assessing the safeness of these extracts and a conclusion will be drawn as an awareness for which plants should our people practicing tradition medicine should be aware of. Scopus, Google Scholar, Web of Science, ScienceDirect, PubMed, and books, as well as local reports and thesis submissions, were used to conduct a broad literature search.

3. Herbs used by the diverse African south African ethnic groups in traditional practices and their scientific safeness discoveries

3.1 *Agapanthus-africanus (L.)*

Agapanthus-africanus belonging to the family *Agapanthaceae* which is found in the Western cape Province mostly from Cape Peninsula towards Swellendam during the favored by the winter rainfall area [4].

The leaves are suberect, strap shaped with flowers deep blue, thick textured and broadly funnel shape (**Figure 3**) [4]. The plant vernacular names used in in the

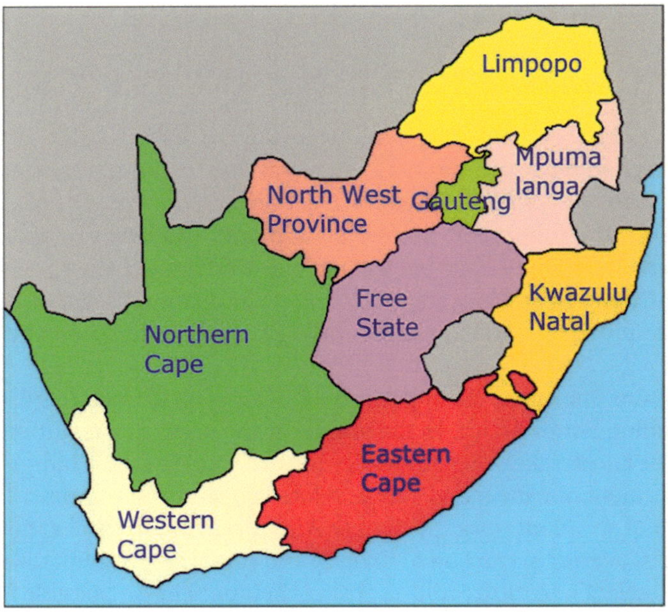

Figure 1.
Map of South Africa showing the different 9 provinces-https://za.pinterest.com/pin/314689092704490764/.

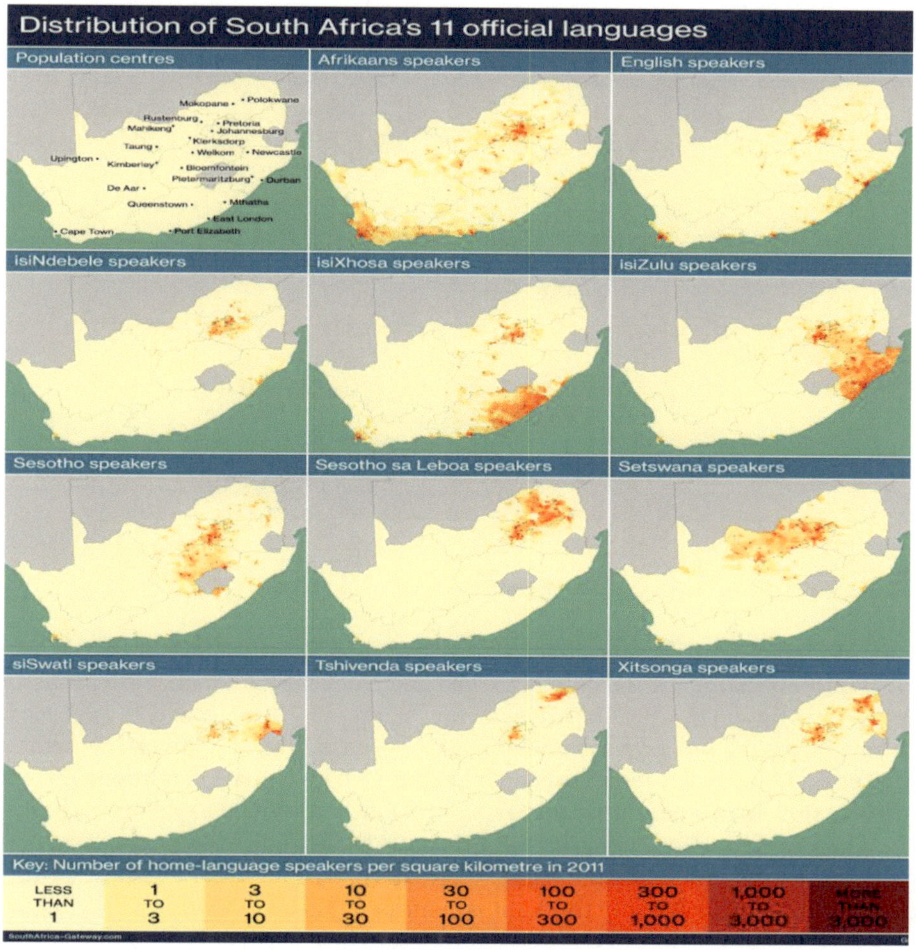

Figure 2.
Distribution pattern of south African 11 languages-https://southafrica-info.com/arts-culture/11-languages-south-africa/ (permission granted by Mary Alexander).

country included Sotho (leta-la-phofu), Zulu (mathunga, icakathi), Xhosa (isilakati), Afrikaans (Haakleli) and English (blue lily). (L.) Hoff manns [4, 5].

Traditionally healers collect and dry the roots of this plant in the sun, once they are dry then that will be followed by extraction method of continuous boiling water until a color change is observed, the aqueous infusion will be orally for the treatment of cancer until the patient is cured [5].

There is no scientific evidence reported on the high toxicity of this plant, the studies have shown low poisonous severity except where other studies have proven parts of the plant like leaves to be poisonous [4, 6].

3.2 *Solanum aculeastrum Dunal*

S. aculeastrum Dunal belong to the family *Solanacease*, is a small tree or shrub native to tropical Africa south to South Africa, in a wide range of soil, terrain and climatic conditions [7]. This taxon can be found in the southern African countries of Swaziland, KwaZulu-Natal, Mpumalanga, Limpopo, and Mpumalanga. In addition to

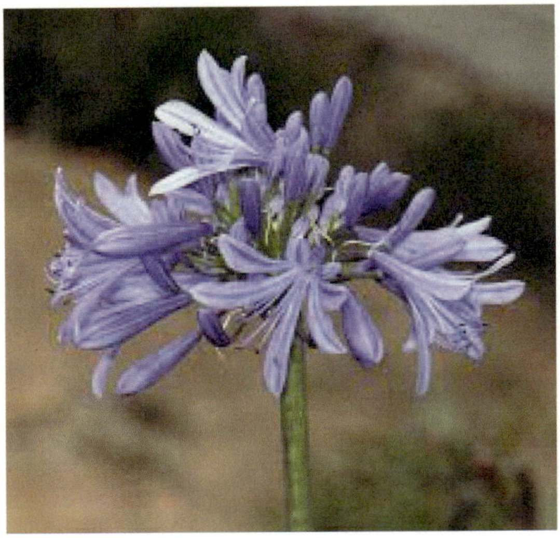

Figure 3.
Agapanthusafricanus-*http://pza.sanbi.org/agapanthus-africanus.*

disturbed areas, *S. aculeastr*um subsp. aculeastrum grows naturally in grassland, woodland, and forest margin. It is highly branched and reaches 1–5 m high, with numerous sharp hooked brown thorns. The leaves are ovate, up to 15 cm long and 13 cm broad, with lobed margins and a downy underside. Its flowering time is between September to July, peaking from November to March in South Africa climate conditions [7]. This shrub contains small smooth, round berries and fade from green to yellow as they ripen. These berries contain high levels of the poisonous alkaloid solanine [8].

The species name *aculeastrum* refers to the thorns that adorn most parts of the shrub (**Figure 4**) (15). Locally the plant is commonly called Zulu (mtuma), Xhosa (umthuma, itunga), Tswana (thola), Venda (murulwa), English (goat bitter-apple, bitter-apple, goat apple, poison apple) and in Afrikaans (bok-bitterappel, bitterappel, bokappel, gifappel) [7].

The zulu's traditional healers and other ethnic groups practices use the fruit fresh, boiled, or charred to make herbal medicine in treating a variety of diseases such as

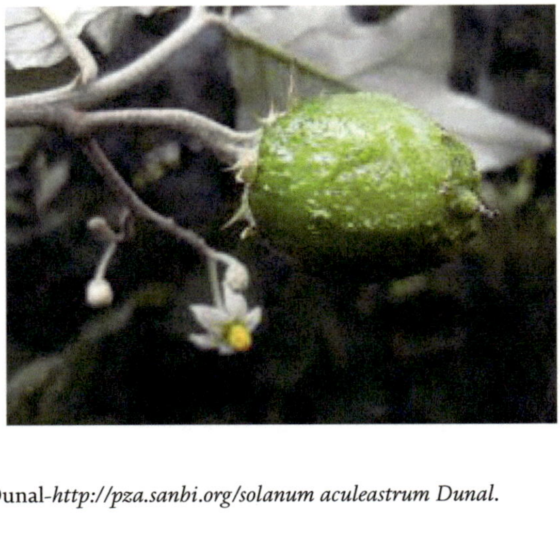

Figure 4.
Solanum aculeastrum Dunal-*http://pza.sanbi.org/solanum aculeastrum Dunal.*

toothaches, ringworms, and cancer [7, 9, 10]. In the Eastern Cape, The Xhosa's, the berries are boiled until this burst into pieces, decoctions prepared from the fruits are taken orally once a day post filtration until the cancer is cured [5, 11].

Scientifically isolated steroid alkaloids from the *Solanaum acueastrum* have been reported to possess anticancer activity [9, 10]. This exceedingly bitter fruit of *S. aculeastrum* is used medicinally (fresh, cooked, or burnt) in a variety of methods for both people and domestic animals, according to Hutchings et al. [9]. Leaf and fruit aqueous extracts were found to possess low activity against cancer cells [12]. Care should be taken in the use of fresh, dried, and boiled berry extracts and they were found to affect organs function in a study done by Aboyade et al. [13]. The deadly alkaloid solanine is present in both adult and immature fruits. Botanist have warned about poisonous nature of this shrub, according to Acocks (1988), this species is an unwelcome plant whose population should be decreased by effective veld management shrub due to the presence of poisonous alkaloid solanine. It's important for traditional healers to take cognisance of this plant and rather use other herbs available at their disposable [14].

3.3 *Leonotis leonurus (L.) R. Br*

L. leonurus (L.) R. Br. belong to the family *Lamiaceae*, the wild dagga with soft-woody fast-growing shrub with 1.5 m wide and almost 3 m tall. When *L. leonurus (L.) R. Br.* leaves are crushed, they release a powerful herby aroma. It consists of flowers varying in color from different shades of orange to vivid orange red, the flower heads are in axillary verticils in clusters of 3–11. The herb has stiff hairs that are prickly when touched. Summer is the season for flowering; in some regions, this occurs from November to January, whereas in others, it occurs from mid-autumn to winter (April to June). There are additional known varieties with apricot, yellow, and white flower (**Figure 5**) (15).

In South African ethnic's groups, the shrub is common named, Sotho (lebake, levake); Zulu (umfincafincane, umcwili, imunyane, utshwala-bezinyoni, Xhosa (utywala-bengcungcu, umfincafincane, umunyamunya), Shona (ibetshule-badala, ilihambambeba), English (wild dagga, lion's ear, leonotis) and Afrikaans (wildedagga, duiwelstabak).

The traditional healers prepare at tea from a handful leaves and flowers each morning and night for the treatment of cancer [15]. Another study at the Eastern Cape South African has supported the anticancer activity from the water extract of both the leaf and the flower [16]. The water extract of the leave was scientifically reported to affect the blood system, kidneys and liver function when tested on the rats [17]. The study done by Dlamini in 2005 on toxicity test in the laboratory (in vitro) found the leaf extract to be non-toxic to the human lympocyets [18]. The scientific studies interchangeable show that even though the leaf and flowers possess anticancer activity care should be taken as it can affect the functioning of other organs of the body.

3.4 *Hypoxis argentea* Harv. Ex baker

Hypoxis argentea Harv. ex Baker belong to the family *Hypoxidaceae*, grows in the Eastern Cape of South Africa on rocky outcrops and grassy areas. It features tiny yellow flowers and slender, ribbed leaves with silky yellowish hairs. A thin, herbaceous perennial plant called Hypoxis argentea can reach heights of 7 to 10 cm and produces a cluster of four to seven grass-like leaves from a tiny, corm-like tuber. The majority

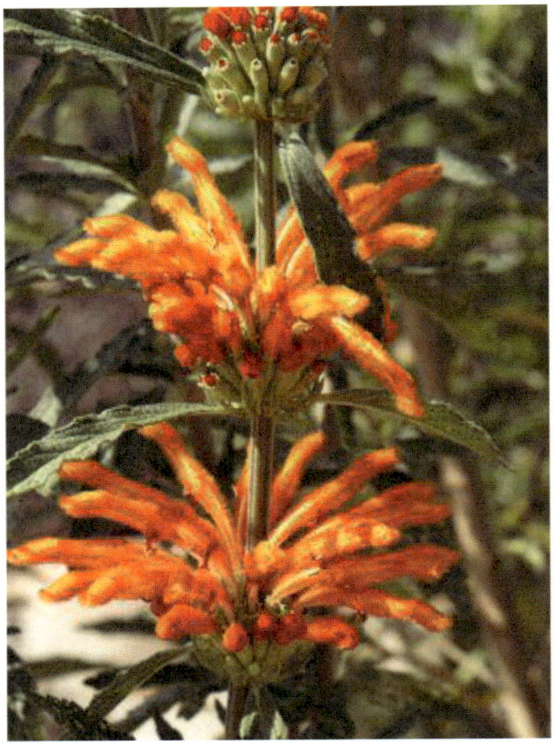

Figure 5.
Leonotis-leonuru-*http://pza.sanbi.org/leonotis-leonurus.*

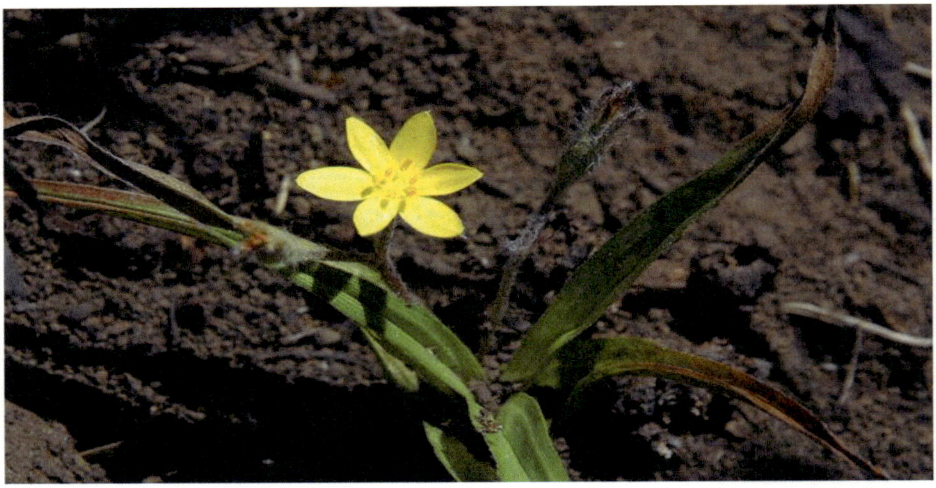

Figure 6.
Hypoxis argentea *Harv. Ex baker - https://www.pacificbulbsociety.org/pbswiki/index.php/ Hypoxis#&gid=1&pid=9.*

of Hypoxis species are severely harmed or killed by even brief frosts because they are often not extremely cold-tolerant plants. Nearly all the S. African species typically thrive in a Mediterranean environment with little to no frost because they are native to regions with summer rainfall and little to no winter rain (**Figure 6**) [19, 20].

The frequently used name by the different ethnic groups is South Africa are Sesotho (Leihlo-khomo le leholo, Leihlo-la-kxomo-le-leholo, letsikitlane), Xhosa(ixalanxa), Zulu (inongwe), English (small silver starflower). Other subspecies of Hypoxidaceae family usend mostly across the country in rural areas included the following hypoxis colchicifolia Bakr (Zulu-iLabatheka; English-broad-leaves hypoxi), hypoxis hemerocallidea Fisch., C.A. Mey. & Ave-Lall (Sesotho-moli kharatsa, lotsane; Tswana-tshuka; Xhosa-inongwe, ilabatheka, ixhalanxa, ikubalo lezithunzela; Zulu-inkomfe, ilabatheka, inkomfe enkulu; English-star flower, yellow star; and Afrikaans-sterblom, geelsterretjie, gifblom) [5].

The plant is harvested from the wild by traditional healers and ordinary people for medicinal use [21]. An aquest decoctions made from crushed buldis orally taken for the treatment of cancer until the patient is cured [5, 22, 23]. No Scientific report on the toxicity of this plants have been documented.

3.5 *Euphorbia ingens* E. Mey. Ex Boiss

E. ingens E. Mey. ex Boiss, a member of the *Euphorbiaceae* family, is a spiny, evergreen, succulent tree with a short trunk [24]. It has a thick bole, gray and coarsely fissured bark, abundant latex, persistent branches from about three meters up, virtually upright, rebranching, and forming a huge, broadly rounded crown [24]. Simple and transitory, the stems' nearly spine-free, green, cactus-like leaves do most of the photosynthesis instead of the leaves themselves. The plant is distributed across the following provinces of South Africa Gauteng, KwaZulu-Natal, Limpopo, Mpumalanga, and North-West [20]. This tree prefers warm areas and can survive in areas that go through long periods of drought or are generally very dry (**Figure** 7) [24].

The vernacular names of the common tree E. ingens E. Mey. ex Boiss are; Sepedi (Mohlohlo-kgomo, Abaphaphi, Mokgoto, Mokgwakgwatha); Tswana (Monkgôpô, Ngôgô, Nkonde, Nkondze.); Zulu (Abaphaphi, Umahetheni, Umhlondlo, Umhlonhlo, Umphapha Umhlondlo, Umpapa, nkondze); Shona (inkonze, mkonde, mukondwe, mukonde); IsiNdebele (Inkonze); English (Cactus Euphorbia, Candelabra Euphorbia, Candelabra Tree, Common Tree Euphorbia, Tree Euphorbia, Giant Euphorbia, Naboom); Afrikaans (Gewone Melkboom, Gewone Naboom, Gewone Melkboom, Gewone Naboom, Kankerbos, Naboom, Noorsboom, Noorsdoring, Noorsdoringboom, Noorsheuning); **Tshivenda (**Mukonde**)**. The vilage **Naboom**spruit (– now Mookgopong), North of Pretoria, took its name from this tree [25].

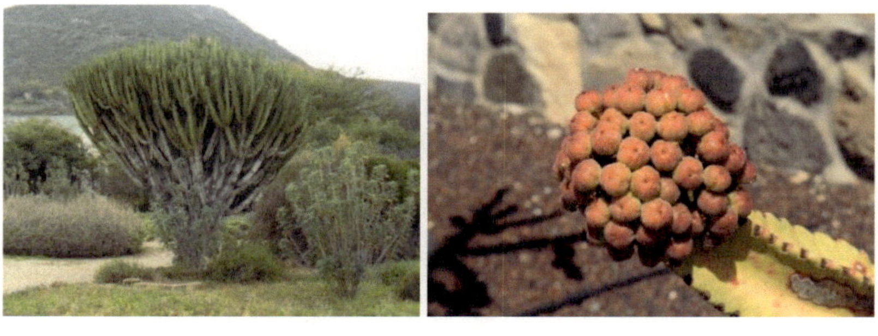

Figure 7.
Euphorbia ingens E. Mey. Ex Boiss-*http://pza.sanbi.org/euphorbia-ingens.*

The plant is harvested by the Bapedi people who use the freshly squeezed juice from the stem and apply it after bathing on the skin topically for the treatment of breast cancer [26]. The Sotho speaking people apply its latex topically for the external cancer on the skin until cancer is cured [5]. The studies shows that other ethnic groups use it for the treatment of cancer [21]. Traditional healers and traditional medicine practicing people at the rural area should be careful when handling this plant, due to the deadly milky sap or latex [25]. It is exceedingly dangerous to use latex because it can cause allergic reactions, blisters, and even blindness [25]. It is advisable burn this tree first to reduce the impact of the toxic fluid before used as a tradition medicine [24, 25].

3.6 *Raphionacme hirsuta* (E. Mey.) R.a. dyer

Raphionacme hiesuta (E. Mey.) R.A. Dyer is a member of the *Apocynaceae* family, a perennial plant that grows to around 200 mm tall, profoundly branched, and has a huge, tuberous rootstock. Its herbaceous, finely hairy stems exude a milky sap. This plant often hibernates during winter and sprouts new growth in the spring. *In a grassland, its blue blossoms are frequently missed because they appear at ground level before the leaves emerge. Once observed, something will always be remembered.* The leaves are 12–50 6–25 mm, hairy or hairless, and have parallel secondary veins and a conspicuous midvein [27]. It forms a very big underground tuber that has many cultural and medicinal attributes. *In savanna and open grassland provinces like Gauteng, Free State, Mpumalanga, KwaZulu-Natal, the Eastern and Northern Cape, North-West, and Limpopo, Raphionacme hirsuta is frequently found on rocky and mountainous terrain* (**Figure 8**) [28].

The vernacular names of the common plant *Raphionacme hirsuta* (E. Mey.) R.A. Dyer are Southern Sotho (Kerentshane), Xhoza (intsema), Zulu (umathanjane, Umathangane), English (false gentian, khadi root), and Afrikaans (Khadiwortel, khadi) [29, 30].

R. hirsuta tubers or roots are traditionally used as a source of yeast to produce beer and as a traditional therapy for maladies and diseases like cancer and chronic ulcers despite being rumored to be poisonous [31, 32]. As early as in the 1960's the Southern Sotho speaking people were using this plant for the treatment of internal tumors [33].

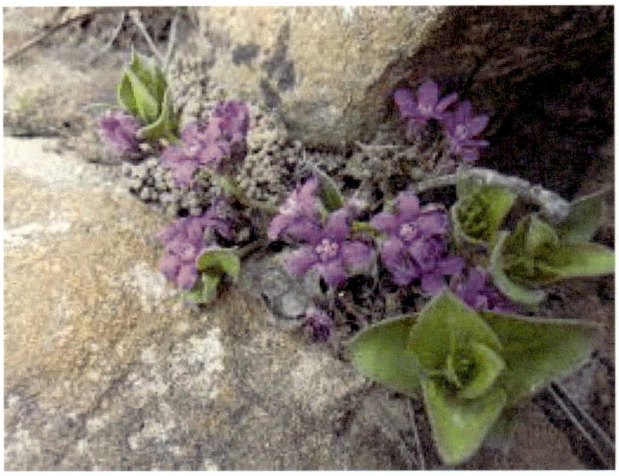

Figure 8.
Raphionacme hirsuta *(E.Mey.) R.a. dyer- http://pza.sanbi.org/raphionacme-hirsuta.*

Scientific study reported that a 50% aqueous methanol was effective to inhibit almost 90% a rodent leukemia (P-388) cancer model [34]. A great caution should be exercised as the roots of this plants are believed to be poisonous [35].

3.7 *Lassertia frutescense (L.)*

Lassertia frutescense is a fast-growing, hardy shrublet in the *fabrica* (*Fabaceae*) family that has been cultivated in gardens for many years. Lessertia frutescens is found in the dry parts of southern Africa. It is found in the Western Cape and up the west coast as far north as Namibia and into Botswana, as well as in the western Karoo and the Eastern Cape including the Mpumalanga and KwaZulu-Natal provices [36]. It is distinguished by its silvery-gray leaves and loose clusters of luminous coral-red pea-shaped flowers that bloom from spring to mid-summer (**Figure 9**) [37]. It is drought-tolerant and prefers well-drained soil. The shrub is native to South Africa and is used to treat illnesses such as cancer, tuberculosis, diabetes, and associated symptoms of HIV/AIDS [38].

The shrub is commonly called Xhoza (Umnwele), English (cancer bush), and Afrokaans (kanerbossie, eendjies, ganbossie) [5]. *Lessertia frutescens* (previously *Sutherlandia frutescens*) is well-known for its medicinal properties, interesting balloon-like fruit capsules and incredibly bitter taste. The shrub became famously known as the 'cancer bush' alludes to its reputation as a potential cure for cancer in South Africa. Although there was no scientific report to support for Lessertia as a cure for cancer as alluded by traditional healers, later there was a proven to boost the immune system and activate the body's resources to combat disease and mental and physical stress of daily life [37].

Traditional healers collect stems, leaves, flowers, and seeds which are then dried, then decoctions from each is administered orally to treat internal cancers. In the case of external cancers decoctions prepared from this shrub are applied topically until the patient is cured [5]. Other traditional healers collect fresh plant materials, dry them, and then stamp or mash them into powder between two stones, as this tradition is practiced by various ethnic groups. The preparation is then typically infused in hot or boiling water, allowed to cool before being administered to the sick person [15, 39, 40].

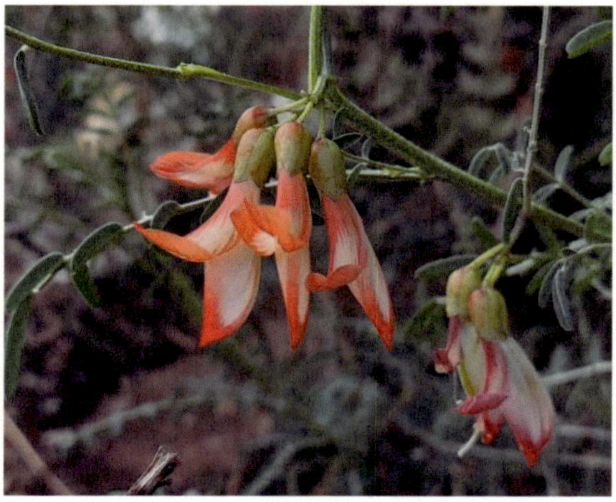

Figure 9.
Lassertia frutescense *https://candide.com/ZA/plants/eaabf98455d9bdfef9c454fdb2d06f99*.

There is scientific evidence that the phenolic, flavonoid, alkaloid, and saponin contents of extracts of in vitro leaves, field leaves, and seeds of the leguminous plant *L. frutescens* were quantified using spectrophotometric and gravimetric methods. Saponins were found to be more abundant in in vitro leaves than in field leaves and seeds, followed by phenolics, flavonoids, and alkaloids. The extracts were also qualitatively examined to determine the presence of additional phytochemicals of medicinal interest. Tannins, phlobatannins, and cardiac glycosides were found in this qualitative analysis [39]. This study clarified and added to the body of knowledge because it is critical for our traditional healers to understand which parts of the shrub contain a variety of ingredients. Another scientific study discovered that our forefathers could even distinguish which decoctions to prepare based on the type of disease indicated by the patient [15]. Other studies reported that the traditional healers prepare this shrub by using its leaves, flowers, stems, and roots to treat various ailments [40]. Furthermore, more studies done globally supported the benefit of this plant in the treatment of cancer and most importantly it was found to induce cell death (apoptosis) and was also reported nontoxic by the different scientific [41–50]. Both the sciences and indigenous knowledge contributed to the identification an honored this plant by calling it cancer bush.

3.8 *Pittosporum viridiflorum Sims*

P. viridiflorum, a *Pittosporaceae* family member, is found throughout the eastern half of South Africa (Eastern, P. viridiflorum, a Pittosporaceae family member, is found throughout the eastern half of South Africa (Eastern), from the Western Cape up into tropical Africa and beyond to Arabia and India [51]. *P. viridiflorum* can grow from a small shrub to a large forest tree up to 30 m tall. The bark is pale brown to grayish, with distinct white dots (lenticels). It has glossy, dark green leaves that are typically wider above the center. In early summer (November to December), small, greenish white, sweetly scented flowers bloom [51]. Following them are small yellow-brown seed capsules. When the capsules are broken open, a slew of small, shiny, orange-red seeds emerge, each encased in a sticky, resinous exudate (**Figure 10**). This cheese wood is frequently confused with white milkwood [51].

The vernacular plant among South African ethnic groups are Southern Sotho (Sesotho) (Mosetlela), Afrikaans (Witboekenhout, Kaarsuur, Bosbeukenhout,

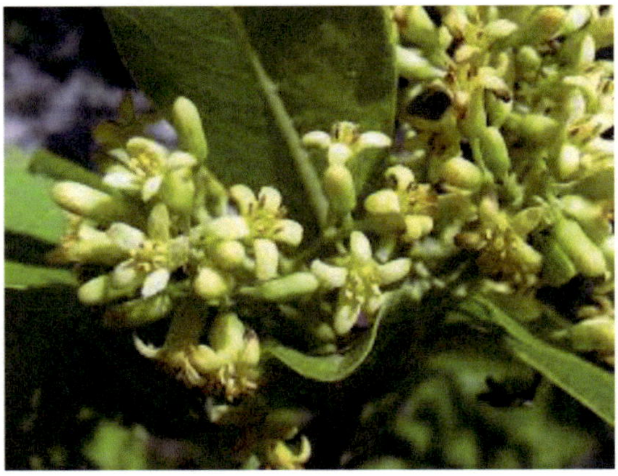

Figure 10.
Pittosporum viridiflorum Sims - http://pza.sanbi.org/pittosporum-viridiflorum.

Bosboekenhout Kersuurboom, Kasuur), English (cheesewood, Umkwenkwe, White Cape Beech), Northern Sotho (Kgalagangwe), Tswana (Mpustinya-poqo, Nkasur), Venda (Mulondwane, Mutanzwakhamelo), Zulu (umfusamvu, Umkhwenkwe, Umphushamvu Umphushane, Umvusamvu), Xhoza (Umgqwengqwe, Umkhwenkwe [52].

Traditionally the root or bark decoctions are administered orally in the Eastern Cape province [5]. Another scientific study has reported that the bitter taste and strong resinous or liquorice smell bark is used medicinally, and it possess positive anticancer activity against human prostate cancer [53]. Dried, powdered root or bark is sometimes added to beer as an aphrodisiac [5]. Traditional healers should practice great caution when using this plant, *P. viridiflorum* has been scientifically found to have moderate to significant toxicity against cancer cells in the laboratory [54–56]. A similar kind of toxicity was observed scientifically when tested Swiss mice study which ranged from low toxicity on bark to killing of the mices in 24 hours by leaf extract [56, 57].

3.9 *Knowltonia capensis (L.) Huth*

Knowltonia capensis (L.) Huth is a slow-growing, stemless perennial herb that grows between 300 and 500 mm tall and belongs to the *Ranunculaceae* family. Flowers are made up of colored sepals rather than petals (this distinguishes it from Ranunculus). In winter and spring, it has a 450 mm long flowering stem with a compound umbel of creamy-green flowers (from June to September). These are followed by fruits, which are small, fleshy berries in dense clusters that are green when ripe and turn black when fully ripe. There is a short rhizome with fleshy roots (**Figure 11**). The tooth-edged, basal leaves are distinctive, being tough, coarse, and leathery in texture. They are usually trifoliately compound, that is, divided into three distinct leaflets, with the middle leaflet being slightly larger than the two on the side. *Anemone knowltonia* is found in coastal bush and forested kloofs and grows along forest margins. This plant is most common in East London, from which it spreads eastward to the KwaZulu-Natal midlands and westward to the Cape Peninsula. Because it has a rhizome, it will most likely be able to withstand frost, and due to its wide distribution range, it can withstand both high and low rainfall [58].

Traditionally healers collect and dry the corms, this normally followed by crushing the corms which will be taken orally with water to treat cancer or in the form of

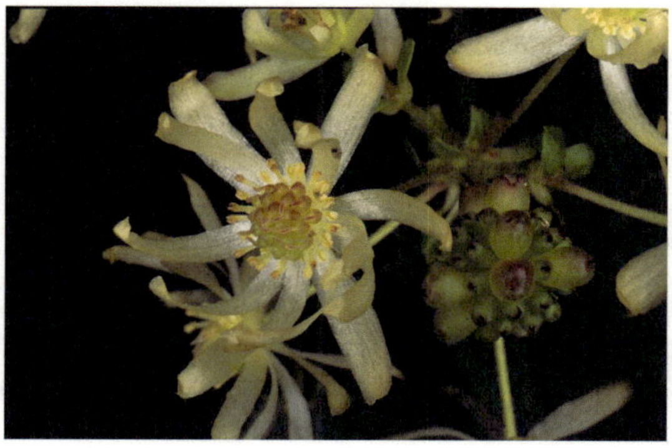

Figure 11.
Knowltonia capensis (L.) Huth-http://pza.sanbi.org/knowltonia-capensis-0.

decoction until the patient is cured [5]. There is no scientific study reported toxicity related to cancer cells on this plant thus far.

3.10 *Celtis Africana Burm.f*

Agapanthus-africanus Celtis Africana is a deciduous shrub or a tree with a spreading crown belong to the family *Ulmacea*. It can grow up to 30 metres tall, rarely to 40 metres. The straight, cylindrical bole can be free of branches for up to 15 metres, though it is often low branching. It is up to 90 cm in diameter, often slightly fluted but usually without buttresses (**Figure 12**) [59].

The common ethnic groups once included Sesotho (modutu, mohatakhomo, modutu, mothibadifate, Northern Sotho (mothibadifate), English (White Stinkwood), Afrikaans (Witstinkhout), Xhosa (umthuma, itunga, mumvumvu), Zulu (Usinga, lwesalukazi), Venda (mpopano), Tswana (modutu) [5].

Traditionally healers collect roots of this plants and sun-dry them, upon confirmation of dryness the aqueous or milk infusion is prepared for the patient can drink until cancer is cure [5]. Studies done on toxicity in the laboratory (*in-vitro*) showed low toxicity to be in general of this plant and no animals (*in-vivo*) reports found in general of this plant.

3.11 Recommended daily use, risk and contraindication of the following herbs used in rural area of South Africa

Most of these plants' extracts are traditionally used daily ranging from 4 teaspoons every morning, a ¼ cup and a 1 cup daily depending on what the traditional healer recommends. There is no specific rule and concentration determined as most are prepared by boiling to a color change in 2 liters of water [59].

3.11.1 Agapanthus-africanus (L)

South African Xhosa tribes revere the *Agapanthus-africanus* for its magical powers according to their indigenous knowledge. *Agapanthus-africanus* is brewed and consumed by pregnant women in their third trimester to help with birth, in the belief

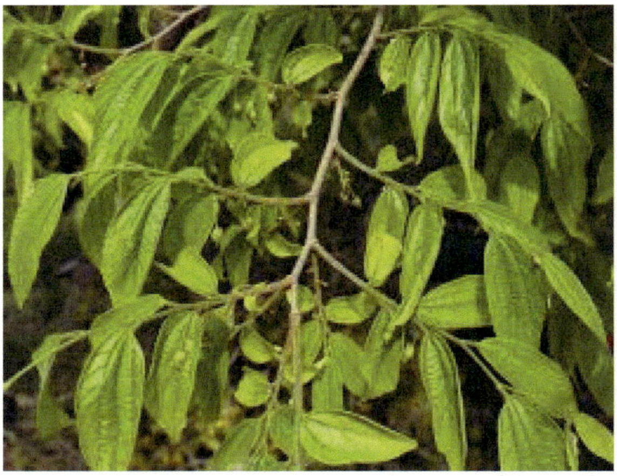

Figure 12.
Celtis Africana Burm.f-*http://pza.sanbi.org/celtis-africana.*

that this will make the child strong and healthy, the newborn is further bathed in a similar concoction on the first day.

The Zulu nation, culturally use *Agapanthus-africanus* to treat flue, paralysis, heart conditions, coughs, chest problems (such as tightness or pains), tired feet (when the plaited leaves are applied as a bandage to the feet) and colds. Significantly, the *Agapanthus-africanus* (including the roots) is considered poisonous to humans, making all these applications rather intriguing given the associated risk [60].

If the clear sticky sap is ingested, symptoms may include nausea, vomiting, abdominal pain, and diarrhea, as well as severe mouth ulceration. When the sap comes into contact with your skin, it can cause burning, irritation, and rashes [61].

3.11.2 Solanum aculeastrum Dunal

S. aculeastrum. Dunal (Solanaceae) is used in traditional medicine to treat various human and animal diseases, specifically stomach disorders and various cancers, in the Eastern Cape, South Africa [11].

A scientific study found that the medicinal use of these plant, on the other hand, poses significant health risks [62]. Berry extracts were nephrotoxic, hepatotoxic, haematotoxic, and fatal at higher doses, according to research into the plant's safety. Another source of concern about the plant's safety is its extracts' non-selectivity in inhibiting carcinoma, actively dividing and un-dividing cells [62, 63]. The effect of processing on the efficacy and safety of the berry as a herbal IV remedy yielded conflicting results [62, 63]. The extract's anti-inflammatory and analgesic activity appeared to improve with processing while its cytotoxic potential appeared to decrease. However, processed extracts were found to be less toxic than fresh extracts. Effect of processing on the efficacy and safety of *Solanum Aculeastrum Dunal* berries [62, 63].

Another study performed on the risk assessment found that the overall changes in biochemical parameters caused by the various extracts of *S. aculeastrum* berries at the different doses suggested that the normal functioning of these organs may be compromised. However, drying and boiling the berries may reduce their toxicity [13]. That is why is important for the indigenous knowledge people need to improve their understanding on the safeness of this plant and it less toxic dose.

3.11.3 Leonotis leonurus (L.) R. Br

The study done on male rats as part of the clinical trisls found that the effects of the aqueous extract of *L. leonurus* leaves on hematological, liver, and kidney functional indices suggest that the extract has parameter and dose-selective effects and will have consequences on the normal functioning of the animals' blood system, kidney, and liver [17]. When consumed daily for 21 days at the low doses, the extract is also unlikely to predispose the animals to cardiovascular risk. As a result, the aqueous extract of *L. leonurus* leaves was not 'safe' as an oral remedy in male rats [17]. High level of caution should be practised when traditional healers used and recommend this herb to their people.

3.11.4 Hypoxis argentea Harv. Ex baker

The study done on *Hypoxis argentea* Harv. ex Baker found that the acclaimed anti-diabetic effects of *H. argentea* could be mediated by its promotion of glucose utilization and preservation of pancreatic beta cell populations while preventing fat accumulation in adipocytes [64].

3.11.5 Euphorbia ingens E. Mey. Ex Boiss

If the latex from this tree is consumed, it can cause severe skin irritation, blindness, and severe illness in both humans and animals. If used correctly, it can be used as a purgative or to treat ulcers. The Basotho and Venda people in South Africa are said to use it as a cancer cure [65].

3.11.6 Raphionacme hirsuta (E. Mey.) R.a. dyer

Raphionacme hirsuta (E. Mey.) R.A. Dyer and Cheilanthes contracta have been used in African anticancer medicines. In some rodent test-systems, extracts of these plants demonstrated antitumor activity [32]. While the tuberous roots are used in the production of alcoholic beverages, the plant is also said to be poisonous [66].

3.11.7 Lassertia frutescense (L.)

Traditionally, S. frutescens has been used to treat fever, wounds, cancer, diabetes, kidney and liver problems, rheumatism, and stomach ailments [67]. *Sutherlandia capsules are commercially available and have been used with apparent positive clinical results in two health facilities in Kwazulu-Natal and the Northern Cape for outpatients living with AIDS* [68].

The safety efficacy of *Lassertia frutescense* was tested on healthy adults, and the results revealed no significant differences in general adverse events, cardiovascular, central nervous system, gastrointestinal tracts, infection, allergy, malaise, or most physical, hematological, biochemical, or physiological parameters ($P > 0.05$). Subjects who consumed *L. frutescens*, on the other hand, reported greater appetite than those in the placebo group (P0.01). Although the treatment group had a lower respiratory rate (P0.04), a higher platelet count (P0.03), MCH (P0.01), MCHC (P0.02), total protein (P0.03), and albumin levels (P0.03) than the placebo group, these differences were within the normal physiological range and were not clinically significant [69]. Canavanine, an *L. frutescens* biomarker, was undetectable in subject plasma. In general, healthy adults tolerated 800 mg/day *L. frutescens* leaf powder capsules well [69]. This indicate that *Lassertia frutescense* can be safely used for human consumption with no adverse events on the patients.

3.11.8 Pittosporum viridiflorum Sims

P. viridiflorum Sims was discovered in a scientific study to be used in traditional medicine to treat tuberculosis, inflammatory disorders, wounds, veterinary ailments, gastrointestinal, sexually transmitted diseases, kidney, circulatory, and malaria. [70]. Toxicological effects have also been reported from this species, that's why safety should be carefully considered when using this herb. Compound(s) with antimalarial, anticancer and acaricidal properties have been isolated from *P. viridiflorum* [70]. There is enough scientific evidence on pharmacological and phytochemical properties of *P. viridiflorum* which gives credibility to the use of this plant species against various diseases in African traditional medicine [70].

3.11.9 Knowltonia capensis (L.) Huth

It was found that when fresh leaves and roots are eaten, a white crystalline compound which is enzymatically changed to a highly toxic oil with an acrid taste that produces the blistering [71]. Traditionally the smoke from burning leaves is inhaled for headaches [71]. These plants' leaf poultices are commonly used in traditional medicine to treat wounds, external cancers, and rheumatism. To relieve toothache, the roots of *Anemone knowltonia* can be applied directly [71].

3.11.10 Celtis Africana Burm.f

The bark extracts of *Celtis Africana Burm.f* have been used as pain-killers, fabrifuges, and during malnutrition, while the leaf extracts was used for the treatment of the eyes infection and pulmonary troubles [72].

Medicinal plant remedies play an important role not only in the treatment of cancer, but also in the treatment of chronic ailments such as hypertension and many others by lay people in rural South Africa. A clear scientific report suggests that there must be awareness on the risks associated with the concurrent use of conventional medication and medicinal plants. Even though this chapter brought both sciences and tradition knowledge together, there is a clear need to educate health practitioners and patients about the potential risks of using both prescribed western drugs and medicinal plants to avid contraindication [73].

4. Conclusions

This chapter brings together traditional knowledge and science to discuss how indigenous plants are widely utilized in South Africa to treat cancer and diseases associated to cancer. The chapter acknowledges the contribution of indigenous knowledge to the body of knowledge to dispel the misconception that African epistemologies are less developed. When the hard sciences and soft social indigenous knowledges are combined, the vertical and horizontal knowledge become less mysterious and less colonized. The plants are common in the many climatic regions of the nation; some are drought-resistant plants that thrive in the provinces of the Western, Eastern, and Northern Cape as well as some parts of KwaZulu-Natal, with differing chemical and genetic compositions in each of these geographical locations. Extensive scientific research is being conducted on the safety, quality, and efficacy of this medicinal plant to validate traditional claims, identify bioactive constituents, and conduct clinical trials. This has created a unique situation in which traditional knowledge and science meet to provide insight into these popular plants as well as safety advice to traditional healers. The chapter demonstrated the relationship between science and indigenous knowledge of traditional healers, local knowledge of people who care for the sick, product development, and the global innovation agenda as it relates to these plants. This chapter demonstrates that there is a growing understanding of phytomedicine and traditional medicines that can potentially be used to treat cancer patients. In selecting plants for cancer treatment, our forefathers' innate knowledge demonstrated true predictions, and our traditional healers should also understand that not all plants and plant parts are safe for human consumption. This chapter demonstrated how a convergence of vertical hardcore sciences and horizontal non formal curriculum indigenous knowledge can contribute to a new decolonized world in which African pedagogies and transformation discourse in society will be permitted. Collaboration between traditional healers and scientists clearly improved understanding of the use, preparation, therapeutic potential, and pharmaceutical make-up of these medicinal plants in the treatment of cancer. In this way, traditional knowledge, and science meet in novel and unexpected ways.

Acknowledgements

I would like to acknowledge the Central University of Technology-Research Office UCDP Grant-for funding the publication.

The CUT Faculty of Health and Environmental Sciences assistance Dean's office: Prof T Makhafola for financial assistance.

The Family, colleagues, and Friends for encouragement.

Thanks to Dr. LF Mogongoa, SD Mokgawa, DE Rampana-Moleleki, D Mathiase, Dr. I Manduna, B Nakedi, A Molelekoa and M Motaung for proof-reading the manuscript and provide constructive comments.

Conflict of interest

The author declares no conflict of interest.

Author details

Pakiso Moses Makhoahle
Faculty of Health and Environmental Sciences, Department of Health Sciences, Biomedical Technology, Central University of Technology-Free State, Bloemfontein, South Africa

*Address all correspondence to: pmakhoahle@cut.ac.za

References

[1] Stats SA. (Statistical South Africa) Republic of South Africa. Available from: https://www.statssa.gov.za/publications/P0302/P03022021.pdf. [Accessed: September 1, 2022]

[2] South African gate way. The 11 languages of South Africa. Available from: https://southafrica-info.com/arts-culture/11-languages-south-africa/. [Accessed: September 1, 2022]

[3] Gideon OA, Ese O, Kola KA, Olanrewaju RO. Indigenous knowledge of herbal medicines among adolescents in Amassoma, Bayelsa state, Nigeria. Global Journal of Health Science. 2016;**8**(1):217-237

[4] *Agapanthus africanus* (L.) Hoffmanns. Available from: http://pza.sanbi.org/agapanthus-africanus. [Accessed: September 1, 2022]

[5] Koduru S, Grierson DS, Afolayan AJ. Ethnobotanical information of medicinal plants used for treatment of cancer in the eastern Cape Province, South Africa. Current Science. 2007;**92**(7):906-908

[6] Veale DJH, Havlik I, Oliver DW, Dekker TG. Pharmacological effects of Agapanthus africanus on the isolated rat uterus. Journal of Ethnopharmacology. 1999;**66**(3):257-262

[7] *Solanum-aculeastrum*. Available from: http://pza.sanbi.org/solanum-aculeastrum. [Accessed: September 14, 2022]

[8] Wanyonyi AW, Tarus PK, Chhabra SC. A novel glycosidic steroidal alkaloid from Solanum aculeastrum. Bulletin of the Chemical Society of Ethiopia. 2003;**17**(1):61-66

[9] Hutchings A, Scott AH, Lewis G, Cunningham A. Zulu Medicinal Plants. Pietermaritzburg: Natal University Press; 1996

[10] Koduru S, Grierson DS, Van de Venter M, Afolayan A. Anticancer activity of steroid alkaloids isolated from Solanum aculeastrum. Pharmaceutical Biology. 2008;**45**:613-618. DOI: 10.1080/13880200701538690

[11] Koduru S, Grierson DS, Afolayan AJ. Antimicrobial activity of Solanum aculeastrum. Pharmaceutical Biology. 2006;**44**(4):283-286. DOI: 0.1080/13880200600714145

[12] Laban LT, Anjili CO, Mutiso JM, Ingonga J, Kiige SG, Ngedzo MM, et al. Experimental therapeutic studies of Solanum aculeastrum Dunal. On Leishmania major infection in BALB/c mice. Iranian Journal of Basic Medical Sciences. 2015;**18**(1):64-71

[13] Aboyade OM, Yakubu MT, Grierson DS, Afolayan AJ. Studies on the toxicological effect of the aqueous extract of the fresh, dried and boiled berries of Solanum aculeastrum Dunal in male Wistar rats. Human & Experimental Toxicology. 2009;**28**(12):765-775

[14] Acocks JPH. Veld Types of South Africa, Edn 3. Memoirs of the Botanical Survey of South Africa. Vol. No. 57. Pretoria: Botanical Research Institute; 1988

[15] Thring TSA, Weitz FM. Medicinal plant use in the Bredasdorp/Elim region of the southern Overberg in the Western Cape Province of South Africa. Journal of Ethnopharmacology. 2006;**103**(2):261-275

[16] Tonis S, Okaiyeto K, Hoppe H, Leonard H, Mabinya V, Nwodo U, et al. Chemical constituents, antioxidant, and cytotoxicity properties of Leonotis leonurus used in the folklore management of neurological disorders in the eastern cape, South Africa. 3 Biotech. 2020;**10**:141. DOI: 10.10.1007/s13205-020-2126-5

[17] Oyedemi SO, Yakubu MT, Afolayan AJ. Effect of aqueous extract of Leonotis leonurus (L.) R. Br. Leaves in male Wistar rats. Human & experimental toxicology. 2010;**29**(5):377-384. DOI: 10.1177/0960327110363864), 10.1177/0960327110363864)

[18] Dlamini ML. Application of some Target Formulations of Active Herbal Plant Components in Reducing Animal Exposure to Mycotoxins and Associated Health Effects [Thesis]. South Africa: University of Johannesburg; 2015

[19] *Leonotis leonurus (L.) R. Br*, Plantzafrica information. Available from: http://pza.sanbi.org/. [Accessed: September 1, 2022]

[20] *Hypoxis argentea* Harv. ex Baker. Available from: http://redlist.sanbi.org/species.php?species=574-193. [Accessed: September 1, 2022]

[21] Sagbo IJ, Otang-Mbeng W. Plants used for the traditional Management of Cancer in the eastern Cape Province of South Africa: A review of ethnobotanical surveys, Ethnopharmacological studies and active phytochemicals. Molecules. 2021;**26**:4639. DOI: 10.3390/molecules26154639

[22] Pooley E. A Field Guide to Wildflowers of Kwa-Zulu Natal and the Easter Region-Exclusive Books. Flora Publications Trust; 1992. Available from: https://www.exclusivebooks.co.za/product/9780620215008. [Accessed: September 1, 2022]

[23] Coopoosamy RM, Naidoo KK. An ethnobotanical study of medicinal plants used by traditional healers in Durban, South Africa. African Journal of Pharmacy and Pharmacology. 2012;**6**:818-823. DOI: 10.5897/AJPP11.700

[24] Euphorbia-ingens. Available from: https://tropical.theferns.info/viewtropical.php?id=Euphorbia+ingens. [Accessed: September 4, 2022]

[25] Euphorbia-ingens. Available from: https://treesa.org/euphorbia-ingens. [Accessed: September 4, 2022]

[26] Semenya S, Maroyi A, Potgieter M, Erasmus L. Herbal medicines used by Bapedi traditional healers to treat reproductive ailments in the Limpopo Province, South Africa. African Journal of Traditional Complement Alternative Medicine AJTCAM. 2013;**10**:331-339

[27] Raphionacme-hirsuta. Available from: http://pza.sanbi.org/raphionacme-hirsuta. [Accessed: September 4, 2022]

[28] Raphionacme-hirsuta. Available from: https://wildflowernursery.co.za/indigenous-plant-database/raphionacme-hirsuta. [Accessed: September 9, 2022]

[29] Raphionacme-hirsuta. Available from: http://llifle.info/Encyclopedia/SUCCULENTS/Family/Asclepiadaceae/32918/Raphionacme_hirsuta. [Accessed: September 9, 2022]

[30] Raphionacme-hirsuta. Available from: 26#:~:text=Raphionacme%20hirsuta%20(E., R.A.Dyer&text=Common%20names%3A%20false%20gentian%2C%20khadi, umathangane%2C%20umathanjana%20(Zul.))

[31] Moteetee A, Wyk B-E. The medical ethnobotany of Lesotho: A review. Bothalia. 2011;**41**:209-228. DOI: 10.4102/abc. v41i1.52

[32] Alexander J. Charlson, antineoplastic constituents of some southern African plants. Journal of Ethnopharmacology. 1980;**2**(4):323-335. DOI: 10.1016/S0378-8741(80)81014-2

[33] Watt J, Breyer-Brandwijk M. The Medicinal and Poisonous Plants of Southern and Eastern Africa: Being an Account of their Medicinal and Other Uses, Chemical Composition, Pharmacological Effects and Toxicology in Man and Animal. 2nd ed. E. & S. Livingstone Ltd.; 1962. Available from: https://www.amazon.com/MEDICINAL-POISONOUS-Composition-Pharmacological-Toxicology/dp/B00CQRBAF4. [Accessed: September 1, 2022]

[34] Charlson AJ. Antineoplastic constituents of some southern African plants. Journal of Ethnopharmacology. 1980;**2**:323-335

[35] Raphionacme-hirsuta. Available from: https://www.operationwildflower.org.za/index.php/albums/bulbs/raphionacme-hirsuta-johannesburg-judd-7-9743. [Accessed: September 17, 2022]

[36] *Lassertia frutescense*. Available from: http://pza.sanbi.org›lessertia-frutescens. [Accessed: September 17, 2022]

[37] *Lassertia frutescense*. Available from: https://candide.com/ZA/plants/eaabf98455d9bdfef9c454fdb2d06f99. [Accessed: September 17, 2022]

[38] Oloyede O. Epistemological issues in the making of an African medicine: Sutherlandia Lessertia frutescens. African Sociological Review. 2010;**14**(2):74-88

[39] Shaik S, Singh N, Nicholas A. Comparison of the selected secondary metabolite content present in the cancer bush Lessertia (Sutherlandia) frutescens L. extracts. African Journal of Traditional, Complementary and Alternative Medicines. 2011;**8**(4):429-434

[40] Ngcobo M. The Biochemical Effects of Sutherlandia frutescens in Cultured H9 Cancerous T Cells and Normal Human T Lymphocytes [Thesis]. South Africa: Department of Physiology, University of KwaZulu-Natal; 2008

[41] Stander A, Marais S, Stivaktas V, Vorster C, Albrecht C, Lottering M-L, et al. In vitro effects of Sutherlandia frutescens water extracts on cell numbers, morphology, cell cycle progression and cell death in a tumorigenic and a non-tumorigenic epithelial breast cell line. Journal of Ethnopharmacology. 2009;**124**:45-60. DOI: 10.1016/j.jep.2009.04.013

[42] Steenkamp V, Gouws M. Cytotoxicity of six south African medicinal plant extracts used in the treatment of cancer. South African Journal of Botany. 2006;**72**:630-633. DOI: 10.1016/J.SAJB.2006.02.004

[43] De Caires SG. An Investigation of the Immunomodulatory Properties of Sutherlandia Frutescens and Hypoxis Hemerocallidea [Thesis]. South Africa: University of Pretoria; 2011

[44] Chinkwo KA. Sutherlandia frutescens extracts can induce apoptosis in cultured carcinoma cells. Journal of Ethnopharmacology. 2005;**98**:163-170. DOI: 10.1016/j.jep.2005.01.016

[45] Ntuli SS, Gelderblom WC, Katerere DR. The mutagenic and antimutagenic activity of Sutherlandia frutescens extracts and marker compounds. BMC Compl. Alternative Med. 2018;**18**(1):93

[46] Korb VC, Moodley D, Chuturgoon AA. Apoptosis-promoting effects of

Sutherlandia frutescens extracts on normal human lymphocytes in vitro. South African Journal of Science. 2010;**106**(1-2):64-69

[47] Chen L, Xu M, Gong Z, Zonyane S, Xu S, Makunga NP. Comparative cardio and developmental toxicity induced by the popular medicinal extract of Sutherlandia frutescens (L.) R. Br. Detected using a zebrafish Tuebingen embryo model. BMC Complementary Alternative Medicine. 2018;**18**(1):273

[48] Zonyane S, Chen L, Xu MJ, Gong ZN, Xu S, Makunga NP. Geographicbased metabolomic variation and toxicity analysis of Sutherlandia frutescens LR Br.–an emerging medicinal crop in South Africa. Industrial Crops and Products. 2019;**133**:414-423

[49] Johnson Q, Syce J, Nell H, Rudeen K, Folk WR. A randomized, double-blind, placebo-controlled trial of Lessertia frutescens in healthy adults. PLoS Clinical Trials. 2007;**2**(4):e16

[50] Van Wyk BE, Albrecht C. A review of the taxonomy, ethnobotany, chemistry and pharmacology of Sutherlandia frutescens (Fabaceae). Journal of Ethnopharmacology. 2008;**119**:620-629. DOI: 10.1016/j.jep.2008.08.003

[51] Pittosporum-viridiflorum. Available from: http://pza.sanbi.org/pittosporum-viridiflorum. [Accessed: September 1, 2022]

[52] *Pittosporum viridiflorum Sims*. Available from: http://redlist.sanbi.org/species.php?species=3479-11[Accessed: September 1, 2022]

[53] Nyongbela KD, Lannang AM, Ayimele GA, Ngemenya MN, Bickle Q, Efange S. Isolation and identification of an antiparasitic triterpenoid estersaponin from the stem bark of Pittosporum mannii (Pittosporaceae). Asian Pacific Journal of Tropical Disease. 2013;**3**:389-392. DOI: 10.1016/S2222-1808(13)60089-4

[54] Otang WM, Grierson DS, Ndip RN. Cytotoxicity of three south African medicinal plants using the Chang liver cell line. African Journal of Traditional, Complementary Alternative Medicine. 2014;**11**(2):324-329

[55] Elisha IL, Dzoyem J-P, Botha FS, Eloff JN. The efficacy and safety of nine south African medicinal plants in controlling bacillus anthracis Sterne vaccine strain. BMC Complementary Alternative Medicine. 2016;**16**:5-12. DOI: 10.1186/s12906-015-0980-1

[56] Muthaura CN, Rukunga GM, Chhabra SC, Omar SA, Guantai AN, Gathirwa JW, et al. Antimalarial activity of some plants traditionally used in Meru district of Kenya. Physiotherapy Research. 2007;**21**:860-867. DOI: 10.1002/ptr.2170

[57] Otang WM, Grierson DS, Ndip N. Assessment of potential toxicity of three south African medicinal plants using the brine shrimp (Artemia salina) assay. African Journal of Pharmacy and Pharmacology. 2013;**7**(20):1272-1279

[58] Anemone-knowltonia. Available from: http://pza.sanbi.org/anemone-knowltonia. [Accessed: September 18, 2022]

[59] Ndhlala AR, Stafford GI, Finnie JF, Van Staden J. Commercial herbal preparations in KwaZulu-Natal, South Africa: The urban face of traditional medicine. South African Journal of Botany. 2011;**77**(4):830-843. DOI: 10.1016/j.sajb.2011.09.002

[60] Agapanthus. Available from: https://www.sa-venues.com/plant-life/agapanthus.php. [Accessed: October 20, 2022]

[61] Agapanthus. Available from: https://www.childrens.health.qld.gov.au/poisonous-plant-agapanthus/#:~:text=Other%3A%20All%20parts%20of%20the,from%20the%20clear%20sticky%20sap. [Accessed: October 20, 2022]

[62] Mayode AO. Effect of Processing on the Efficacy and Safety of Solanum Aculeastrum Dunal Berries [thesis]. South Africa: University of Fort Hare; 2009

[63] Solanum Aculeastrum Dunal berries. Available from: http://vital.seals.ac.za:8080/vital/access/manager/Repository/vital:11302?site_name=GlobalView. [Accessed: October 20, 2022]

[64] Akinrinde A, Koekemoer T, Venter MV, Bradley G. In vitro investigation of potential anti-diabetic activity of the corm extract of Hypoxis Argentea Harv. Ex baker. Acta Pharmaceutica. 2018;**68**(4):389-407. DOI: 10.2478/acph-2018-0023

[65] Euphorbia-ingens. Available from: http:/pza.sanbi.org/euphorbia-ingens. [Accessed: October 20, 2022]

[66] Raphionacme-hirsuta. Available from: https://www.operationwildflower.org.za/index.php/albums/bulbs/raphionacme-hirsuta-johannesburg-judd-7-9743. [Accessed: October 20, 2022]

[67] Gibson D. Ambiguities in the making of an African medicine: Clinical trials of Sutherlandia frutescens (L.) R. Br 1 (Lessertia frutescens). African Sociological Review. 2011;**15**(1):124-137

[68] Gericke N. Sutherlandia and AIDS patients. Australian Journal of Med Herbalism. 2001;**13**(1):17-189

[69] A Safety Study of Lessertia Frutescens in Adults. Available from: https://clinicaltrials.gov/ct2/show/NCT00376415. [Accessed: September 20, 2022]

[70] Madikizela B, Mcgaw L. Pittosporum viridiflorum Sims (Pittosporaceae): A review on a useful medicinal plant native to South Africa and tropical Africa. Journal of Ethnopharmacology. 2017;**205**:217-230. DOI: 10.1016/j.jep.2017.05.005

[71] Anemone-knowltonia. Available from: [Accessed: October 20, 2022]

[72] Anemone-knowltonia. Available from https://plants.jstor.org/stable/10.5555/al.ap.upwta.5_376. [Accessed: October 20, 2022]

[73] de Wet H, Ramulondi M, Ngcobo ZN. The use of indigenous medicine for the treatment of hypertension by a rural community in northern Maputaland. South Africa, South African Journal of Botany. 2016;**103**:78-88. DOI: 10.1016/j.sajb.2015.08.011

Chapter 11

Nutritional Values and Therapeutical Effects of Mediterranean Herbs, Spices, and Medicinal Plants

Anita Trajkovska-Broach and Anka Trajkovska Petkoska

Abstract

This chapter highlights the traditional use of Mediterranean edible plants, frequently used as herbs and spices in Mediterranean cuisine, and medicinal plants, used as natural therapeutics among the people in the Mediterranean region. The high phytonutrient content and diversity of these edible and nonedible wild plants in the Mediterranean are emphasized and their folk use is reviewed. The herbs, spices, and medicinal plants are vital constituents of the Mediterranean dietary pattern and lifestyle, known as the Mediterranean diet (MD). They significantly contribute to high antioxidant and anti-inflammatory character of the diet and its health and well-being benefits.

Keywords: herbs, spices, medicinal plants, bioactive compounds, Mediterranean diet

1. Introduction

In the 70s and 80s of the last century, the western world embraced low-fat, energy-dense, and calorie-counting diets; however, obesity, metabolic syndrome, and other noncommunicable diseases (NCDs) were on rise. Strong scientific evidence has linked the disorders related to metabolic syndrome and cardiovascular diseases, as well as the risks for many types of cancer and other diseases, to unhealthy diets and lifestyles besides genetics and other factors [1, 2]. To address the question if the most pressing diseases of modern society could be overcome by adopting traditional diets, many researchers studied the nutritive attributes and the health benefits of traditional diets and found that using raw (or less-processed) nutrient-dense food choices, like those consumed in the traditional diets, could improve the human health and well-being. In other words, the research proved that it is possible to live as Hippocrates said many years ago, "*Let food be thy medicine and medicine be thy food*" [3–6].

Mediterranean diet (MD) is one of the traditional diets that has attracted the attention of the scientific and medical community worldwide. MD is a nutrient-packed, mainly plant-based dietary pattern, emphasizing consumption of minimally-processed seasonal fruits and vegetables, whole grains, nuts, legumes, and seeds, followed by moderate consumption of fish, poultry, fermented dairy products, and extra virgin olive oil (EVOO) as the main source of healthy fats, while the consumption of processed red meat products and refined sugars is limited. In addition, plenty of water, fruit juices, herb teas, and soups are also frequently consumed, and a moderate amount of red wine is usually taken with the meals.

People adhering to MD have been associated with a reduced risk of developing chronic diseases, including cancer, metabolic syndrome (obesity), depression, and cardiovascular and neurodegenerative diseases, as well as better cognitive health and increased longevity [7–9]. MD is also one of the most sustainable diets in the world and easy to follow outside the Mediterranean region. MD, if adopted widely, could reduce the high carbon footprint due to the current production of processed food and foods of animal origin, could lead to zero hunger and could lower the burden of noncommunicable and other "modern" diseases [10, 11].

When MD was originally promoted in the form of the Mediterranean diet pyramid, the herbs and the spices, often consumed within this dietary pattern, did not get their fair share. Years later, with the new proposed Mediterranean diet pyramids, herbs and spices were included and recognized to play an important role in Mediterranean cuisine and lifestyle. Examples of a diet pyramid and a lifestyle pyramid along with the MD health benefits are given in **Figure 1**. As reported before [8], the socializing aspect of MD, that is, the set of lifestyle habits and behaviors of the people in the Mediterranean, such as preparation and consumption of food together with family and friends, daily physical and leisure activities, festivities, the conviviality (the sense of being a part of the community), and adequate rests, are distinct features of the Mediterranean way of living, and are responsible for the health benefits. Furthermore, the regions around the Mediterranean sea are characterized by high biodiversity of plants, which have a long tradition of being used as herbs and spices in traditional Mediterranean cuisines, but also in folk medicine to treat different ailments and injuries. Due to the unique region's climate and geography, such as high mountains and coastal areas, some of the herbs, spices, and medicinal plants are indigenous, and some are even endemic, while some of them have been introduced in the region by the people migration, by trade activities and/or by the region's occupation by other nations.

In this chapter, Mediterranean herbs, spices, and medicinal plants will be presented with an emphasis on their diversity and richness with bioactive components. In particular, the objectives of this study are as follows: to highlight the knowledge about the traditional Mediterranean edible and medicinal plants, often used as herbs, spices, and remedies for different ailments; to contribute toward the preservation of this traditional knowledge; to inspire the readers to search for their roots, heritage, and folk wisdom; and to encourage those involved in botanical and medical research to look closely in specific Mediterranean plants, which might help in the development of natural-based treatments for various injuries and diseases.

2. Mediterranean herbs and spices

Herbs and spices have been used for both, culinary and medicinal purposes, since the beginning of human history. They have been used mainly for food and beverage flavoring and coloring, but also for food preservation. The wide use of some herbs and spices as remedies to treat different ailments has been most likely due to their high

DOI: http://dx.doi.org/10.5772/intechopen.108838

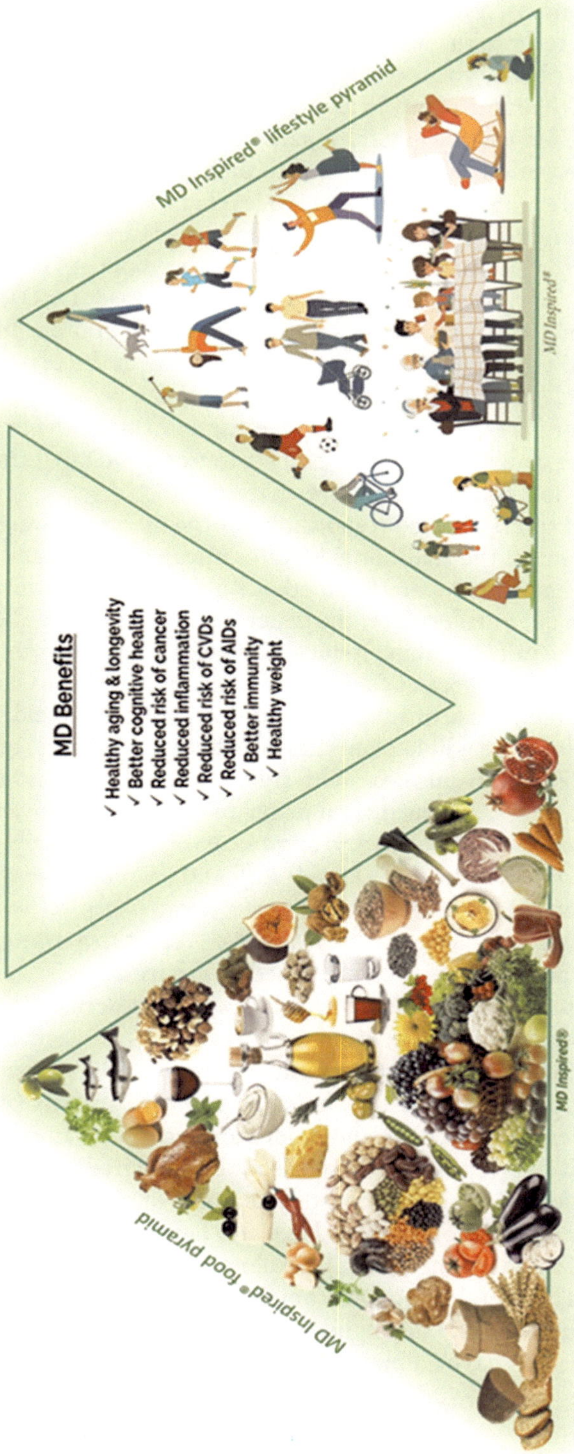
MD Inspired® lifestyle pyramid
MD Inspired®
MD Benefits
✓ Healthy aging & longevity
✓ Better cognitive health
✓ Reduced risk of cancer
✓ Reduced inflammation
✓ Reduced risk of CVDs
✓ Reduced risk of AIDs
✓ Better immunity
✓ Healthy weight
MD Inspired® food pyramid
MD Inspired®

Figure 1.
MD inspired® food and lifestyle pyramids with the associated health benefits.

content of various bioactive compounds, such as phenylpropanoids, terpenes, isoflavones, flavonoids, and anthocyanins [2, 12–14].

Herbs usually refer to the leafy parts of the plant, while spices are derived from other parts of the plants, viz. roots, stems, bulbs, barks, or seeds. Herbs and spices may derive from the same plant; in any case, both represent highly-concentrated sources of phytochemicals. The traditional MD emphasizes a high consumption of wild greens, spices, and herbs, which due to their high content of polyphenols and other bioactive, are responsible for the high level of dietary antioxidants consumed by the people adhering to the MD. Some herbs and spices are being categorized as functional foods (or nutraceuticals) yielding health properties beyond basic nutrition, like reduction of the risks related to cardiovascular disease (CVD), cancer, obesity, diabetes, Alzheimer's disease, etc. [15, 16]. Moreover, the borderline between herbs, spices, and remedies, sometimes, is not obvious; some of the plants, like the *Allium* family (viz. garlic, onion, leek, shallots, and chives) can be used in all these categories, as a whole plant or part of it. These bioactive components in the herbs and spices used in the MD are also contributing to the two attributes of MD that this diet is known for —its antioxidant and anti-inflammatory character.

The herbs and spices are also responsible for the unique character, flavorful taste, and excellent aroma of the traditional Mediterranean dishes in addition to the raw ingredients used and the preparation methods utilizing minimum cooking, in mainly, extra-virgin olive oil. Furthermore, the generous use of herbs and spices in MD, also replaces part of the salt, and thus, reduces the sodium intake in those adhering to the MD. In addition, the plethora of flavors and tastes of MD dishes contribute to the feeling of satiety (i.e., sense of fullness), and thus, yield less incidents of over-eating.

In the text below, the edible plants, such as herbs and spices, often used in traditional Mediterranean cuisine and lifestyle are described. A nonexclusive list of the most used herbs, spices, and medicinal plants in the Mediterranean region is given below: *garlic, onion, leek, mint, parsley, oregano, basil, rosemary, thyme, dill, fennel, marjoram, rosemary, lavender, bay (laurel) leaf, sage, cumin, paprika, hot (chili) pepper, coriander, marjoram, purslane, nettle, cinnamon, clove, ginger, saffron, chamomile, linden, dandelion, calendula, lavender, St. John's Wort, echinacea, chicory, milk thistle, red clove, and others.* Some of them are presented in **Figure 2**.

Due to their importance, *Allium* vegetables will be described in more detail. *Allium* vegetables are frequently used in Mediterranean cuisine as vegetables, but also as herbs and flavoring spices. The genus includes approx. 500 species among which are onions (*A. cepa*), garlic (*A. sativum*), leeks (*A. porrum*), shallots (*A. ascalonicum*), and chives (*A. schoenoprasum*). Garlic and onions are accounted among the oldest cultivated plants in the world; they both are also the key ingredients in the Mediterranean dietary pattern yielding the specific taste and aroma of many traditional savory dishes. From ancient times, garlic and onions have also been used for preparation of numerous remedies in folk medicine [16–18]. Shallots, which are closely related to onions, are characterized by their less pungent onion flavor, while scallions are also referred as green onions. The chives are distinguished by their edible green parts with mild onion flavor, while the leeks have edible green leaf sheaths and white flesh with a characteristic flavor.

Allium vegetables are rich in various bioactive constituents, including organosulfur compounds, flavonoids, saponins, and many other polyphenol compounds, with a spectrum of biological activities, including antimicrobial, antihypertensive, antidiabetic, and anticarcinogenic effects, among others. A summary of the nutrients, vitamins, and minerals in the *Allium* vegetables is given in **Tables 1–3**

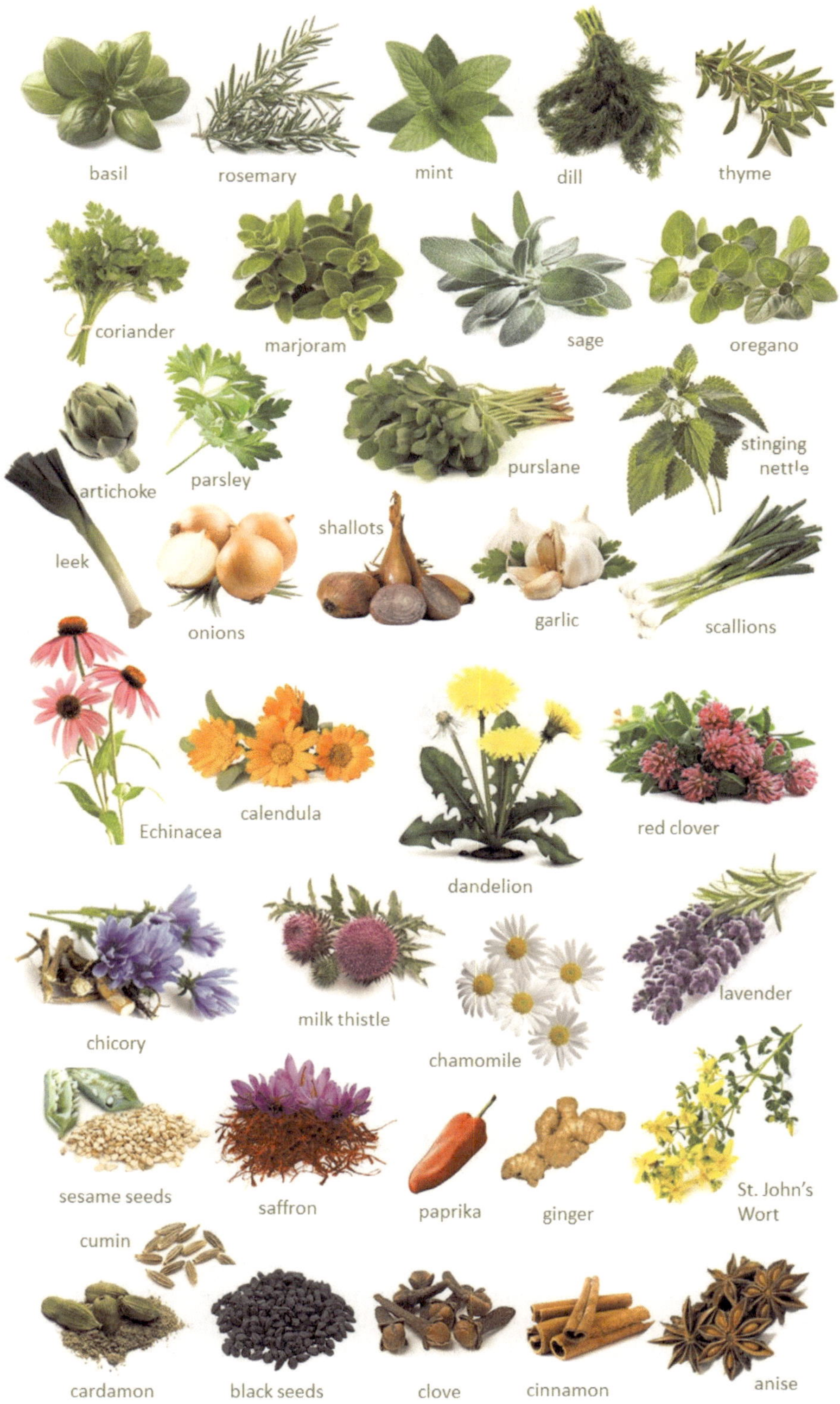

Figure 2.
Herbs, spices, and medicinal plants are often used in the Mediterranean region.

	Garlic	Onions	Leeks	Chives	Shallots
Total lipids [g]	0.5	0.1	0.3	0.7	0.1
Total sugars [g]	1.0	4.2	3.9	1.9	7.9
Proteins [g]	6.4	1.1	1.5	3.3	2.5
Dietary fibers [9]	2.1	1.7	1.8	2.5	3.2

Table 1.
Nutritional value of several allium *genus per 100 g [19].*

	Garlic	Onions	Leeks	Chives	Shallots
Calcium [mg]	181.0	23.0	59.0	92.0	37.0
Magnesium [mg]	25.0	10.0	28.0	42.0	21.0
Potassium [mg]	401	146	180	296	334
Zinc [mg]	1.2	0.2	0.1	0.6	0.4
Phosphorus [mg]	153	29	35	58	60
Iron [mg]	1.7	0.2	2.1	1.6	1.2

Table 2.
Minerals in several allium *genus per 100 g [19].*

	Garlic	Onions	Leeks	Chives	Shallots
Ascorbic acid [mg]	31.0	7.0	12.0	58.1	8.0
Vitamin B6 [mg]	1.235	0.12	0.233	0.138	0.345
Folate [μg]	3.0	19.0	64.0	105.0	34.0
Riboflavin [mg]	0.11	0.027	0.03	0.115	0.02
Niacin [mg]	0.70	0.116	0.400	0.647	0.200
Vitamin A [IU]	9.0	2.0	1.667	4.353	4.0
Vitamin E [mg]	0.1	0.0	0.9	0.2	0.0
Vitamin K [μg]	1.7	0.4	47.0	217.7	0.8 g

Table 3.
Vitamins in several allium *genus per 100 g [19].*

[18–22]. Low in fats and sugars, *Alliums* are rich sources of minerals, such as calcium, potassium, phosphorous, magnesium, and vitamins, for example, vitamin C and some of the *Alliums* are rich in vitamins B, K, and A.

The beneficial properties of the *Allium* genus are mainly attributed to the presence of a number of *organosulfur compounds*, such as alliin, allicin, dimethyl disulfide, methyl propenyl disulfide, propyl propenyl disulfide, dimethyl trisulfide, methyl propyl trisulfide, methyl propenyl trisulfide, S-methyl cysteine sulfoxide, S-propyl cysteine sulfoxide, S-propenyl cysteine sulfoxide, and N-γ(−glutamyl)-S-(E-1-propenyl) cysteine. Moreover, the characteristic flavors and odors of *Allium* vegetables arise from these sulfur-containing compounds [23, 24]. Several of the organosulfur compounds found in the *Alliums* are given in **Table 4**. Among numerous benefits, *Alliums* could affect many biological processes, which modify and reduce cancer risks [25–29]. In fact, it has been found that *Alliums* have effects on each stage

Compound	Chemical structure
Alliin	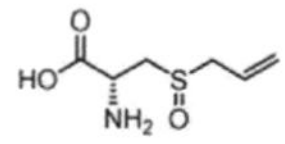
Allicin	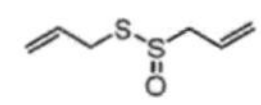
Diallyl sulfide	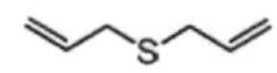
Diallyl disulfide	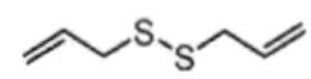
Diallyl trisulfide	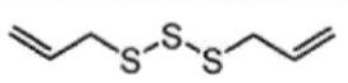
Allyl methyl sulfide	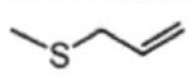
Ajoene	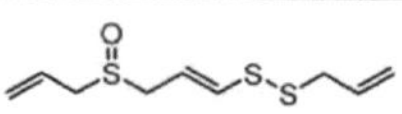

Table 4.
Organosulfur compounds in allium *vegetables.*

of carcinogenesis. As for many other *Alliums'* benefits, the anticancerogenic effects have been attributed mainly to the sulfur-containing, which besides the antimicrobial activities, contribute to reduced bioactivation of carcinogens. Among the protection against cancers and tumors, the most reported benefit of *Alliums* consumption has been related to gastric cancer. This is most likely because *Alliums* have shown inhibitory effects on the growth of *Helicobacter pylori; H. pylory* infection has been identified as one of the risk factors for gastric cancer [28, 30, 31]. The protective effects of *Allium* plants have been also reported against prostate and breast cancers [29]. The *Alliums*' organosulfur components have been also shown to inhibit several proinflammatory enzymes, such as cyclooxygenase and lipoxygenase [28].

Garlic (*Allium sativum* L.) is a bulbous plant, which is commonly used as a spice to add flavor not only in the Mediterranean but also in many other traditional cuisines around the globe. Like the other *Allium* plants, garlic is rich in organosulfur and polyphenolic compounds, both categories of compounds resulting in its strong antioxidant, anti-inflammatory, anticancerogenic, and other beneficial activities. The major garlic thiosulfinate produced is allicin (thio-2-propene-1-sulfinic acid S-allyl ester). Allicin and its oil-soluble metabolites are largely responsible for the garlic's odor. However, allicin is unstable and breaks down further to ajoene, vinyldithiins, and sulfides, including diallyl sulfide (DAS), diallyl disulfide (DADS), and diallyl trisulfide. Various sulfur compounds, including allicin, DAS, DADS, and ajoene derivatives (**Table 4**) also contribute to garlic's antimicrobial properties. Allicin is considered as a natural antibiotic, which does not appear to create resistant bacteria strains, and in combination with the other sulfur compounds in garlic, has been shown to be deadly for many viruses and bacteria [25–38]. Antifungal properties of garlic have been reported, too [17]. Diallyl disulfide, diallyl trisulfide, S-allyl-mercapto cysteine, S-allyl-L-cysteine, and others have been shown to exert potent anti-inflammatory, antifibrotic, antioxidative, and antimetastatic effects [28]. Furthermore, garlic has been recommended as beneficial for patients with dyslipidemia and diabetes. In traditional Mediterranean medicine, garlic has been used for boosting the immune system. A remedy prepared with honey and garlic cloves has been used for respiratory infections, for example, to relieve bronchitis, influenza, and lung infections, while a remedy prepared with garlic and milk is being used to treat fever and croup [24, 29]. Garlic has been also used to fight fungal (yeast) infections, such as candida.

Aged garlic extract and fresh garlic extract have been compared and found that both have anticancer effects. Namely, aged garlic has cytotoxic effects on cancer cells by causing oxidative stress in the mitochondria, while fresh garlic extract suppresses cancer cell proliferation. Aged garlic extract had a blood pressure-lowering effect, and thus, might be a safe adjunct treatment in addition to conventional antihypertensive therapy. Garlic significantly lowers systolic blood pressure and diastolic blood pressure and could act as an anticoagulant. It also reduces the level of C-reactive protein, and thus, has anti-inflammatory activity [28, 37].

Onion (*Allium cepa* L.) has been consumed in traditional Mediterranean cuisine as both, a vegetable and a flavoring spice, due to its pronounced and characteristic flavor. The bulbs and leaves of various types of onions have a variety of flavors and textures responsible for the palatability of traditional Mediterranean dishes. Onion consumption varies in the region, but onions are typically consumed in larger quantities than garlic, chives, shallots, or leeks. Onion consumption has increased significantly over the years and might be among the most consumed vegetables. Onions are rich in flavonoids and organosulfur compounds. Onion bulbs are among the richest sources of dietary flavonoids and might be the largest contributor to the overall intake of flavonoids in the diet. Two flavonoid subgroups are found in onions, anthocyanins, which impart a red/purple color to some varieties, and flavanols (e.g., quercetin and its derivatives) responsible for the yellow and brown skins of other onion varieties. The organosulfur compounds are the flavor precursors, which, when cleaved by the enzyme alliinase, generate the characteristic odor and taste of the onion. The downstream products are a complex mixture of compounds, which include thiosulfinates, thiosulfonates, mono-, di-, and tri-sulfides. These compounds found in onions have been reported to have a range of health benefits, including anticarcinogenic properties, cardioprotective, antiplatelet, and antithrombotic activities, as well as anti-asthmatic and antibiotic effects [17, 39–49]. Onions have also been used in traditional medicine to treat different ailments, such as helping the body to release toxins, and as a remedy for cold and flu. Besides being an expectorant, it is also used as a diuretic and can facilitate muscle relaxation and improve blood circulation.

Leek (*Allium ampeloprasum* L. *var. porrum* or *Allium porrum* L.) is known for its high nutritional value, but also for its wide spectrum of biological activities, primarily a high antioxidant content and specific taste. Leeks show a wide spectrum of biological activities, among which are antimicrobial, cardio-protective, hypocholesterolemic, hypoglycemic, and anticancer activities. The anti-inflammatory, gastroprotective, and cytotoxic activities of organosulfate compounds have been well documented for leek. In addition, antimicrobial activity has been reported; in fact, leeks have been used to treat wounds and respiratory diseases [23]. The most important biologically-active compounds in the leek are polyphenols, glucosinolates, S-alkenyl-L-cysteine sulfoxides, and pectic polysaccharides, each showing immune-boosting activity. The polyphenol content in some leek types is comparable with the shallot and significantly exceeds that of garlic, chive, and onion. Kaempferol is the main flavonoid aglycone in the leek. Polyphenols along with vitamin C significantly affect plant antioxidant activity. The nutritional value of leek is also correlated with the high content of potassium and iron [49, 50]. Leek consumption is known to improve liver and gastrointestinal tract functioning, quicken metabolic processes, reduce blood pressure, protect against anemia, enhance brain activity, and inhibit platelet aggregation, but is also useful in rheumatism treatment. Moreover, consumption of leek reportedly reduces the risk of prostate, colon, stomach, and breast cancers. Antimicrobial effects of leek have been reported for both, against gram-positive (e.g., *Streptococcus pneumonia and Staphylococcus aureus*) and gram-negative bacteria (e.g., *Escherichia coli and Proteus vulgaris*); antifungal activity has been reported, too [49, 51]. Epidemiological studies have linked the reduction of the risk of prostate, colorectal, stomach, and breast cancer to leek consumption. In traditional medicine, leek has been used to ease the sting of insect bites, as a diuretic and a stimulant, remedy for respiratory problems, such as sore throat and cough, while warm juices of its leaves and bulb have been used for earaches [49–51].

Basil (*Ocimum basilicum* L.) is known as a royal herb, derived from "basileus" (meaning "king" in Greek), and is one of the most widely used herbs in Mediterranean cuisine. Extract from basil contains rosmarinic acid and catechin, which could protect against metabolic syndrome, anemia, osteoporosis, vitamin A, and iron deficiency. The antidiabetic effects of basil extract are most likely due in part to the rosmarinic acid content since rosmarinic acid has been found to inhibit a-glucosidase, a-amylase, and aldose reductase *in vitro*. Advanced glycation end products (AGEs) are usually a consequence of oxidative stress. It is known that polyphenols are potent antioxidants, thus, the anti-AGE effects of basil are associated with its relatively high polyphenol content. In addition, basil is also strong anti-inflammatory and antimicrobial plant, and has also favorable effects on blood pressure [52–56].

Mint (*Mentha sp.*) belongs to the genus *Mentha* of the Lamiaceae family; *M. spicata* L., *M. pulegium* L., and *M. rotundifolia* L. are some of the species that belong to this family. In general, mint is used for the preparation of herbal teas and as a spice in the Mediterranean. Species of the genus *Mentha* contain a range of components, including cinnamic acids and aglycon, glycoside, and/or acylated flavonoids, particularly flavones and flavanones. Luteolin and its derivatives are the main flavones found in Mentha; however, phenolic acids, like caffeic acid and its derivatives, chlorogenic and rosmarinic acid, and salvianolic acids have also been found in *Mentha* plants. The most recognized properties of the mint are antioxidant, antimicrobial, antiviral, anti-inflammatory, neuroprotective, cardiovascular, and antitumor properties [17, 57].

Peppermint (*Mentha piperita* L.), a member of the *Mentha sp*. family has the strongest flavor when compared to other members of the mint family. Compounds found in peppermint leaves are fatty acids—linoleic, linolenic, and palmitic acid, then triterpenoids and steroids, and different pigments, such as xanthophylls, chlorophylls, and carotenes [57].

Coriander (*Coriandrum sativum* L.) leaves and seeds are the edible parts of this plant and are often used in Mediterranean cuisine. Coriander leaves (or cilantro) are usually used in bean dishes, stews, dips, and salsas. The most potent compounds in the coriander are essential oils, flavonoids (quercetin, kaempferol, and acacetin), phenolic acids (vanillic acid, p-coumaric acid, syringic acid, cis-ferulic acid, and trans-ferulic acid), and polyphenols. It is also rich in vitamins, such as vitamins C and K [23]. Coriander seed extract significantly reduces serum glucose and increased insulin secretion by pancreatic b-cells compared to diabetic controls. Oral administration of coriander seed extract also reduces total cholesterol and increased HDL in diabetic rats. Coriander seeds are also hypolipidemic—they could mitigate atherosclerosis development by reducing circulating cholesterol, cholesterol synthesis, and facilitating cholesterol excretion [58]. It is also reported for its antibacterial and antifungal properties [53].

Parsley (*Petroselinum crispum* (Mill)) leaves are often used to add flavor to sauces, soups, and savory dishes, but also as a garnish for traditional Mediterranean dishes. The extract from parsley is high in flavonoid apigenin. Parsley extract has been shown to reverse hyperglycemia and protein glycation associated with diabetes. The mechanism for the antidiabetic action of parsley extract may be via inhibiting absorption of glucose by a-glucosidase. In addition, parsley has anti-inflammatory potential and greater parsley consumption, which may be beneficial in the treatment of hypertension, iron deficiency, anemia, and osteoporosis [58–60].

Rosemary (*Rosmarinus officinalis* L.) belongs to the *Lamiaceae* family and is usually used to flavor meat dishes, soups, and stews in the Mediterranean region. The leaves are used to prepare herbal teas, or steeped in vinegar and/or oil are used to flavor sauces. Rosmarinic acid is one of the major components of rosemaryit is a phenolic compound having pronounced anti-inflammatory, hepatoprotective, and antihyperlipidemic properties [14, 16, 17, 61, 62]. Namely, rosemary possesses therapeutic properties, such as hepatoprotective, antifungal, antioxidant, and antibacterial [53]. It also protects against hypertension and can be hypolipidemic. In addition, rosemary extract shows both subacute and acute antidiabetic potential. Rosemary also exhibits NO-scavenging activity, it could be used in cases of low blood pressure, anemia, iron deficiency, and gallbladder problems [55, 58, 63–69].

Sage (*Salvia officinalis* L.) is used to flavor meat, stews, and sausages. In dry or fresh state, sage leaves are steeped in water to make herbal teas. Sage is rich in polyphenols, particularly rosmarinic acid, caffeic acid, α- and β-pinene, limonene, thymol, carvacrol, and others [14, 58]. Sage has strong antioxidant, antibacterial, and antiviral activities. The sage extract can reduce hyperglycemia associated with diabetes after acute or sub-acute treatment; it can also exhibit an antidiabetic effect [58]. In addition, anti-inflammatory activity and beneficial effects on the blood lipid profile are found for sage. Sage has been suggested for novel natural treatment for cure of many serious diseases, such as depression, dementia, obesity, lupus, heart disease, and cancer. In Mediterranean traditional medicine, it has been used for the treatment of flu, fever, colds, and digestive problems [14, 58, 63].

Thyme (*Thymus vulgaris* L.) is the most widely used plant from the *Thymus* genus as a culinary herb in many savory dishes and as a medicinal plant. Fresh thyme is high in rosmarinic acid, thymol, carvacrol, p-cymene, and luteolin. The health effects of thyme and its constituents, particularly thymol and carvacrol, include antioxidant, antimicrobial, anti-inflammatory, respiratory, and neurological effects [53]. Regarding inflammation, thyme extract was found to significantly inhibit metabolic activity, neutrophil adhesion, and superoxide production in a dose-dependent manner. Thyme extract can also be hypolipidemic, but also could help with anemia, iron deficiency, bronchitis, flu, etc. Traditional remedies utilizing thyme include alleviation of depression, epilepsy, and nightmares, as well as treatments of headaches and coughs [14, 53, 55, 66].

Oregano (*Origanum vulgare* L.) is usually used as dried in many dishes in the Mediterranean region, such as soups, meat and vegetable dishes, and pizza. Leaves and flowering tops of oregano are also used in preparation of tea drinks. It has a high content of polyphenols, among which rosmarinic acid is the most representative compound found in it. Oregano and oregano oil have strong antibacterial, antifungal, and antiviral properties [53]. Oregano extract exhibits a wide range of antidiabetic and hypolipidemic effects. It has been shown that oregano alleviates oxidative stress, decreases markers of inflammation *in vitro*, and helps with throat infections, coughs, and headaches [14, 54, 55, 58, 66].

Marjoram (*Origanum majorana* L.) leaves are commonly used to flavor Mediterranean dishes, but also for flavoring vinegar and oils. Phenolic acids found in this plant are trans-2-hydroxycinnaminic acid, rosmarinic acid, and biflavone amentoflavone as its most prevalent flavonoid. The plant exhibits antioxidant, antidiabetic, and anti-inflammatory potential, which lowers fasting glucose and glycated hemoglobin, and improves oral glucose tolerance compared to the diabetic control. *In vitro*, marjoram extract prevents hemoglobin, albumin, and LDL glycation, but it may also protect against diabetic nephropathy [58, 70, 71].

Cayenne pepper (*Capsicum annum* L.) is found in a wide range of spiciness, which originates from the pepper's active ingredient, capsaicin. Capsaicin is an alkaloid that accounts for ~50–70% of the total capsaicinoids, dihydrocapsaicin accounts for 20–25%, while cryptoxanthin, which is a carotenoid, acts as a pigment and it gives the pepper its red color. In addition, cayenne pepper also contains nonpungent compounds called capsinoids (e.g., capsiate and dihydrocapsiate). Cayenne peppers exhibit antioxidant and anti-inflammatory effects, can exhibit control over blood glucose, and decrease the risk of CVD and cancers, but also are beneficial for gut health and management of satiety and weight. It is also known to possess protective activities against asthma, cancer, and diabetes. In addition, capsaicin has been also used to treat cancer; more recent findings revealed that it has an effect on promoting apoptosis and inhibiting tumor growth [17, 23, 72]. Cayenne pepper can also help with ulcers causing internal pain. Although people often associate spicy foods with stomach upset, but capsaicin aids in helping reduce ulcers by restricting the growth of an ulcer-causing bacteria (*H. pylori*), reducing excess stomach acid and increasing blood flow; the antimicrobial activity has been highlighted by its inhibitory effects against *H. pylori* and other bacteria and fungi.

Long pepper (*Piper longum* L.) is a spice, where the whole plant is used as it is and is known to yield many biologically-important compounds, such as piperine, piperlongumine, and piperinic acid. They are known for their benefits in the treatment of inflammation-mediated diseases (cancer, lupus, arthritis, and asthma) due to their ability to supress pro-inflammatory cytokines (TNF-α and IL-6 induce the expression of anti-inflammatory cytokine IL-10). Paprika, a commonly used spice in the Mediterranean, is usually made from dried and ground red peppers from the *Capsicum annuum* family, but also from the Longum group of peppers, which includes chili peppers [17].

Saffron (*Crocus sativus* L.) belongs to the Iridaceae family. The interest in saffron, that is, in the stigmas of the flower of *Crocus sativus*, is due to its content of many bioactive molecules with health-promoting properties, including crocin, crocetin, picrocrocin, and safranal. The spice saffron is actually made from the dried stigmas of the plant. The main use of saffron is in cooking, due to its ability to impart color, flavor, and aroma to variety of foods and beverages. Among the various therapeutic properties it possesses, the most notable are its antidepressant, anti-inflammatory, and antitumor effects. Among different compounds, safranal is the constituent primarily responsible for the aroma of saffron and exhibits antioxidant and gastroprotective effects. Saffron has been also found to help with improving mood, treatment of depression, reducing PMS symptoms and CVD risks, and weight management [17, 73–77]. The *Crocus sativus* L. plant contains various compounds belonging to different classes of secondary metabolites, such as carotenoids, monoterpenoids, flavonoids, and anthocyanins. Carotenoids are the most important components of saffron stigmas, responsible for the colorant features of this spice; they include both, fat-soluble carotenoids, such as lycopene, α- and β-carotene, zeaxanthin, and water-soluble C20 apocarotenoid, crocetin, and its ester derivatives. Several minor components have been also isolated from stigmas and other plant parts, such as petals and corms; terpenoids are the most often components, while the crocusatins, present in stigmas and petals, show significant antityrosinase activity. A series of flavonoids, all glycosidic derivatives of kaempferol, have been characterized in the stigmas of saffron and together with picrocrocin are responsible for the bitter taste of saffron [78].

Purslane weed (*Portulaca oleracea* L.) is popular in many regions around the Mediterranean sea. Studies have confirmed that the plant is a rich source of phytochemicals, such as flavonoids, alkaloids, terpenoids, proteins, carbohydrates, vitamins (A, C, E, and B), carotenoids, and minerals (phosphorus, calcium, magnesium, and zinc). It is particularly very important due to the presence of a very high concentration of omega-3- fatty acids, especially α-linolenic acid, gamma-linolenic acid, and linoleic acid. Purslane is one of the richest source of omega-3 fatty acids, alpha-linolenic acid (ALA), and gamma-linolenic acid (LNA), among many green leafy vegetables. Omega-3 fatty acids are known to protect against cardiovascular disease, cancers, and other chronic diseases. Moreover, purslane has shown anti-inflammatory, antidiabetic, antitumor, hepatoprotective, anticancer, antioxidant, anti-insomnia, analgesic, gastroprotective, neuroprotective, wound healing, and antiseptic properties [79–81].

Bay leaf (*Laurus nobilis* L.) is often used in a variety of MD-style cooking and preservation processes of sweet and savory dishes. The extract of bay leaves contains minerals, vitamins, and essential oils, such as cineol, eugenol, chavicol, acetyl eugenol, methyl eugenol, and ß-pinene, various flavonoids, such as quercetin and kaempferol, as well as various sesquiterpenes. Bay leaf exhibits a wide array of antioxidant, anti-inflammatory, antidiabetic, diuretic, and appetite-stimulating effects. Several *in vivo* studies support the hypolipidemic effect of the bay leaf, that is, lowering the plasma total cholesterol, triglycerides, and glucose [17, 58].

Dill (*Anethum graveolens* L.) is a spice used for seasoning traditional Mediterranean fish and vegetable dishes. Fresh dill has a high content of quercetin and isorhamnetin. The dill extract has antidiabetic potential, as well as can be hypolipidemic. It could also help with the issues of immune deficiency, kidney stones, osteoporosis, and vitamin A deficiency. Dill seeds have been used in the folk to treat insomnia, respiratory disorders, calm down allergies, and boost immunity [58].

Fennel (*Foeniculum vulgare* Mill.): bulbs, leaves, flowers, and seeds are all considered edible parts and used for preparation of many dishes consumed within the Mediterranean dietary pattern. Bulbs are usually used raw in salads, seeds are used for flavoring sausages and bread, while the leaves are cooked with fish, or used for preparation of herbal teas. The most prevalent flavonoid in polar extract of fennel leaves is quercetin. The potential health benefits of fennel have been reported to be antidiabetic, anti-inflammatory effects have been related to the consumption of fennel seed extract, and antihyperlipidemic have been associated with the fennel bulb. In particular, the fennel bulb extract has been reported to manage the total cholesterol, triglycerides, and LDL levels, as well as prevent lipid accumulation in the coronary artery and decrease the hepatic total cholesterol and triglycerides. It also possesses antimicrobial properties [53, 58].

Black pepper (*Piper nigrum* L.), commonly known as pepper, is considered to be the "king of spices," because of its high trade share in the global market. Black pepper is principally used as a seasoning ingredient to enhance food flavor, as well as in food preserving. Black pepper contains a number of bioactive ingredients, such as essential oils and the alkaloid piperine. Many studies on the biological properties of piperine have revealed its antioxidant, anticarcinogenic, anti-inflammatory, antiulcer, antithyroid, and antimicrobial effects with some potential to modulate immune responses [53]. Apart from its culinary uses, *P. nigrum* is also used as an insecticide [82–85].

Sesame seeds (*Sesamum indicum* L.) belong to the *Pedaliaceae* family and exhibit medicinal properties, such as anticancer, hepatoprotective, and antihypertensive. They contain various bioactive compounds, including lignans, tocopherol homologs, phytosterols, and others. Based on their medicinal and pharmacological properties, the most important lignans are sesamin, sesamol, sesamolin, and sesamol, but also α-, γ-, and δ-tocopherols. In addition, sesame is an important source of phytosterols, phytates, polyunsaturated fatty acids, and bioactive peptides [17, 86–91].

Cumin seeds (*Cuminum cyminum* L.) are usually ground and used in herb rubs for meat dishes, as well as to flavor sauces, pickles, and bread. They are rich in phenolic acids, including chlorogenic acid and flavonoids, particularly apigenin. Cumin seeds have antidiabetic effects *in vivo*; cumin extract/ground cumin administered orally reduced blood glucose and glycosylated hemoglobin in diabetic rats. The seeds also reduced triglycerides and total cholesterol in plasma, liver, kidney, intestines, and pancreas of diabetic animals [17, 58, 92–95]. Cumin also exhibits antimicrobial properties [53].

Black seeds or **black cumin** (*Nigella sativa* L.) are totally unrelated to cumin seeds (*C. cyminum*); numerous preclinical and clinical trials have investigated their efficacy using the seed oil, essential oil, and its main constituent thymoquinone. Antidiabetic, anti-allergic, antimicrobial, immune-modulatory, anti-inflammatory, and antitumor effects have been observed for black cumin. It possesses gastroprotective, hepatoprotective, nephroprotective, and neuroprotective activities [96–98].

Clove (*Syzygium aromaticum* L.) is a spice that has been used as a food preservative and to add flavor to traditional dishes. The spice is derived from flower buds. It is rich in phenolic compounds, such as eugenol, eugenol acetate, and gallic acid, with great potential for pharmaceutical, cosmetic, food and agricultural applications [99]. Clove is also rich in manganese, potassium, vitamin K, and beta-carotene. Clove has been used mainly for oral health and treatment of gingivitis but also has antidiabetic, anti-inflammation, and antimicrobial activity [53, 100]. Clove also protects the stomach from ulcers and provides better liver function. Eugenol, the main component of clove oil, has strong antioxidant activity, as well [99, 101–104].

Cinnamon (*Cinnamomum* L.) spice is derived from the innermost bark of the cinnamon tree. Cinnamon's key components are essential oils and other derivatives, such as cinnamaldehyde, cinnamic acid and cinnamate, cinnamon oil, cinnamyl alcohol, cinnamyl acetate, eugenol, and water-soluble polyphenols, for example, catechin, epicatechin, procyanidin, quercetin, kaempferol, polyphenolic polymers, and various coumarins, which all contribute to its overall flavor and aroma [17, 100, 105]. In addition to its common culinary use as a condiment and flavoring spice, cinnamon is widely known for its antidiabetic and glucose-lowering effects [100]. Extracts of cinnamon and its major components (cinnamaldehyde and eugenol) have been shown to attack major respiratory and gastrointestinal tract pathogens *in vitro*. It has also beneficial effects on chronic salmonella infection. *In vitro* studies have suggested that cinnamon may have some bactericidal activity against *H. pylori*. Cinnamon has also shown anti-inflammatory, antimicrobial, and antioxidant effects; its polyphenol extracts suppressed inflammation processes through the regulation of anti- and proinflammatory gene expression *in vitro* [17, 53]. Studies showed that cinnamon supplementation significantly reduced blood triglycerides and total cholesterol concentrations [106]. Consumption of cinnamon has been also associated with notable reductions in systolic and diastolic blood pressure, as well as showed blood glycose control and hepatoprotective and neuroprotective effects. Moreover, cinnamon may have protective effects against different metabolic syndrome aspects [17].

Ginger (*Zingiber officinale*) is a root or rhizome-based spice derived from the ginger plant, a member of the turmeric family (*Zingiberaceae*). It is a culinary additive —a hot and fragrant spice, as well as a folk medicine well-known for its use to treat nausea. Many components found in ginger have been found to have anti-inflammatory, antibacterial, antipyretic, antilipidemic, antitumorigenic, and antiangiogenic effects [53]. Ginger's flavor and aroma come from its volatile oils and nonvolatile pungent oleoresins. A variety of active components have been identified in the oleoresins of ginger, including zingerone, gingerols, and shogaols. Gingerols (e.g., 6-gingerol) are the major pungent components in the fresh ginger rhizome, while in dried ginger, the quantity of shogaols is significantly increased [17, 100, 105]. In general, ginger has been reported to have anti-inflammatory, antioxidant, antiplatelet, antihypertensive, and hypolipidemic effects. It could improve joint and muscle health, as well as has weight management potential and neuroprotective effects. Clinical trials have shown that ginger is safe and effective for decreasing nausea and vomiting during pregnancy or induced by chemotherapy. Ginger and its extracts (6-gingerols and 6-shogaol) exhibits substantial free-radical scavenging activities and inhibits the production of inflammatory mediators [17].

Anise (*Pimpinella anisum* L.) is a seed spice derived from a flowering plant belonging to the family Apiaceae, which is native to the eastern Mediterranean region. The distinctive licorice flavor and aroma from anise come from anethole—a phenylpropene derivative. Anethole exists in both a cis and a trans isomer. In Mediterranean countries, the popularity of alcoholic and nonalcoholic anise-flavored beverages has led to much greater consumption of trans-anethole. However, anethole is also used in medicines as an expectorant, an antitussive, and an antispasmodic for treating gastrointestinal tract illnesses; as a result, anise is found in a number of pharmaceutical products [105]. It has been used in traditional medicine due to its antimicrobial, anti-inflammatory, and antioxidant properties as well as antidiabetic [100].

3. Mediterranean medicinal plants

Mediterranean folk medicine has used local plants to treat different ailments since ancient times. A wide range of nonedible wild plants, characteristic in the Mediterranean region, has been used as natural remedies and therapeutics for curing fever, cold, and flu, for treatment of injuries, such as bruises, cuts, and insect bites, or simply to help with some neurological functions, such as reducing anxiety, stress, and improve sleep. Medicinal plants prepared in a form of extracts, tinctures, oil macerates, herbal infusions and teas, ointments, and balms are among the most used ones.

In recent decades, Mediterranean medicinal plants have been studied and some of them have been proven to be great alternatives and additions to the conventional drug treatments of severe diseases, such as cancer, without the side effects often associated with synthetic drugs. In the text below, a brief review of Mediterranean plants being used as natural therapeutics for treatment of different ailments is presented.

Dandelion (*Taraxacum officinale*) is a member of the *Asteraceae* family [107–110]. It is a nontoxic herb that has been exploited for its choleretic, diuretic, anti-rheumatic, and anti-inflammatory properties. It has also gained a lot of scientific attention due to its antioxidant activity and its beneficial effects against the development of obesity, cancer, and numerous CVD risk factors. Dandelion contains several phenylpropanoids yielding inflammation-modulating effects, inulin having immune-stimulatory functions, and terpenoids and polysaccharides having roles in immune regulation and platelet anti-aggregation activity, hepatoprotective effects, and antitumoral activity. Vitamins (A, B, C, D, and E), inositol, lecithin, minerals, and oligo-elements (calcium, potassium, sodium, magnesium, iron, silicon, copper, phosphorus, zinc, and manganese) are found in dandelion. Dandelion's bitterness is due to its sesquiterpene lactones (eudesmanolide and germacranolide types), which are unique to this plant and yield anti-inflammatory and anticancer functions. In particular, dandelion flowers are rich in phenolic compounds (phenolic acids and flavonoids), the roots contain terpenes (sesquiterpene lactones, triterpenes, and phytosterols), phenolic compounds (phenolic acids and coumarins), and carbohydrate (inulin), while the other aerial parts (leaves and stems) are rich in terpenes, phenolic compounds (phenolic acids, flavonoids, and coumarins) [110]. In addition to its uses in traditional medicine, dandelion has been used as a vegetable in preparation of fresh saladsalone or in combination with other plants, such as lettuce, shallots, and chives. A comparison of its nutritional composition with similar vegetables, such as lettuce and spinach, shows that dandelion has a higher content of dietary fiber and proteins, as well as a variety of amino acids, vitamins, and minerals. It also contains lipids and has high proportions of unsaturated fatty acids (oleic, palmitoleic, linoleic, and linolenic acids). Dandelion is also one of the richest green-vegetable sources of beta-carotene. The health benefits of dandelion are summarized as anti-inflammatory and antimicrobial properties, reduced cholesterol absorption, immuno-stimulatory properties, effects on cardiovascular system, prebiotic activity, and antioxidant properties.

Chicory (*Cichorium intybus* L.) is a perennial plant common in the Mediterranean region and is used as forage for livestock, as supplement to the human diet, or for preparation of folk remedies—all uses are due to its medicinal, culinary, and nutritional qualities. Inulin, coumarins, tannins, monomeric flavonoids, chichoric acid, phenolic acids, and sesquiterpene lactones are some of the major phyto-compounds found in chicory. Chicory is also a source of biologically-relevant elements, such as potassium, iron, calcium, and vitamins A, B1, B2, and C. In folk medicine, it is usually used against constipation and displays choleretic and digestion-promoting effects, but also for its appetite-increasing effects, and anti-inflammatory, antifungal, antiviral, and antibacterial activities. It also shows anticarcinogenic, antimutagenic, anthelmintic, immune-stimulating, antihepatotoxic, and antioxidative qualities. Chicory is among the plants, which have been investigated for its potential effects against SARS-CoV-2 [111–114]. Apart from its phytochemical applications, chicory is used in gastronomy as a coffee substitute, and food or drink additive [112, 115]. Namely, chicory's inulin, which belongs to the category of soluble dietary fiber, is a prebiotic ingredient that selectively stimulates the growth of bifidobacteria in the large intestine. As a dietary fiber, chicory inulin is resistant to digestion and absorption in the upper digestive system but is being partially or totally fermented in the large intestine. Chicory's inulin also ameliorates type 2 diabetes mellitus [114].

Milk thistle *(Silybum marianum* (L.) Gaertn.) is a plant that has been used traditionally as a herbal treatment for liver and biliary tract diseases. According to traditional knowledge, it has been used for liver disorders, such as hepatitis, liver cirrhosis, and gallbladder diseases [116–118]. *Silymarin* is the main component derived from the fruits and seeds of milk thistle, which has been found to exhibit antioxidant, lipid-lowering, antihypertensive, antidiabetic, anti-atherosclerotic, anti-obesity, and hepatoprotective effects [119]. Silymarin is a mixture of flavonolignans containing silibinin, isosilybin, silychristin, and silydianin, but also some minor fractions of other flavanols, such as quercetin and kaempferol, among the others. Studies have shown that silymarin has potential hepatoprotective effects due to its antioxidant and anti-inflammatory effects. Milk thistle is used for treatment of a wide range of disorders of the liver, heart, kidney, and nervous system. Metabolic syndrome, nephropathy, hepatitis, viral infections, cancer, and diabetes have been also reported to benefit from this plant's use. In addition, antimicrobial, anticancer, antidiabetic, skin-protective, heparoprotective, cardioprotective, and neuroprotective effects (Alzheimer's, Parkinson's, ischemia, multiple sclerosis, aging, and depression) have been associated with the use of milk thistle.

Chamomile (*Chamaemelum nobile* L., *Matricaria chamomilla* L.) is one of the widely used medicinal plants; it has been used for preparation of herbal infusions, teas, balms, ointments, and other application forms with numerous healing benefits. It is a member of the daisy family (*Asteraceae* or *Compositae*). It contains a variety of bioactive, among which the flavanoids (apigenin, luteolin, patuletin, and quercetin), coumarins (herniarin and umbelliferone), terpenoids, and mucilage are considered to be the major bioactive compounds. Chamomile is usually used to treat wounds, ulcers, eczema, gout, skin irritations, bruises, burns, canker sores, neuralgia, sciatica, rheumatic pain, hemorrhoids, and mastitis in folk medicine. In the form of an aqueous extract (herbal infusions and teas), it has been used as a mild sedative to calm nerves and reduce anxiety, to treat hysteria, nightmares, insomnia, and other sleep problems. It is also effective in reducing pains associated with arthritis, bedsores and stomach cramps, and back pain. Scientific evidence has also pointed to its anti-inflammatory and anticancer activity, reducing the risks of CVDs, efficacy in the treatments of diarrhea, eczema, sore throat, hemorrhoids, and inhibitory effects on the bacteria that contribute to stomach ulcers (*H. pylori*) [120–122].

Lavender (*Lavandula spica* L.) has been traditionally used in treating parasitic infections, burns, insect bites, and spasms due to its therapeutic properties, as well as treating neurological disorders due to its anxiolytic, mood stabilizing, sedative, analgesic, and anticonvulsive and neuroprotective properties. Lavender oil is usually produced from the flowers of *Lavandula* angustifolia by steam distillation and is composed of many beneficial compounds, such as linalyl acetate, linalool, lavandulol, lavandulyl acetate, and camphor, among others [123–125]. Lavender inhalation aromatherapy is widely used to impart a hypnotic effect, where lavender acts as a mood stabilizer, or enhances the positive feelings, for example, of mothers toward their infants, etc. [126–128]. Aromatherapy massage with lavender essential oil was found to be effective in relieving the pain in patients with knee osteoarthritis [129], but also reducing the severity of primary dysmenorrhea. Other beneficial activities of lavender essential oil are antibacterial, antioxidant, analgetic, and anti-inflammatory effects. There has been also reported a potential wound healing activity of lavender oil in the early phase by acceleration of formation of granulation tissue, tissue remodeling by collagen replacement and wound contraction [130–135].

Linden (*Tilia platyphyllos*, *Tilia cordata* Mill.) is a popular medicinal plant in the Mediterranean region, because of its effects on the central nervous system. Its flowers are usually consumed as herbal infusions or teas, and are widely known for their tranquilizing and analgesic properties, but linden also exhibits hepatoprotective and antioxidant effects. Linden is also a great source of phenolic components, viz. flavonoids, phenolic acids, and others [136, 137]. Linden leaves are usually used for treatment of colds, stuffy nose, sore throat, breathing problems (bronchitis), headaches, and fever. Linden has also been used for treatments of rapid heartbeat, high blood pressure, excessive bleeding (hemorrhage), nervous tension, trouble sleeping (insomnia), problems with bladder control, and muscle spasms.

Nettle (*Urtica dioica* L.), also known as "stinging nettle," contains a significant number of bioactive compounds. In particular, the leaves are rich sources of terpenoids, carotenoids, fatty acids, essential amino acids, chlorophyll, vitamins, tannins, carbohydrates, sterols, polysaccharides, isolectins, and minerals. Extracts from the aerial parts of nettles are rich sources of polyphenols, while the roots contain oleanol acid, sterols, and steryl glycosides. Nettles show noticeable activity against both gram-positive and gram-negative bacteria. Due to their rich content of phytonutrients, nettles are suitable for a range of possible applications, such as functional foods, dietary supplements, and pharmacological formulations. This plant is also used as a preservative in foods for both human and animal consumption, but also it has been used in traditional medicine, such as treating the problems associated with hair loss [138–142].

Calendula (*Calendula officinalis* L.) is a plant also known as pot marigold, belonging to the daisy family Asteraceae, which includes approx. 20 herbaceous annual or perennial species. Triterpene alcohols (α-amyrin, β-amyrin, and lupeol), triterpene saponins (calendulosides), flavonoids (quercetin and isorhamnetin), coumarins, carotenoids (flavoxanthin, zeaxanthine, and lutein), and polysaccharides are some of the major classes of phytoconstituents of this plant [143]. Some species of this genus have medicinal values. For instance, *Calendula officinalis Linn*. has been traditionally used in the treatment of various skin tumors, dermatological lesions, ulcers, swellings, and nervous disorders. The aerial parts are used for the treatment of kidney stones and gallstones. The field marigold has been used as disinfectant, antispasmodic, and diuretic agent. In folk medicine, the plant is used as an anti-inflammatory, anticancer, and antipyretic agent. It is known to have wound-healing properties; crushed leaves are usually topically applied on wounds, or are used for treatment of burns. The dried flower heads have been used due to their antipyretic, antitumor, and cicatrizing effects. Topical application of infusion of flowers is used as antifungal and antiseptic in wounds, marks, freckles, sprain and conjunctivitis. Calendula tea is used as eyewash, gargle, or for treatment of diaper rashes and other inflammatory conditions of the skin and mucous membranes [143, 144].

Echinacea (*Echinacea purpurea* (L.) Moench.) is a genus of herbaceous flowering plants in the daisy family (*Asteraceae; Compositae*) and is commonly called coneflower. It has been used for treatment of respiratory tract infections and inflammatory conditions, including common cold, coughs, bronchitis, and inflammation of the mouth and pharynx. Fresh or dry herbs, dried rhizome and roots, and alcoholic extracts are usually used alone or combined with ginseng, goldenseal, or garlic. Echinacea is also known as an immune stimulant, and there are studies supporting its positive effects on both, innate and adaptive immunity. Furthermore, strong antimicrobial activities have also been reported for echinacea [145, 146].

Feverfew (*Tanacetum parthenium* (L.) Sch. Bip.) is a medicinal plant with numerous bioactive constituents, including sesquiterpene lactones, flavonoid glycosides, and pinenes. It has multiple pharmacologic properties, such as anticancer, anti-inflammatory, cardiotonic, and antispasmodic, as well as has been used as an emmenagogue or as an enema for worms. In folk medicine, feverfew has been used for the treatment of fevers, migraine headaches, rheumatoid arthritis, stomach aches, toothaches, insect bites, infertility, and problems with menstruation and labor during childbirth. Feverfew has also been used for treatments of psoriasis, allergies, asthma, tinnitus, dizziness, nausea, and vomiting [147–150].

St. John's Wort (*Hypericum perforatum* L.) is a herbaceous perennial plant of Hypericeae family [151]. It is well known as a medicinal plant and its extracts are used as a healing and anti-inflammatory agent. St. John's wort extracts contain a number of constituents with biological activity, including phenolic acids, a broad range of flavonoids, naphthodianthrones, and phloroglucinols. The antidepressant activity of *H. perforatum* is mainly attributed to the naphthodianthrones hypericin, pseudohypericin, protohypericin, and protopseudohypericin, but also to the flavonoids. In addition, naphthodianthrones have been discovered to act as an antiviral agent and to inhibit the growth of a variety of neoplasmatic cell types, while hyperforin has been shown to display antibacterial activity. It has been reported that it also acts as a novel anticancer drug, due to its activity to inhibit apoptosis [151, 152]. Moreover, antidiabetic [153] and anti-inflammatory activities [154, 155], have been also reported.

Red clover (*Trifolium pratense* L.) is a wild flowering plant, which belongs to the family of peas and beans. It is rich in isoflavones and is known for its use in traditional medicine, like for treatment of high blood pressure, arthritis, or used by women in menopause [156–158].

Elderberry (*Sambucus nigra* L.) is a plant that has been used in traditional medicine to heal wounds and burns, as well as for treatment of fever and rheumatism. Also, elderberries are known to boost immunity and have been used for treatment of viral infections, such as influenza A and B, and other respiratory infections. The plant is rich in dietary fibers, polyphenols, and vitamins C and A [159–161].

A brief overview of the use of some Mediterranean plants in folk medicine is given in **Table 5**.

Herb, spice, medical plant		Uses in folk medicine
Dandelion (*Taraxacum Officinale*)	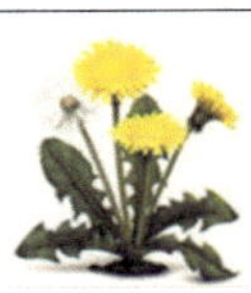	• Reduces cholesterol and triglycerides' levels.
		• Lowers blood pressure.
		• Treats constipation (root); stimulates urination, diuretic.
		• Treats poor digestion, and increases appetite.
		• Improves liver function.
		• Supports production of red blood cells in the body, anti-anemia (leaves).
Oregano (*Origanum Vulgare*)	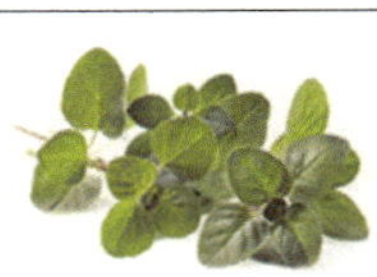	• Relieves inflammation and joint pain, rheumatism, toothaches, fevers, and menstrual cramps.
		• Soothes menstrual cramps, toothaches, and fevers.
		• Regulates digestion.
		• Helps alleviating flatulence and stomach aches.
		• Has antiseptic and antifungal properties
Echinacea (*Echinacea Purpurea*)	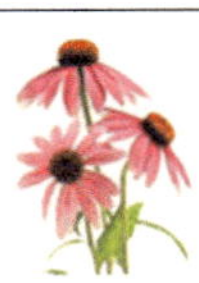	• Helps treating respiratory and urinary tract infections (antimicrobial)
		• Disinfects and sanitizes open wounds and prevents infections.
		• Relieves upper respiratory infections (cough, cold, and throat irritation).
		• Enhances immunity; anti-inflammatory properties.

Herb, spice, medical plant		Uses in folk medicine
Feverfew *(Tanacetum Parthenium)*	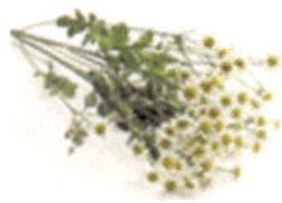	• Reduces inflammatory pain, fights arthritis, and rheumatism.
		• Relieves migraine pains and severe headaches.
		• Treats menstrual cramps.
		• Helps lowering fever and high body temperature.
Lavender *(Lavandula Angustifolia)*	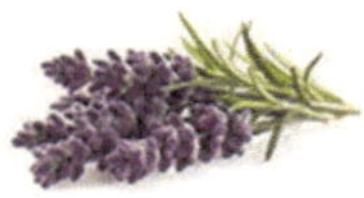	• Helps relieve stress, induces relaxation, and sleep (sedative properties).
		• Sanitizes superficial wounds, burns, and scraps, and treats acne, eczema, and other skin problems.
		• Alleviates tension headaches (as inhaled or rubbed into the skin)
Basil *(Ocimum Basilicum)*	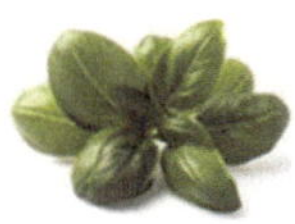	• Relieves indigestion, flatulence, and stomach discomfort.
		• Heals gastric infections, food poisoning, and improves stomach flu.
		• Prevents blood cloths and anticoagulant properties.
		• Relieves mosquito bites' itching, swelling, and redness of insect bites (basil poultice).
Bay leaves *(Laurus Nobilis)*	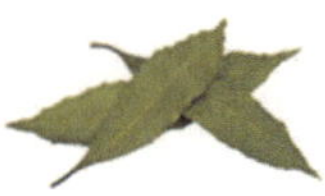	• Settles stomach discomfort and treats diarrhea.
		• Alleviates cough.
		• Eliminates mucus from the respiratory tract in infectious processes.
Chicory *(Cichorium Intybus)*	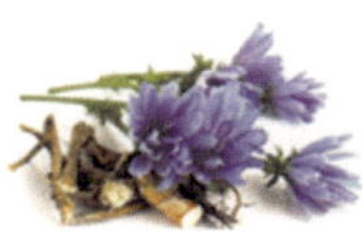	• Prevents fungal growth on the skin (topically-applied raw crushed leaves).
		• Fights sinus infection and gallstones.
		• Prevents liver damage and intestinal parasites and bacterial infections (tincture of chicory leaves and roots macerated in alcohol).
Valerian *(Valeriana Officinalis)*	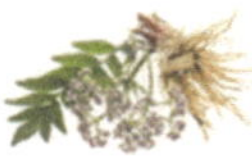	• Treats insomnia.
		• Lowers anxiety.
		• Helps with menopause symptoms.
Red clove *(Trifolium Pratense)*	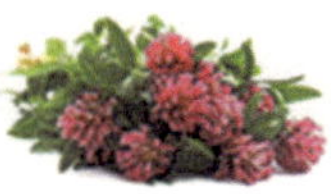	• Helps with asthma, whooping cough, and gout.
		• Soothes skin inflammation.
		• Treats female hormonal imbalances, menopause symptoms, and menopausal discomforts.
Sage *(Salvia Officinalis)*	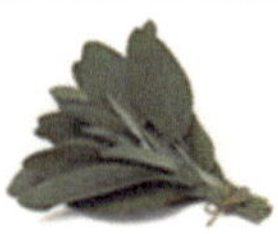	• Improves digestion and soothes indigestion and diarrhea.
		• Reduces night sweats and hot flashes, among other menopause symptoms.
		• Improves memory and cognition.
St John's Wort *(Hypericum Perforatum)*	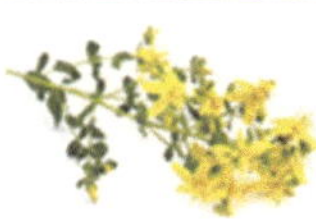	• Soothes anxiety and moderates the symptoms of panic disorder.
		• Treats minor or moderate depression.

Herb, spice, medical plant		Uses in folk medicine
		• Soothes skin injuries.
		• Alleviates sleep disorders and insomnia.
Dill *(Anethum Graveolens)*	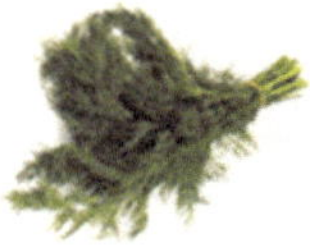	• Relieves stomach cramps, suppress muscle spasms and soothes stomach pain and irritation.
		• Treats flatulence.
		• Supports the immune system in fighting against pathogens.
Calendula *(Calendula Officinalis)*	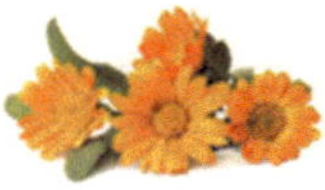	• Treats bacterial infections.
		• Relieves pain and has analgesic properties.
		• Promotes eye health and prevents AMD.
		• Uses as dry skin remedy (calendula petals-ointment); Heals bruises, cuts, and wounds.
Nettle *(Urtica Dioica)*	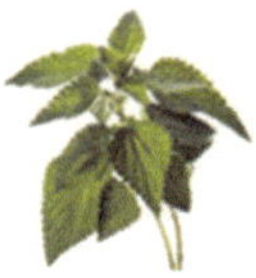	• Relives allergies symptoms.
		• Helps reduce internal inflammation, skin swelling, and irritation (leaves).
		• Has diuretic properties (nettle root).
		• Promotes hair growth.
		• Has anti-anemia properties and boosts production of red blood cells in the body (leaves).
Linden *(Tilia)*	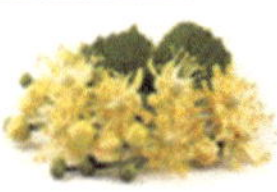	• Treats sleep disorders, including insomnia (linden flowers prepared as tea).
		• Soothes airways and helps clear airways in congested sinuses.
		• Relieves muscle cramps or spasms, especially in arms and legs.
		• Helps digestive functions and relieves indigestion.
Rosemary *(Rosmarinus Officinalis)*	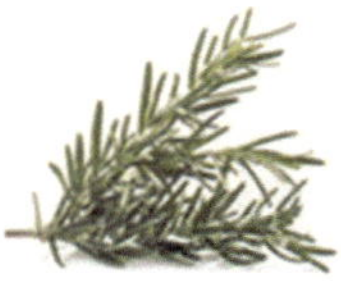	• Treats stomach aches and renal colics.
		• Relieves respiratory disorders and muscle spams.
		• Acts as a stimulant, dilating blood vessels, and aiding circulatory health.
		• Reduces joint pain caused by inflammatory diseases, for example, arthritis (topically-applied rosemary essential oil).
		• Fights hair loss and stimulates hair growth.
		• Improves memory and overall brain function (tea).
Milk thistle *(Silybum Marianum)*	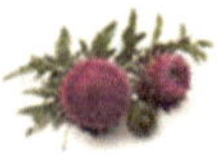	• Relieves jaundice.
		• Manages Hepatitis B and C.
		• Protects liver.

Table 5.
Mediterranean plants used in traditional medicine in the Mediterranean region.

4. Conclusions

This chapter highlighted the traditional use of spices and herbs in Mediterranean cuisine, and the medicinal plants used as natural remedies in the Mediterranean region. The study also emphasized their diversity and richness in phytonutrients, which greatly contribute to the health and well-being benefits of the Mediterranean diet and lifestyle, recognized worldwide as a highly antioxidant and anti-inflammatory diet; the bioactive compounds in the Mediterranean herbs, spices, and medicinal plants have notable anticancerogenic, antidiabetic, antihyperlipidemic, antihypertensive, and cardio-protective effects. In fact, they act as "*natural health promoters.*" If consumed regularly, they significantly reduce the risks of number of diseases and help maintain good health. Furthermore, the Mediterranean medicinal plants, used for centuries to treat different ailments among the indigenous people in the Mediterranean basin, are rich sources of bioactive compounds and represent nontoxic alternatives and supplements to synthetic drugs, which is in line with the modern trends of using natural products for disease treatment without the side effects of synthetic drugs. Conditions associated with metabolic syndrome, diabetes, inflammation, hyperlipidemia, hypertension, respiratory diseases, anxiety, sleep disorders, and others, have been shown to improve significantly with the use of medicinal plants.

Despite the tremendous scientific advancements in the areas of phytochemical and medical research, this chapter is believed to contribute toward the promotion of the traditional knowledge about Mediterranean herbs, spices, and medicinal plants, used for centuries among the people in the Mediterranean region. These plants along with the Mediterranean dietary pattern and lifestyle could indeed result in a healthier society with reduced incidences of NCDs, cancers, and CVDs.

Acknowledgements

The authors sincerely acknowledge the support of MD Inspired, LLC for promoting the Mediterranean diet and lifestyle outside the Mediterranean region.

Author details

Anita Trajkovska-Broach[1,2] and Anka Trajkovska Petkoska[3*]

1 MD Inspired. LLC, Virginia, USA

2 CSI: Create. Solve. Innovate. LLC, Virginia, USA

3 Faculty of Technology and Technical Sciences, University St. Kliment Ohridski-Bitola, Veles, N. Macedonia

*Address all correspondence to: anita@createsolveinnovate.com; anka.trajkovska@uklo.edu.mk

References

[1] Mentella MC, Scaldaferri F, Ricci C, Gasbarrini A. Giacinto abele Donato Miggiano. Cancer and Mediterranean diet: A review. Nutrients. 2019;**11**:2059. DOI: 10.3390/nu11092059

[2] Baselga-Escudero L, Souza-Mello V, Pascual-Serrano A, Rachid T, Voci A, Demori I, et al. Beneficial effects of the Mediterranean spices and aromas on nonalcoholic fatty liver disease. Trends in Food Science & Technology. 2017;**61**: 141e159

[3] Yeung SSY, Kwan M, Woo J. Healthy diet for healthy aging. Nutrients. 2021; **13**:4310

[4] Dominguez LJ, Di Bella G, Veronese N, Barbagallo M. Impact of Mediterranean diet on chronic non-communicable diseases and longevity. Nutrients. 2028;**2021**:13

[5] Yiannakou I, Singer MR, Jacques PF, Xanthakis V, Ellison RC, Moore LL. Adherence to a Mediterranean-style dietary pattern and cancer risk in a prospective cohort study. Nutrients. 2021;**13**:4064

[6] Miguel A. Martínez-González, Alfredo Gea, Miguel Ruiz-Canela, The Mediterranean diet and cardiovascular health, a critical review. Circulation Research. 2019; **124**(5):779-798

[7] Trajkovska-Broach A, Trajkovska PA. Mediterranean diet ingredients: Their antioxidant and anti-inflammatory potential. Austin Journal of Biotechnology Bioengineering. 2021;**8**(2):1114

[8] Trajkovska Petkoska A, Broach AT. Mediterranean way of living as an optimal lifestyle and a dietary pattern for healthy gut and strong immunity, EC. Nutrition. 2021;**16**(1):141-171

[9] Valeria Tosti, Beatrice Bertozzi, Luigi Fontana, Health benefits of the Mediterranean diet: Metabolic and molecular mechanisms. The Journals of Gerontology: Series A. 2018;**73**(3): 318-326

[10] Maggi S, Rogoli D, Ecarnot F. Healthy aging in the context of the Mediterranean diet–health-environment trilemma. Aging and Health Research. 2021;**1**:100015

[11] Trajkovska Petkoska A, Trajkovska-Broach A. Mediterranean diet: A nutrient-packed diet and a healthy lifestyle for a sustainable world. Journal of the Science of Food and Agriculture. 2020;**101**(7):2627-2633. DOI: 10.1002/JSFA.10907

[12] Otunola GA. Culinary spices in food and medicine: An overview of Syzygium aromaticum (L.) Merr. And L. M. Perry [Myrtaceae]. Frontiers in Pharmacology. 2021;**12**:793200. DOI: 10.3389/fphar.2021.793200

[13] Ibourki M, Ait Bouzid H, Bijla L, et al. Mineral profiling of twenty wild and cultivated aromatic and medicinal plants growing in Morocco. Biological Trace Element Research. 2022;**200**: 4880–4889. DOI: 10.1007/s12011-021-03062-w

[14] Giacometti J, Kovačević DB, Putnik P, Gabrić D, Bilušić T, Krešić G, et al. Extraction of bioactive compounds and essential oils from mediterranean herbs by conventional and green innovative techniques: A review. Food Research International. 2018;**113**:245-262

[15] Sikalidis AK, Kelleher AH, Kristo AS. Mediterranean Diet. Encyclopedia. 2021; **1**:371-387

[16] Alan Jiang T. Health benefits of culinary herbs and spices. Journal of AOAC International. 2019;**102**(2):17A-19A. DOI: 10.1093/jaoac/102.2.17A

[17] Kunnumakkara AB, Rana V, Parama D, Banik K, Girisa S, Henamayee S, et al. COVID-19, cytokines, inflammation, and spices: How are they related? Life Sciences. 2021;**284**:119201

[18] Quesada I, de Paola M, Torres-Palazzolo C, Camargo A, Ferder L, Manucha W, et al. Effect of Garlic's active constituents in inflammation, obesity and cardiovascular disease. Current Hypertension Reports. 2020;**22**: 6. DOI: 10.1007/s11906-019-1009-9

[19] Putnik P, Gabrić D, Roohinejad S, Barba FJ, Granato D, Mallikarjunan K, et al. Danijela Bursać Kovačević, an overview of organosulfur compounds from *allium* spp.: From processing and preservation to evaluation of their bioavailability, antimicrobial, and anti-inflammatory properties. Food Chemistry. 2019;**276**:680-691. DOI: 10.1016/j.foodchem.2018.10.068

[20] Rouf R, Uddin SJ, Sarker DK, Islam MT, Ali ES, Shilpi JA, et al. Anti-viral potential of garlic (*Allium sativum*) and it's organosulfur compounds: A systematic update of pre-clinical and clinical data. Trends in Food Science & Technology. 2020;**104**:219-234. DOI: 10.1016/j.tifs.2020.08.006

[21] Ekşi G, Özkan AMG, Koyuncu M. Garlic and onions: An eastern tale. Journal of Ethnopharmacology. 2020; **253**:112675. DOI: 10.1016/j.jep.2020.112675

[22] El-Saber Batiha G, Magdy Beshbishy A, Wasef LG, Elewa YHA, Al-Sagan AA, Abd El-Hack ME, et al. Chemical constituents and pharmacological activities of garlic (*Allium sativum* L.): A review. Nutrients. 2020;**12**:872. DOI: 10.3390/nu12030872

[23] Tighe-Neira R, Alberdi M, Arce-Johnson P, Romero-Romero JL, Reyes-Díaz M and Inostroza-Blancheteau C. Foods with functional properties and their potential uses in human health. In: Superfood and Functional Food - An Overview of Their Processing and Utilization. InTechOpen. 2017. DOI: 10.5772/67077

[24] Wan Q, Li N, Liang D, Zhao R, Yi M, Qiushi X, et al. Allium vegetable consumption and health: An umbrella review of meta-analyses of multiple health outcomes. Food Science & Nutrition. 2019;**7**:2451-2470

[25] Dorrigiv M, Zareiyan A, Hosseinzadeh H. Garlic (*Allium sativum*) as an antidote or a protective agent against natural or chemical toxicities: A comprehensive update review. Phytotherapy Research. 2020:1-28

[26] Mondal A, Banerjee S, Bose S, Mazumder S, Haber RA. Mohammad Hosein Farzaei and Anupam Bishayee, garlic constituents for cancer prevention and therapy: From phytochemistry to novel formulations. Pharmacological Research. 2021;**175**:105837. DOI: 10.1016/j.phrs.2021.10583

[27] De Greef D, Barton EM, Sandberg EN, Croley CR, Pumarol J, Wong TL, et al. Anticancer potential of garlic and its bioactive constituents: A systematic and comprehensive review. Seminars in Cancer Biology. 2020;**73**:219-264. DOI: 10.1016/j.semcancer.2020.11.020

[28] Shang A, Cao S-Y, Xiao-Yu X, Gan R-Y, Tang G-Y, Corke H, et al. Bioactive compounds and biological functions of garlic (*Allium sativum* L.). Food. 2019;**8**: 246. DOI: 10.3390/foods8070246

[29] Kiesel VA, Stan SD. Diallyl trisulfide, a chemopreventive agent from allium vegetables, inhibits alpha-secretases in breast cancer cells. Biochemical and Biophysical Research Communications. 2017;**484**:833e838

[30] Bhatwalkar SB, Mondal R, Krishna SBN, Adam JK, Govender P, Anupam R. Antibacterial properties of organosulfur compounds of garlic (*Allium sativum*). Frontiers in Microbiology. 2021;**12**: 613077. DOI: 10.3389/fmicb.2021.613077

[31] Gowsala P. Sivam. Protection against helicobacter pylori and other bacterial infections by garlic. Recent Advances on the Nutritional Effects Associated with the Use of Garlic as a Supplement. 2001; **131**(3s):1106S-8S. DOI: 10.1093/jn/131.3.1106S

[32] Magryś A, Olender A, Tchórzewska D. Antibacterial properties of Allium sativum L. against the most emerging multidrug-resistant bacteria and its synergy with antibiotics. Archives of Microbiology. 2021;**203**:2257-2268. DOI: 10.1007/s00203-021-02248-z

[33] Forma A, Chilimoniuk Z, Januszewski J, Sitarz R. The potential application of allium extracts in the treatment of gastrointestinal cancers. Gastroenterology Insights. 2021;**12**:136-146. DOI: 10.3390/gastroent12020012

[34] Borlinghaus J, Albrecht F, Gruhlke MCH, Nwachukwu ID, Slusarenko AJ. Allicin: Chemistry and biological properties. Molecules. 2014;**19**:12591-12618. DOI: 10.3390/molecules1908 12591

[35] Borlinghaus J, Foerster J, Kappler U, Antelmann H, Noll U, Gruhlke MCH, et al. Allicin, the odor of freshly crushed garlic: A review of recent Progress in understanding Allicin's effects on cells. Molecules. 2021;**26**:1505. DOI: 10.3390/molecules26061505

[36] Ankri S, Mirelman D. Antimicrobial properties of allicin from garlic. Microbes and Infection. 1999;**2**:125-112

[37] Santhosha SG, Prakash Jamuna SN, Prabhavathin. Bioactive components of garlic and their physiological role in health maintenance: A review. Food Bioscience. 2013;**3**:59-74

[38] Marchese A, Barbieri R, Sanches-Silva A, Daglia M, Nabavi SF, Jafari NJ, et al. Antifungal and antibacterial activities of allicin: A review. Trends in Food Science & Technology. 2016;**52**:49-56. DOI: 10.1016/j.tifs.2016.03.010

[39] Zhao X-X, Lin F-J, Li H, Li H-B, Wu D-T, Geng F, et al. Recent advances in bioactive compounds, health functions, and safety concerns of onion (*Allium cepa* L.). Frontiers in Nutrition. 2021;**8**: 669805. DOI: 10.3389/fnut.2021.669805

[40] Galavi A, Hosseinzadeh H, Razavi BM. The effects of *Allium cepa* L. (onion) and its active constituents on metabolic syndrome: A review. Iranian Journal of Basic Medical Sciences. 2021; **24**:3-16. DOI: 10.22038/ijbms.2020.46956.10843

[41] Marefatia N, Ghorania V, Shakeric F, Boskabadye M, Kianiang F, Rezaeeh R, et al. A review of anti-inflammatory, antioxidant, and immunomodulatory effects of *Allium cepa* and its main constituents. Pharmaceutical Biology. 2021;**59**(1):287-302. DOI: 10.1080/13880209.2021.1874028

[42] Dorrigiv M, Zareiyan A, Hosseinzadeh H. Onion (*Allium cepa*) and its Main constituents as antidotes or protective agents against natural or chemical toxicities: A comprehensive review. Iranian Journal of

Pharmaceutical Research. 2021;**34**(8): 1770-1797. DOI: 10.1002/ptr.6645

[43] Zamri N. Hazrulrizawati Abd Hamid, comparative study of onion (*Allium cepa*) and Leek (Allium ampeloprasum): Identification of Organosulphur compounds by UPLC-QTOF/MS and anticancer effect on MCF-7 cells. Plant Foods for Human Nutrition. 2019;**74**:525–530. DOI: 10.1007/s11130-019-00770-6

[44] Marrelli M, Amodeo V, Statti G, Conforti F. Biological properties and bioactive components of *Allium cepa* L.: Focus on potential benefits in the treatment of obesity and related comorbidities. Molecules. 2019; **24**:119

[45] Nicastro HL, Ross SA, Milner JA. Garlic and onions: Their cancer prevention properties. Cancer Prevention Research (Philadelphia, Pa.). 2015;**8**(3):181-189

[46] Slimestad R, Fossen T. Ingunn Molund Vågen, onions: A source of unique dietary flavonoids. Journal of Agricultural and Food Chemistry. 2007; **55**:10067-10080

[47] Griffits G, Trueman L, Crowther T. Brian Thomas and Brian smith onions—A global benefit to health. Phytotherapy Research. 2002;**16**:603-615

[48] Puccinelli MT, Silvia D. Stan dietary bioactive Diallyl Trisulfide in cancer prevention and treatment. International Journal of Molecular Sciences. 2017;**18**: 1645

[49] Golubkina NA, Seredin TM, Antoshkina MS, Kosheleva OV, Teliban GC, Caruso G. Yield, quality, antioxidants and elemental composition of new Leek cultivars under organic or conventional Systems in a Greenhouse. Horticulturae. 2018;**4**:39

[50] Shahrajabian MH, Sun W, Qi Cheng A. Review of Leek (*a. ampeloprasum* L.), an important vegetable and food ingredient with remarkable pharmaceutical activities. Pharmacognosy Communications. 2021; **11**(1):9-12

[51] Mikaili P, Maadirad S, Moloudizargari M, Aghajanshakeri S, Sarahroodi S. Therapeutic uses and pharmacological properties of garlic, shallot, and their biologically active compounds. Iranian Journal of Basic Medical Sciences. 2013;**16**:1031-1048

[52] Raclariu-Manolica AC, Anmarkrud JA, Kierczak M, Rafati N, Thorbek BLG, Schrøder-Nielsen A, et al. DNA Metabarcoding for quality control of basil, oregano, and paprika. Frontiers in Plant Science. 2021;**12**:665618. DOI: 10.3389/fpls.2021.665618

[53] Liu Q, Meng X, Li Y, Zhao C-N, Tang G-Y, Li H-B. Antibacterial and antifungal activities of spices. International Journal of Molecular Sciences. 2017;**18**:1283. DOI: 10.3390/ijms18061283

[54] Sakkas H, Papadopoulou C. Antimicrobial activity of basil, oregano, and thyme essential oils. Journal of Microbiology and Biotechnology. 2017; **27**(3):429-438. DOI: 10.4014/jmb.1608.08024

[55] do Nascimento LD, de Moraes AAB, da Costa KS, Galúcio JMP, Taube PS, Costa CML, et al. Bioactive natural compounds and antioxidant activity of essential oils from spice plants: New findings and potential applications. Biomolecules. 2020;**10**:988. DOI: 10.3390/biom10070988

[56] Sestili P, Ismail T, Calcabrini C, Guescini M, Catanzaro E, Turrini E, et al. The potential effects of Ocimum

basilicum on health: A review of pharmacological and toxicological studies. Expert Opinion on Drug Metabolism & Toxicology. 2018;**10**(7): 988. DOI: 10.1080/17425255.2018.1484450

[57] Fatiha Brahmi, Madani Khodir, Chibane Mohamed and Duez Pierre. Chemical composition and biological activities of Mentha species. In book: Aromatic and Medicinal Plants - Back to Nature. London, UK: InTech; 2017

[58] Bower A, Marquez S, de Mejia EG. The health benefits of selected culinary herbs and spices found in the traditional Mediterranean diet. Critical Reviews in Food Science and Nutrition. 2016;**56**(16) 2728-2746. DOI: 10.1080/10408398.2013.805713

[59] Farzaei MH, Abbasabadi Z, Ardekani MRS, Rahimi R, Farzaei F. Parsley: A review of ethnopharmacology, phytochemistry and biological activities. Journal of Traditional Chinese Medicine. 2013;**33**(6):815-826

[60] Karimi MH, Ebadi P, Amirghofran Z. Parsley and immunomodulation. Expert Review of Clinical Immunology. 2012;**8** (4):295-297. DOI: 10.1586/eci.12.12

[61] Ahmed Z et al. Phytochemical screening and mineral profiling of wild and cultivated rosemary (Rosmarinus officinalis L.) from Taounate region (northern Morocco). PhOL. 2021;**2**: 576-582

[62] Zeroual A et al. Effects of extraction technique and solvent on phytochemicals, antioxidant, and antimicrobial activities of cultivated and wild rosemary (Rosmarinus officinalis L.) from Taounate region (northern Morocco). Biointerface Research in Applied Chemistry. 2022;**12**(6): 8441-8452

[63] Eva Ivanišová, Miroslava Kačániová, Tatsiana A. Savitskaya and Dmitry D. Grinshpan. Medicinal herbs: Important source of bioactive compounds for food industry. In book: Herbs and Spices - New Processing Technologies. London, UK: InTechopen; 2021

[64] González-Vallinas M. Guillermo Reglero & Ana Ramírez de Molina (2015): Rosemary (*Rosmarinus officinalis* L.) extract as a potential complementary agent in anticancer therapy. Nutrition and Cancer. 2015. DOI: 10.5772/intechopen.98819

[65] Fernández-Ochoa Á, Borrás-Linares I, Pérez-Sánchez A, Barrajón-Catalán E, González-Álvarez I, Arráez-Román D, et al. Phenolic compounds in rosemary as potential source of bioactive compounds against colorectal cancer: In situ absorption and metabolism study. Journal of Functional Foods. 2017;**33**: 202-210

[66] Vallverdú-Queralt A, Regueiro J, Martínez-Huélamo M, Alvarenga JF, Leal LN, Lamuela-Raventos RM. A comprehensive study on the phenolic profile of widely used culinary herbs and spices: Rosemary, thyme, oregano, cinnamon, cumin and bay. Food Chemistry. 2014. DOI: 10.1016/j.jff.2017.03.046

[67] Habtemariam et al. The therapeutic potential of rosemary (Rosmarinus officinalis) Diterpenes for Alzheimer's disease. Hindawi Publishing Corporation. Evidence-based Complementary and Alternative Medicine. 2016;**2016**:2680409

[68] Petiwala SM, Johnson JJ. Diterpenes from rosemary (*Rosmarinus officinalis*): Defining their potential for anti-cancer activity. Cancer Letters. 2015;**367**(2): 93-102

[69] Allegra et al. Anticancer activity of Rosmarinus officinalis L.: Mechanisms of action and therapeutic potentials. Nutrients. 2020;**12**:1739. DOI: 10.3390/nu12061739

[70] Bina F, Rahimi R, Marjoram S. A review of Ethnopharmacology, Phytochemistry, and biological activities. Journal of Evidence-Based Complementary & Alternative Medicine. 2017;**22**(1):175-185

[71] Cala A, Salcedo JR, Torres A, Varela RM, Molinillo JMG, Macías FA. A study on the phytotoxic potential of the seasoning herb Marjoram (Origanum majorana L.) leaves. Molecules. 2021;**26**:3356. DOI: 10.3390/molecules26113356

[72] Sahin TK, Bilir B, Kucuk O. Modulation of inflammation by phytochemicals to enhance efficacy and reduce toxicity of cancer chemotherapy. Critical Reviews in Food Science and Nutrition. 2021;**26**(11):3356. DOI: 10.1080/10408398.2021.1976721

[73] M. Moshiri, M. Vahabzadeh, H. Hosseinzadeh. Clinical applications of Saff Ron (*Crocus sativus*) and its constituents: A review. DOI: 10.1055/s-0034-1375681 Published online: 2014 Drug Res. Georg Thieme Verlag KG Stuttgart · New York ISSN 2194-9379

[74] Mousavi SZ, Bathaie SZ. Historical uses of saffron: Identifying potential new avenues for modern research. Avicenna Journal of Phytomedicine. 2011;**1**(2):57-66

[75] Shafiee M, Arekhi S, Omranzadeh A, Sahebkar A. Saffron in the treatment of depression, anxiety and other mental disorders: Current evidence and potential mechanisms of action. Journal of Affective Disorders. 2018. DOI: 10.1016/j.jad.2017.11.020

[76] Pourmasoumi M, Hadi A, Najafgholizadeh A, Kafeshani M, Sahebkar A. Clinical evidence on the effects of saffron (*Crocus sativus* L.) on cardiovascular risk factors: A systematic review meta-analysis. Pharmacological Research. Journal of Afective Disorders. 2018;**227**:330-337. DOI: 10.1016/j.phrs.2018.11.038

[77] Rahmani J, Manzari N, Thompson J, Clark CCT, Villanueva G, Varkaneh HK, et al. The effect of saffron on weight and lipid profile: A systematic review, meta-analysis, and dose–response of randomized clinical trials. Phytotherapy Research. 2019;**139**:348-359

[78] Gresta F, Lombardo GM, Siracusa L, Ruberto G. Saffron, an alternative crop for sustainable agricultural systems. A review. Agronomy for Sustainable Development. 2008;**28**:95-112

[79] Kumar A, Sreedharan S, Kashyap AK, Singh P, Ramchiary N. A review on bioactive phytochemicals and ethnopharmacological potential of purslane (Portulaca oleracea L). Heliyon. 2022;**8**:e08669

[80] Dehghan F, Soori R, Gholami K, Abolmaesoomi M, Yusof A, Muniandy S, et al. Purslane (Portulaca oleracea) seed consumption and aerobic training improves biomarkers associated with atherosclerosis in women with type 2 diabetes (T2D). Scientific Reports. Heliyon. 2022;**8**(1):e08669. DOI: 10.1016/j.heliyon.2021.e08669

[81] Uddin M, Juraimi AS, Hossain MS, Nahar M, Ali M, and Rahman MM. Purslane weed (*Portulaca oleracea*): A prospective plant source of nutrition, Omega-3 fatty acid, and antioxidant attributes. Hindawi Publishing Corporation. Vol. 2014. 2016. Article ID: 951019. DOI: 10.1155/2014/951019

[82] Takooree H, Aumeeruddy MZ, Rengasamy KRR, Venugopala KN, Jeewon R, Zengin G, et al. A systematic review on black pepper (Pipernigrum L.): From folk uses to pharmacological applications. Critical Reviews in Food Science and Nutrition. 2019. DOI: 10.1007/s40200-021-00783-6

[83] Turrini E, Sestili P, Fimognari C. Overview of the anticancer potential of the "king of spices" Piper nigrum and its Main constituent Piperine. Toxins. 2020; **59**(Sup 1):S210-S243. DOI: 10.3390/toxins12120747

[84] Chavarria D, Silva T, Magalhães e Silva D, Remião F, Borges F. Lessons from black pepper: Piperine and derivatives thereof. Expert Opinion on Therapeutic Patents. 2015;**12**(12): 747. DOI: 10.1517/13543776.2016.1118057

[85] Shityakov S, Bigdelian E, Hussein AA, Hussain MB, Tripathi YC, Khan MU, et al. Phytochemical and pharmacological attributes of piperine: A bioactive ingredient of black pepper. European Journal of Medicinal Chemistry. 2019;**176**:149e161

[86] Pathak N, Bhaduri A, and Rai AK. Sesame: Bioactive compounds and health benefits. In: Mérillon JM, Ramawat KG, editors. Bioactive Molecules in Food, Reference Series in Phytochemistry. 2019;**176**:149-161. DOI: 10.1007/978-3-319-54528-8_59-1

[87] Moazzami AA. Sesame Seed Lignans Diversity, Human Metabolism and Bioactivities. Doctoral thesis. Swedish University of Agricultural Sciences Uppsala. Springer, Cham. 2018

[88] Pathak N, Rai AK, Kumari R, Bhat KV. Value addition in sesame: A perspective on bioactive components for enhancing utility and profitability. Pharmacognosy Reviews. 2014; **Vol 8**(16)

[89] Namiki M. Nutraceutical functions of sesame: A review. Critical Reviews in Food Science and Nutrition. 2007;**47**(7): 651-673. DOI: 10.1080/10408390600 91911

[90] Kim S, Yang HY, Lee HJ, Ju J. In vitro antioxidant and anti-colon cancer activities of Sesamum indicum L. leaf extract and its major component, Pedaliin. Food. 2021;**10**:1216. DOI: 10.3390/foods10061216

[91] Majdalawieh AF, Mansour ZR. Sesamol, a major lignan in sesame seeds (Sesamum indicum): Anti-cancer properties and mechanisms of action. European Journal of Pharmacology. 2019;**10**(6):1216. DOI: 10.1016/j.ejphar.2019.05.008

[92] Allaq AA, Sidik NJ, Abdul-Aziz A, Ahmed IA. Cumin (*Cuminum cyminum* L.): A review of its ethnopharmacology, phytochemistry. Biomedical Research and Therapy. 2020;**855**:75-89

[93] Sowbhagya HB. Chemistry, technology, and nutraceutical functions of cumin (cuminum cyminum L): An overview. Critical Reviews in Food Science and Nutrition. 2013;**53**(1):1-10. DOI: 10.15419/bmrat.v7i9.634

[94] Mnif S, Aifa S. Cumin (*Cuminum cyminum* L.) from traditional uses to potential biomedical applications. Chemistry & Biodiversity. 2015;**53**(1): 1-10

[95] Zhang Y, Ma H, Liu W, Yuan T, Seeram NP. New Antiglycative compounds from cumin (*Cuminum cyminum*) spice. Journal of Agricultural and Food Chemistry. 2015;**63**:10097-10102. DOI: 10.1002/cbdv.201400305

[96] Srinivasan K. Cumin (*Cuminum cyminum*) and black cumin (*Nigella sativa*) seeds: Traditional uses, chemical constituents, and nutraceutical effects. Food Quality and Safety. 2018;**2**:1-16. DOI: 10.1021/acs.jafc.5b04796

[97] Yimer EM, Tuem KB, Karim A, Ur-Rehman N, Anwar F. *Nigella sativa* L. (black cumin): A promising natural remedy for wide range of illnesses. Evidence-based Complementary and Alternative Medicine. 2019;**2**(1):1–16. DOI: 10.1093/fqsafe/fyx031

[98] Hannan MA, Rahman MA, Sohag AAM, Uddin MJ, Dash R, Sikder MH, et al. Black cumin (*Nigella sativa* L.): A comprehensive review on Phytochemistry, health benefits, molecular pharmacology, and safety. Nutrients. 2021;**13**:1784. DOI: 10.3390/nu13061784

[99] Alfikri FN, et al. Yield, quality, and antioxidant activity of clove (*Syzygium aromaticum* L.) bud oil at the different phenological stages in young and mature trees. 2021;**13**(6):1784. DOI: 10.1155/2020/9701701

[100] Akhter S. Low to no cost remedies for the management of diabetes mellitus; global health concern. Journal of Diabetes and Metabolic Disorders. 2021;**20**:951-962

[101] Cortés-Rojas DF, de Souza CR, Oliveira WP. Clove (Syzygium aromaticum): A precious spice. Asian Pacific Journal of Tropical Biomedicine. 2014;**4**(2):90-96. DOI: 10.1016/S2221-1691(14)60215-X

[102] Kothiwale SV, Patwardhan V, Gandhi M, Sohoni R, Kumar A. A comparative study of antiplaque and antigingivitis effects of herbal mouthrinse containing tea tree oil, clove, and basil with commercially available essential oil mouthrinse. Journal of Indian Society of Periodontology. 2014;**18**(3):316-320. DOI: 10.4103/0972-124X.134568

[103] Ghaffar S, Afridi SK, Aftab MF, Murtaza M, Hafizur RM, Sara S, et al. Clove and its active compound attenuate free fatty acid-mediated insulin resistance in skeletal muscle cells and in mice. Journal of Medicinal Food. 2017;**20**(4):335-344. DOI: 10.1089/jmf.2016.3835 Epub 2017 Mar 24

[104] Irahal IN, Guenaou I, Lahlou FA, Hmimid F, Bourhim N. Syzygium aromaticum bud (clove) essential oil is a novel and safe aldose reductase inhibitor: in silico, in vitro, and in vivo evidence. Hormones (Athens, Greece). 2022;**20**(4):335-344. DOI: 10.1089/jmf.2016.3835. DOI: 10.1007/s42000-021-00347-6

[105] Vázquez-Fresno R, Rosana ARR, Sajed T, Onookome-Okome T, Wishart NA, Wishart DS. Herbs and spices-biomarkers of intake based on human intervention studies - a systematic review. Genes & Nutrition. 2019;**21**(2):229-240. DOI: 10.1186/s12263-019-0636-8

[106] Maierean SM et al. The effects of cinnamon supplementation on blood lipid concentrations: A systematic review and meta-analysis. Journal of Clinical Lipidology. 2019;**14**:18

[107] Yang Y, Li S. Dandelion extracts protect human skin fibroblasts from UVB damage and cellular senescence. Oxidative Medicine and Cellular Longevity. 2015;**11**:(6):1393-1406. DOI: 10.1016/j.jacl.2017.08.004

[108] Yang Y, Ying G, Shanshan W, Fengtian W, Chen Z. In vitro inhibition effects of hepatitis B virus by dandelion and taraxasterol. Infectious Agents and Cancer. 2020;**15**:44

[109] Wirngo FE, Lambert MN, Jeppesen PB. The physiological effects of dandelion (*Taraxacum Officinale*) in type 2 diabetes. The Review of Diabetic Studies. 2016;**13**(2–3). DOI: 10.1186/s13027-020-00309-4

[110] Marta González-Castejón, Francesco Visioli, and Arantxa Rodriguez-Casado. Diverse biological activities of dandelion. DOI 10.1900/RDS.2016.13.113. Nutrition Reviews, 2012

[111] Nwafor IC, Shale K, Achilonu MC. Chemical composition and nutritive benefits of chicory (*Cichorium intybus*) as an ideal complementary and/or alternative livestock feed supplement. Scientific World Journal. 2017;**70**(9): 534-547. DOI: 10.1155/2017/7343928

[112] Janda K, Gutowska I, Geszke-Moritz M, Jakubczyk K. The common Cichory (*Cichorium intybus* L.) as a source of extracts with health-promoting properties—A review. Molecules. 2021; **26**:1814. DOI: 10.3390/molecules26061814

[113] Micka A, Siepelmeyer A, Holz A, Theis S, Schön C. Effect of consumption of chicory inulin on bowel function in healthy subjects with constipation: A randomized, double-blind, placebo-controlled trial. International Journal of Food Sciences and Nutrition. 2016;**26**(6):1814. DOI: 10.1080/09637486.2016.1212819

[114] Marteau P, Jacobs H, Cazaubiel M, Signoret C, Prevel J-M, Housez B. Effects of chicory inulin in constipated elderly people: A double-blind controlled trial. International Journal of Food Sciences and Nutrition. 2011;**62**(2):164-170

[115] Perović J, Šaponjac VT, Kojić J, Krulj J, Moreno DA, García-Viguera C, et al. Chicory (*Cichorium intybus* L.) as a food ingredient – Nutritional composition, bioactivity, safety, and health claims: A review. Food Chemistry. 2021;**336**:127676

[116] Marmouzi I, Bouyahya A, Ezzat SM, El Jemli M, Kharbach M. The food plant *Silybum marianum* (L.) Gaertn.: Phytochemistry, Ethnopharmacology and clinical evidence. Journal of Ethnopharmacology. 2021;**265**:113303

[117] Wang X, Zhang Z, Shuai-Cheng W. Health benefits of Silybum marianum: Phytochemistry, pharmacology, and applications. Journal of Agricultural and Food Chemistry. 2020:113303. DOI: 10.1016/j.jep.2020.113303

[118] Vostálová J, Tinková E, Biedermann D, Kosina P, Ulrichová J, Svobodová AR. Skin protective activity of Silymarin and its Flavonolignans. Molecules. 2019;**24**: 1022. DOI: 10.3390/molecules24061022

[119] Tajmohammadi A, Razavi BM, Hosseinzadeh H. *Silybum marianum* (milk thistle) and its main constituent, silymarin, as a potential therapeutic plant in metabolic syndrome: A review. Phytotherapy Research. 2018;**24**(6):1-17

[120] Srivastava JK, Shankar E, Gupta S. Chamomile: A herbal medicine of the past with bright future. Molecular Medicine Reports. 2010;**3**(6):895-901. DOI: 10.3892/mmr.2010.377

[121] Taia Y, Linga C, Wanga C, Wanga H, Sua L, Yanga L, et al. Analysis of terpenoid biosynthesis pathways in German chamomile (*Matricaria recutita*) and Roman chamomile (*Chamaemelum nobile*) based on co-expression networks. Genomics. 2020;**112**:1055-1064

[122] Kolodziejczyk-Czepas J, Bijaka M, Saluka J, Ponczeka MB, Zbikowskaa HM, Nowaka P, et al. Radical scavenging and antioxidant effects of Matricaria chamomilla polyphenolic–polysaccharide

conjugates. International Journal of Biological Macromolecules. 2015;**72**: 1152-1158

[123] Dehkordi ZR, Baharanchi FSH, Bekhradi R. Effect of lavender inhalation on the symptoms of primary dysmenorrhea and the amount of menstrual bleeding: A randomized clinical trial. Complementary Therapies in Medicine. 2014;**22**:212-219

[124] Koulivand PH, Ghadiri MK, Gorji A. Lavender and the nervous system. Evidence-based Complementary and Alternative Medicine. 2013;**2014**: 681304. DOI: 10.1016/j.ctim.2013.12.011

[125] López V, Nielsen B, Solas M, Ramírez MJ, Jäger AK. Exploring pharmacological mechanisms of lavender (*Lavandula angustifolia*) essential oil on central nervous system targets. Frontiers in Pharmacology. 2017;**8**:280. DOI: 10.3389/fphar.2017.00280

[126] Chen S-L, Chen C-H. Effects of lavender tea on fatigue, depression, and maternal-infant attachment in sleep-disturbed postnatal women. Worldviews on Evidence-Based Nursing. 2015;**12**(6): 370-379

[127] Afshar MK, Moghadam ZB, Taghizadeh Z, Bekhradi R, Montazeri A, Mokhtari P. Lavender fragrance essential oil and the quality of sleep in postpartum women. Iranian Red Crescent Medical Journal. 2015;**17**(4):e25880

[128] Lillehei AS, Halco'n LL, Savik K, Reis R. Effect of inhaled lavender and sleep hygiene on self-reported sleep issues: A randomized controlled trial. The Journal of Alternative and Complementary Medicine. 2015;**21**(7):430-438

[129] Nasiri A, Mahmodi MA, Nobakht Z. Effect of aromatherapy massage with lavender essential oil on pain in patients with osteoarthritis of the knee: A randomized controlled clinical trial. Complementary Therapies in Clinical Practice. 2016;**25**:75e80

[130] Nikjou R, Kazemzadeh R, Rostamnegad M, Moshfegi S, Karimollahi M, Salehi H. The effect of lavender aromatherapy on the pain severity of primary dysmenorrhea: A triple-blind randomized clinical trial. Annals of Medical and Health Sciences Research. 2016;**6**(4):75-80. DOI: 10.1016/j.ctcp.2016.08.002

[131] Bakhtshirin F, Abedi S, Zoj PY, Razmjooee D. The effect of aromatherapy massage with lavender oil on severity of primary dysmenorrhea in Arsanjan students. Iranian Journal of Nursing and Midwifery Research. 2015; **20**(1):211-215

[132] da Silva GL, Luft C, Lunardelli A, Amaral RH, da Silva Melo DA, et al. Antioxidant, analgesic and anti-inflammatory effects of lavender essential oil. Anais da Academia Brasileira de Ciências. 2015; **87**(2 Suppl):156

[133] Cardia GFE, Silva-Filho SE, Silva EL, Uchida NS, et al. Effect of lavender (Lavandula angustifolia) essential oil on acute inflammatory response. Evidence-based Complementary and Alternative Medicine. 2018;**2018**:1397-408. DOI: 10.1590/0001-3765201520150056

[134] Hossain S, Heo H, De Silva BCJ, Wimalasena SHMP, Pathirana HNKS, Heo G-J. Antibacterial activity of essential oil from lavender (Lavandula angustifolia) against pet turtle-borne pathogenic bacteria. Laboratory Animal Research. 2017;**33**(3):195-201. DOI: 10.5625/lar.2017.33.3.195

[135] Mori H-M, Kawanami H, Kawahata H, Aoki M. Wound healing potential of lavender oil by acceleration of granulation and wound contraction through induction of TGF-β in a rat model. BMC Complementary and Alternative Medicine. 2016;**16**:144. DOI: 10.1186/s12906-016-1128-7

[136] Ça K, ğgatay Selvi. Investigating the influence of infrared drying method on Linden (Tilia platyphyllos Scop.) leaves: Kinetics, color, projected area, modeling, Total phenolic, and flavonoid content. Plants. 2020;**9**:916. DOI: 10.3390/plants9070916

[137] Yayalacı Y, Celik I, Batı B. Hepatoprotective and antioxidant activity of Linden (*Tilia platyphyllos* L.) infusion against ethanol-induced oxidative stress in rats. The Journal of Membrane Biology. 2014;**247**:181-188

[138] Dorota Kregiel ID, Pawlikowska E, Antolak H. Urtica spp.: Ordinary plants with extraordinary properties. Molecules. 2018;**23**:1664. DOI: 10.3390/molecules23071664

[139] Mahlangeni NT, Moodley R, Jonnalagadda SB. Nutritional value, antioxidant and antidiabetic properties of nettles (*Laportea alatipes* and *Obetia tenax*). Scientific Reports. 2020;**10**:9762. DOI: 10.1038/s41598-020-67055-w

[140] Ibrahim M, Rehman K, Razzaq A, Hussain I, Farooq T, Hussain A, et al. Investigations of phytochemical constituents and their pharmacological properties isolated from the genus Urtica: Critical review and analysis. Critical Reviews in Eukaryotic Gene Expression. 2018;**28**(1):25-66

[141] Mahlangeni NT, Moodley R, Jonnalagadda SB. The distribution of macronutrients, anti-nutrients and essential elements in nettles, Laportea peduncularis susp. Peduncularis (river nettle) and Urtica dioica (stinging nettle). Journal of Environmental Science and Health, Part B. 2016;**51**(3): 160-169. DOI: 10.1080/03601234.2015.1108806

[142] Hodroj MH, al Hoda Al Bast N, Taleb RI, Borjac J, Rizk S. Nettle tea inhibits growth of acute myeloid leukemia cells In vitro by promoting apoptosis. Nutrients. 2020;**12**:2629. DOI: 10.3390/nu12092629

[143] Bittner Fialová S, Rendeková K, Mučaji P, Nagy M, Slobodníková L. Antibacterial activity of medicinal plants and their constituents in the context of skin and wound infections, considering European legislation and folk medicine—A review. International Journal of Molecular Sciences. 2021;**22**: 10746. DOI: 10.3390/ijms221910746

[144] Arora D, Rani A, Sharma A. A review on phytochemistry and ethnopharmacological aspects of genus calendula. Pharmacognosy Reviews. 2013;**22**(19):10746

[145] Susan S. Percival, use of Echinacea in medicine. Biochemical Pharmacology. 2000;**60**:155-158

[146] Catanzaro M, Corsini E, Rosini M, Racchi M, Lanni C. Immunomodulators inspired by nature: A review on curcumin and Echinacea. Molecules. 2018;**23**:2778. DOI: 10.3390/molecules23112778

[147] Pareek A, Suthar M, Rathore GS, Bansal V. Feverfew (Tanacetum parthenium L.): A systematic review. Pharmacognosy Reviews. 2011;**5**(9): 103-110

[148] Wider B, Pittler MH, Ernst E. Feverfew for preventing migraine.

Cochrane Database of Systematic Reviews 2015, Issue 4. Art. No.: CD002286. DOI: 10.4103/0973-7847.79105

[149] Pourianezhad F, Tahmasebi S, Abdusi V, Nikfar S, Mirhoseini M. Review on feverfew, a valuable medicinal plant. Journal of HerbMed Pharmacology. 2016;**5**(2):45-49

[150] Zhang F, Zhou J, Shi Y, Karaisz K. Identification of Antioxidative ingredients from feverfew (Tanacetum Parthenium) extract substantially free of Parthenolide and other alpha-unsaturated gamma-lactones. Open Journal of Analytical and Bioanalytical Chemistry. 2019;**3**(1):076-082. DOI: 10.17352/ojabc.000015

[151] Tatsis EC, Boeren S, Exarchou V, Troganis AN, Vervoort J, Gerothanassis IP. Identification of the major constituents of *Hypericum perforatum* by LC/SPE/NMR and/or LC/MS. Phytochemistry. 2007;**68**:383-393

[152] Süntar IP, Akkol EK, Yılmazer D, Baykal T, Kırmızıbekmezc H, Alper M, et al. Investigations on the in vivo wound healing potential of Hypericum perforatum L. Journal of Ethnopharmacology. 2010;**127**:468-477

[153] Galeotti N, Maidecchi A, Mattoli L, Burico M, Ghelardini C, St. John's wort seed and feverfew flower extracts relieve painful diabetic neuropathy in a rat model of diabetes. Fitoterapia. 2014;**92**: 23-33

[154] Novelli M, Menegazzi M, Beffyc P, Porozova S, Gregorelli A, Giacopelli D, et al. John's wort extract and hyperforin inhibit multiple phosphorylation steps of cytokine signaling and prevent inflammatory and apoptotic gene induction in pancreatic cells. The International Journal of Biochemistry & Cell Biology. 2016;**81**:92-104

[155] Apaydin EA, Maher AR, Shanman R, Booth MS, Miles JNV, Sorbero ME, et al. A systematic review of St. John's wort for major depressive disorder. Systematic Reviews. 2016;**5**:148

[156] Ghazanfarpour M, Sadeghi R, Latifnejad Roudsari R, Khorsand I, Khadivzadeh T, Muoio B. Red clover for treatment of hot flashes and menopausal symptoms: A systematic review and meta-analysis. Journal of Obstetrics and Gynaecology. 2015;**5**(1):148. DOI: 10.1186/s13643-016-0325-2

[157] Kanadys W, Baranska A, Jedrych M, Religioni U, Janiszewska M. Effects of red clover (Trifolium pratense) isoflavones on the lipid profile of perimenopausal and postmenopausal women - a systematic review and meta-analysis. Maturitas. 2019;**36**(3):1-11. DOI: 10.3109/01443615.2015.1049249

[158] Kanadys W, Baranska A, Błaszczuk A, Polz-Dacewicz M, Drop B, Kanecki K, et al. Evaluation of clinical meaningfulness of red clover (*Trifolium pratense* L.) extract to relieve hot flushes and menopausal symptoms in Peri- and post-menopausal women: A systematic review and meta-analysis of randomized controlled trials. Nutrients. 2021;**13**:1258

[159] Hawkins J, Baker C, Cherry L, Dunne E. Black elderberry (Sambucus nigra) supplementation effectively treats upper respiratory symptoms: A meta-analysis of randomized, controlled clinical trials. Complementary Therapies in Medicine. 2018;**13**(4):1258. DOI: 10.3390/nu13041258

[160] Macknin M, Wolski K, Negrey J, Mace SE. Elderberry extract outpatient influenza treatment for emergency room patients ages 5 and above: A randomized,

double-blind, placebo-controlled trial. Journal of General Internal Medicine. 2020;**42**:361-365. DOI: 10.1016/j.ctim.2018.12.004

[161] Zakay-Rones Z, Thom E, Wollan T, Wadstein J. Randomized study of the efficacy and safety of Oral elderberry extract in the treatment of influenza a and B virus infections. Journal of International Medical Research. 2004; **32**(2):132-140

Chapter 12

Trace Element Determination in Medicinal Plant Samples by ED-XRF Analysis

Archana A. Yelmate, Sanjay S. Thonte and Kranti L. Satpute

Abstract

The main objective of this study is to determine the concentration of trace elements in selected medicinal plants which are used for the treatment of dermal diseases. The trace element analysis was carried out in *Trigonella foenum-graecum, Azadirachta indica, Vitex nigundo, and Argemone mexicana,* using ED-X-ray Florescence (XRF) technique. The experiments were carried out using 3MV pelletron accelerator. The elements K, Ca, Cr, Mn, Fe, Cu, Zn, Rb, Sr., and Pb were identified in the sample. The elements K and Ca were present in maximum quantities. The relative concentrations of different elements in these medicinal plants have been given. All four plants contain trace elements of different concentrations in medicinal plants selected for this study. It is believed that the various trace elements present in the plants play an important role in the management of skin diseases. The present information will be helpful to prescribe the type of extract, dose, and mixture of these plants. The results justify that usage of these plants in the traditional systems of medicine for the treatment of skin diseases contains appropriate amounts of Fe, Zn, Cu, etc.

Keywords: ED-XRF, *Argemone Mexicana* Linn, *Trigonella foenum-graecum*, *Azadirachta indica*, *Vitex nigundo*

1. Introduction

Many plants are well known for the medicinal value and are used in herbal formulations. These plants are taken for elemental analysis using XRF. The medicinal action of these medicinal plants totally depends on the chemical constituents present in these plants. Herbal drugs are being used as remedies for various diseases and disorders throughout the world [1].

Nowadays more interest has been focused on phytomedicines or Ayurvedic medicines as they are safe and cost-effective as well as more compatible with the human body. These plants are used for the manufacturing of various synthetic drugs. It has been reported that the trace elements present in the plants are responsible for the development of different chemical constituents. Also, plant nutrients, including potassium (K), phosphorus (P), and sulfur (S), play an important role in regulating various processes, such as photosynthesis, carbon respiration, tissue building, etc [2]. However, most of the studies have been done on constituents present in plants like essential oils, vitamins, glycosides, and other organic components but very little has been reported about the elemental composition of the plants [3].

A literature survey revealed a significant role played by the trace elements in the treatment of various diseases and disorders. It has been documented that alteration of trace elemental in an organism has a direct relation with different pathological conditions. Hence, the screening of the bioactive elements present in the plants and determination of the elemental composition of widely used medicinal plants is highly essential and also in identifying potentially hazardous trace metals in plants. In this study, attention has been focused on the specific biological significance of these trace elemental compositions of plants, which is crucial for the development of new drugs based on natural sources. The present investigation is an attempt to gain insight into the trace elemental composition analysis of some medicinal plants [4, 5].

For this study, X-Ray Fluorescence (XRF) analysis technique has been employed which is a fast technique for the identification and determination of elements. XRF is a powerful technique for nutrient plant analysis to estimate trace elemental concentrations.

XRF has been successfully applied in studies on the element composition analysis of plants, soil contamination, and agriculture out of which most of them applied pressed powder pellets to perform XRF analysis. The X-ray fluorescence method (EDXRF) uses loose powder, which decreases time and analysis costs [6, 7].

The main objective of this study is to determine the concentration of trace elements in selected medicinal plants, which are used for the treatment of dermal diseases by the tribal people. The four plants were selected for the present study mentioned here *Azardirachta indica, Vitex nigundo, Argemone mexicana,* and *Trigonella fornum graecum* [5, 6].

2. Toxic effects of heavy metals on plants and the human body

Heavy metal poisoning is caused by the accumulation of certain metals in the body due to exposure through food, water, industrial chemicals, or other sources. While your body needs small amounts of some heavy metals to function normally, such as zinc, copper, chromium, iron, and manganese toxic amounts are harmful. Iron, cobalt, copper, manganese, molybdenum, and zinc are required by humans in adequate amounts. In the human body, these heavy metals are transported and compartmentalized into body cells and tissues binding to proteins, nucleic acids destroying these macromolecules and disrupting their cellular functions. Heavy metals disrupt metabolic functions in two ways: They accumulate and thereby disrupt function in vital organs and glands such as the heart, brain, kidneys, bone, liver, etc. They displace the vital nutritional minerals from their original place, thereby, hindering their biological function. The study on the absorption and accumulation of heavy metals lead, zinc, copper, and cadmium by various plant species around a smelter showed that the accumulation of the metals by plants differed with plant species and their parts [7].

Heavy metals can accumulate and migrate in the soil environment. Metal pollutants in soil may be absorbed by the plants through their roots and vascular system. Once in the body, heavy metals can accumulate over time in your bones, liver, brain, kidneys, and heart. Having excess heavy metals in the body can damage vital organs, and cause behavioral changes and difficulties with thinking and memory. The heavy metals most commonly associated with the poisoning of humans are lead, mercury, arsenic, and cadmium. Heavy metal poisoning may occur as a result of industrial exposure, air or water pollution, foods, medicines, improperly coated food containers, or the ingestion of lead-based paints. Zinc reduces the amount of copper your body absorbs, and high doses of zinc can cause a copper deficiency. Gastrointestinal and kidney dysfunction, nervous system disorders, skin lesions, vascular damage, immune system dysfunction, birth defects, and cancer are examples of the complications of heavy metals toxic effects. Heavy metal intoxication is another reason for liver disease, it has great importance due to unnoticed intake of heavy metals by humans and because heavy metals can be present in drinking water, food, and the environment or workplace of affected people. A person who lost his vision and even suddenly became color blind turned out to have an unusual cause for the problems: thallium poisoning. Thallium is a metal that can be absorbed through a skin and can cause neurological problems [7, 8].

Essential and non-essential heavy metals generally produce common toxic effects on plants, such as low biomass accumulation, chlorosis, inhibition of growth and photosynthesis, altered water balance and nutrient assimilation, and senescence, which ultimately cause plant death.

To minimize the detrimental effects of heavy metal exposure and its accumulation, plants have evolved detoxification mechanisms. Such mechanisms are mainly based on chelation and subcellular compartmentalization. Chelation of heavy metals is a ubiquitous detoxification strategy described in wide variety of plants. Among the most significant heavy metals from the point of view of health are mercury, lead, cadmium, nickel, and zinc [6, 7].

3. Materials & methods

Medicinal plant samples for the study were collected from different areas of Maharashtra with the help of experts and subjected to authentication at by a botanist. All the samples were washed under running tap water and also rinsed with deionized water to remove any earthy matter before drying in an oven at 60°C for near about 2–3 days. Milling of the plant materials was done in a grinder (**Table 1**). Experiments were performed with dried samples of medicinal plants No. 1 – No. 4, (No. 1 – *Azardirachta indica*, No. 2 – *Vitex nigundo*, No. 3 – *A. mexicana*, No. 4 – *Trigonella fornum graecum*,)

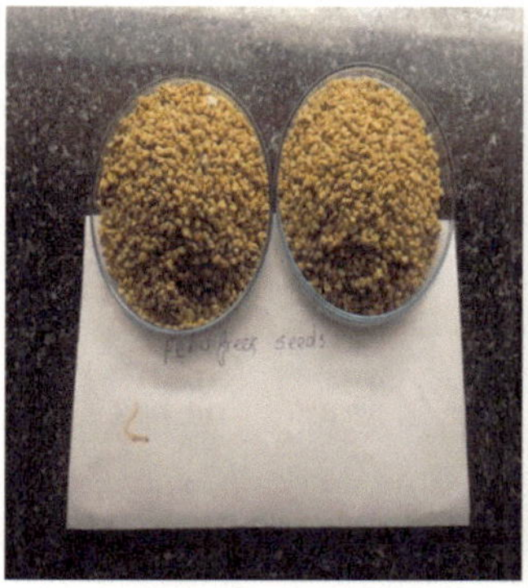

Trigonella foenum graecum

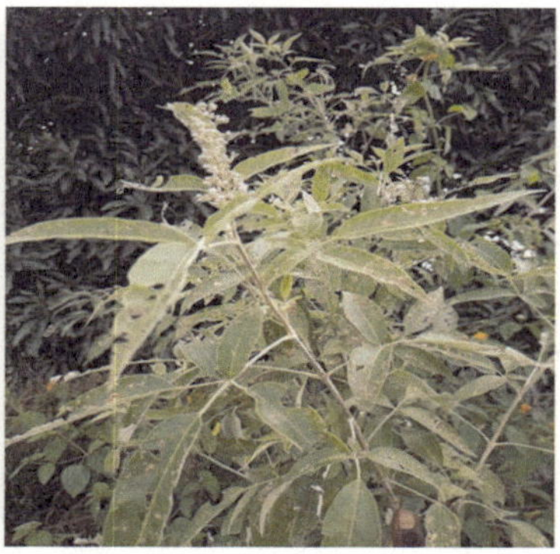

Vitex nigundo linn

Sr.No	Local name	English name	Scientific name	Family	Part used	Medicinal uses
1	Methi	Fenugreek	*Trigonellafoenumgraecum*	Fabaceae	Seed	Diabetes, Asthma, Anemia.
2	nirgudi	Five leaved chaste tree	*Vitexnigundo*Linn	Verbenaceae	Leaves	Anti-inflammatory, analgesic, antihistaminic property, astringent.
3	Satyanashi	Mexican poppy	*Argemonemexicana*	Papaveraceae	Leaves	relieve toothache, skin diseases, Leprosy.
4	Kadunimb	Neem tree	*Azardirachtaindica*	Meliaceae	Leaves	Malaria, tuberculosis, rheumatism, arthritis, jaundice and intestinal worms, and skin diseases.

Table 1.
Selected plants information.

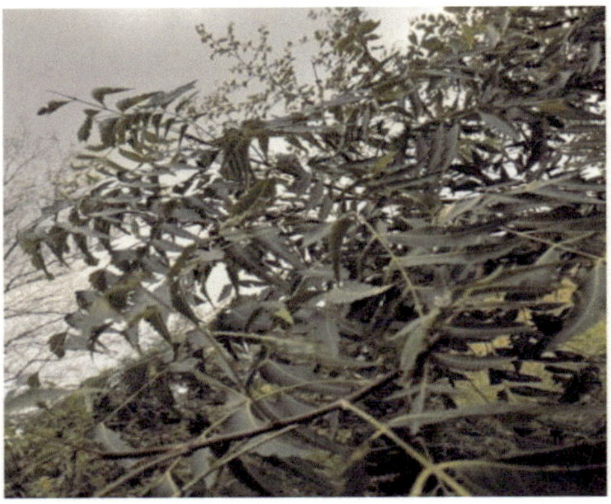

Azardirachta indica

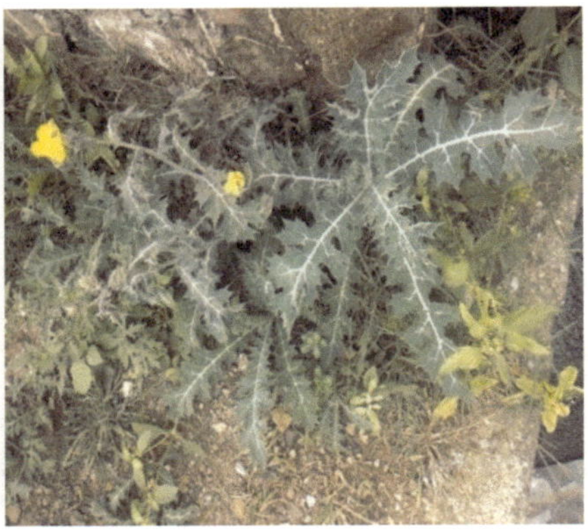

Argemone Mexicana

4. Authentification of plants

According to WHO, the best source of medicines are medicinal plants. The herbs under study are easily available throughout the year and in almost all parts of India. They are cheap and can be easily procured from wild sources also. Since whole plants do not stay stable and potent for a longer duration, they were used freshly dried specific parts of plants. We have selected *A. indica* Linn leaves, *Vitex nigundo* Linn leaves, seeds of *Trigonella foenum graecum* Linn, and A. mexicana Linn leaves. Selection of plants based on an extensive literature survey, the literature reveals that the selected plants were used traditionally for curing various skin diseases. The selected plant parts contain different phytoconstituents responsible for antimicrobial and anti-inflammatory activities. In the ayurvedic system of medicines, these plants are used traditionally. Also, these plants have been reported in CHARAK SAMHITA ancient and authoritative textbook of Ayurveda and Unani [6, 7]. *A. indica* leaves, *Vitex nigundo* Linn leaves were collected from the local region of Latur in the month of July and August, seeds of *Trigonella foenum graecum* Linn and were collected from the local market of Latur in the month of august, *A. mexicana* Linn leaves, in the month of October respectively and authenticated under the supervision of expert botanist by submitting herbarium of each sample. Authenticated plant parts were evaluated for its morphological characteristics such as color, odor, taste, size, shape, and nature of outer and inner surfaces as per guidelines of WHO. The plant parts were shade dried for a month and powdered in mechanical grinder and stored in airtight container [8].

5. Standardization of plants

In order to produce reproducible quality of final product the quality of starting material is very important. Therefore, standardization of plant samples under study was performed as per the comprehensive guidelines of WHO monographs. World health organization emphasized the need of ensuring quality of herbal drugs by using different modern techniques and by applying suitable standards. The following parameters were used for standardization [8, 9].

6. Extractive values

The extractive value of drug helps to determine the amount of soluble constituents in a medicinal plant material, after extraction with solvents. The extraction of any crude drug with a particular solvent gives a solution containing different chemical constituents, which are soluble in that solvent only. The composition of these chemical constituents in a solvent depends upon the nature of phytoconstituents and their solubility in solvent used for extraction [8, 9].

7. Water soluble extractive

Accurately weighed 5 gm of crude drug sample of *Argemone Mexicana* Linn, *Vitex nigundo* Linn, *Azardirachta indica* Linn leaves and seeds of *Trigonella foenum graecum* Linn taken in a weighing bottle and then transfer it to each different dry 250 ml. conical flask. Each flask was filled to the delivery mark with the chloroform water for water soluble extractives. Tightly packed all flasks and kept a side for 24 hours. Then it was filtered, when sufficient filtrate has collected, takes 25 ml of the filtrate and transferred to a thin porcelain dish. Evaporated to dryness on a water bath and subjected for drying in an oven at 100^0c. Cool in desiccators and of percentage water soluble extractive was calculated (**Table 2**) [8–10].

8. Alcohol soluble extractive

Accurately weighed 5 gm of each *Argemone Mexicana* Linn, *Vitex nigundo* Linn, *Azardirachta indica* Linn leaves, and seeds of *Trigonella foenum graecum* Linn powder drug taken in a weighing bottle and transfer it to separate dry 250 ml. conical flasks.

Each flask was filled to the delivery mark with the solvent (90% alcohol). Tightly packed all flasks and kept aside for 24 hours, then it was filtered rapidly in order to

Evaluation parameters	Name of plants			
	Azadirachta indica Linn	*Vitex nigundo* Linn	*Trigonella foenum graecum* Linn	*Argemone Mexicana* Linn
Foreign matter	0.2	0.3	0.3	o.2
Ash values	7.9	0.35	9.5	16.7
Acid insoluble ash	1.89	0.29	1.3	2.9
Water soluble ash	16.4	12.45	8.2	4.8
Alcohol soluble extractive	13.21	10.20	10.31	17.3
Water soluble extractive	21.4	33.21	22.32	26.0
Moisture and volatilities	5.4	6.2	9.2	8.2

Table 2.
Results of standardization of plant materials.

prevent the loss of alcohol. When sufficient filtrate has collected, take 25 ml. of the filtrate and transferred to thin porcelain dish. Evaporated to dryness on a water bath and subjected for drying in an oven at 100^0c. Cool in desiccators and of Percentage ethanol soluble extractive was calculated [8–10].

Ash values: Ash value means residue remained after incineration of crude drugs. It is inorganic mixture of metallic salts and silica. It helps in determining the quality and purity of crude drugs, especially in the powdered form of crude drugs. The objective of ash value is to remove all traces of organic matter which may interfere in an analytical determination. Ash contains inorganic like phosphates, carbonates, silicates of sodium, potassium, magnesium, calcium, etc. Sometimes, inorganic variables like calcium oxalate carbonate content of drug affects "Total ash value"(139).

The different Types of ash values are as follows:

Total Ash: It is the total mixture of physiological ash and non-physiological ash. Water Soluble Ash: If a total ash is treated with chloroform water then the resulting ash is known as water- soluble ash. Sulfated Ash: It involves the treatment of drug with dil. Sulfuric acid before ignition. In this all oxides and carbonates are converted to sulfates and ignition is carried out at a higher temperatures in a muffle furnace. Acid Insoluble Ash: If a total ash is treated with dil. HCL then the resulting ash is known as acid insoluble ash. This value mainly represents contamination with materials like sand. Weighed and ignited flat thin porcelain dish or a tarred silica crucible was taken. 2 g of the powdered drug were weighed and taken in the dish /crucible. Support the dish on a triangle placed on the ring of the retort stand. Heated with a burner using a flame till vapors almost ceases to be evolved then lower the dish and heat more strongly until all the carbon is burnt off and placed the silica crucible in a desiccator for cooling. After cooling weight, the ash and calculated the percentage [8–10].

Acid Insoluble Ash: Using 25 ml of dil. HCL washed the ash obtained from the dish used for determination of total ash value into 100 ml beaker. Boiled for 5 minutes over a Bunsen burner and filtered the above solutions through an ash less filter paper, washed the residue twice with hot water, ignite a crucible in a flame, cool, and weighed. Cooled the silica crucible in desiccator weighed the residue and calculated the acid insoluble ash value [8–11].

Water soluble ash: Total ash obtained was boiled for five minutes with 25 mL of distilled water. Cooled and collected the insoluble matter on an ash less filter paper, washed with hot water and again ignited for 15 minutes at temperature not exceeding 450°C and percentage of water soluble ash was calculated [12, 13].

Sulfated ash: Heated empty silica crucible to redness for 10 minutes. Allowed to cooled and weighed. Placed one gram of powder of plants in a silica crucible, treated with Sulfuric acid, ignited again moistened with sulfuric acid, and ignited at about 800°C in a muffle furnace, cooled and weighed. The percentage of sulfated ash was calculated.

Moisture and Volatilities: About 5 – 6 g of *A. indica* Linn leaves, *vitex nigundo* Linn leaves, *Argemone Mexicana* Linn leaves, and *Trigonella foenum graecum* Linn seeds were accurately weighed in a petri dish and kept in a hot air oven at 110°C for 4 hours. After cooling in a desiccator, the loss in weight was recorded in each case. This procedure was repeated until a constant weight was obtained.

Moisture and Volatilities (%) = Loss in weight x 100 W, W = Weight of the leaves in grams.

Determination of foreign organic matter in plant samples: Foreign organic matter means the material not collected during collection from an original plant source. Insects, molds, or any other contaminated material is considered as foreign organic matter. Procedure: 500 gm of crude collected drug taken and evenly spread on a clean tile. Then visually inspect the sample with eyes and separate the foreign matter if any [14–17].

Morphologic evaluation: After authentification, all plants are subjected for morphological parameters like color, odor, taste, size, shape, etc. The results are recorded in **Table 3**.

Sr. No	Characters	Name of plant samples			
		Azadirachta indica **Linn**	***Vitex nigundo*** **Linn**	***Trigonella foenum graecum*** **Linn**	***Argemone Mexicana*** **Linn**
1	Color	Dark green	Green, dark reddish brown.	Yellowish or yellowish brown	Green-brown
2	Odor	Typical, Characteristi cs	None, when crushed strong smell	Characteristi cs, Pungent Spicy	Slightly pleasant
3	Taste	Intensely Bitter	None	Bitter and mucilaginous	Non Characteristics
4	Size	1–3 cm in diameter, 2 – 8 cm in length	Variable	3–6 mm length, 2 – 4 mm width.	1.5–2 cm in diameter, 3–5 cm length
5	Shape	Lanceolate	Ovoid, tears	Rectangular to round	Elliptical ovoid
6	Extra features	Compound	Transparent , glossy	Solid- rhomboidal	Smooth

Table 3.
Morphological observation of selected plants.

Elements	*Trigonella Foenum Graecum* Linn (seed)	*Vitex nigundo*Linn	*Argemone Mexicana* Linn	*Azardirachta indica*
Fe	2.022%	5.387%	2.467%	1.977%
Mn	0.466%	0.561%	0.225%	0.371%
Zn	0.411%	0.204%	0.049%	0.047%
Cu	0.162%	0.054%	0.030%	0.024%
V	0.00%	0.051%	0.076%	0.107%
Si	0.00%	0.227%	0.000%	0.213%
P	4.669%	1.628%	1.195%	0.966%
S	5.184%	1.910%	1.619%	1.733%
Cl	8.138%	2.611%	3.971%	5.733%
K	56.797%	31.975%	35.399%	20.825%
Ca	21.827%	54.418%	54.450%	67.265%
Ti	0.176%	0.842%	0.385%	0.391%
Br	0.033%	0.000%	0.022%	0.186%
Rb	0.074%	0.019%	0.040%	0.007%
Sr	0.042%	0.07%	0.056%	0.154%

Table 4.
Trace element concentrations of the selected medicinal plants.

Experiments were performed with dried samples of medicinal plants No. 1 – No. 4, (No. 1 – *Azardirachta indica,* No. 2 – *Vitex nigundo*, No. 3 – *A. mexicana*, No. 4 – *Trigonella fornum graecum*,)

Total 19 number of elements, such as phosphorus, sulfur, potassium, calcium, scandium, titanium, vanadium, manganese, iron, cadmium, iodine etc. were detected from the four medicinal plant samples of *Arardirachta indica, vitex nigundo* Linn, *Argemone Mexicana* Linn, leaves and *T. foenum-graecum* Linnseed by ED-XRF. The detected concentrations found in the samples are presented in **Table 4** (**Figures 1–5**).

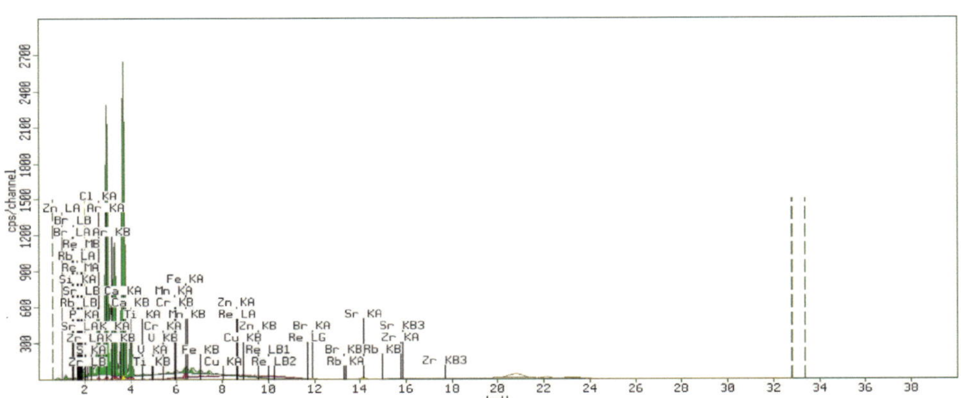

Figure 1.
ED-XRF analysis of Arardirachta indica.

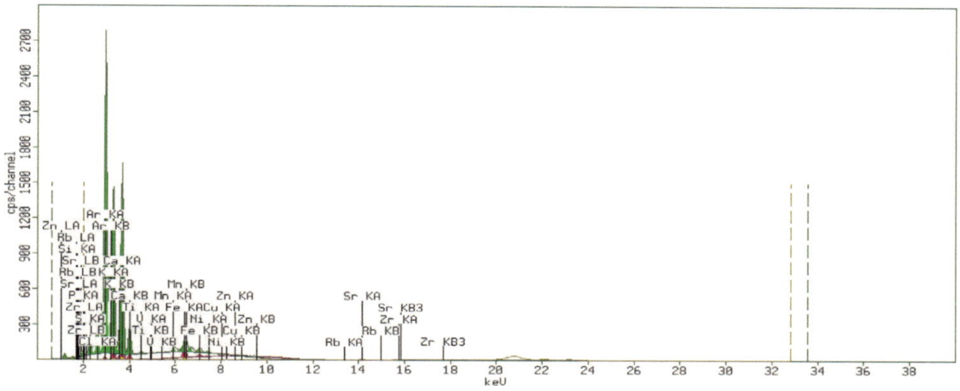

Figure 2.
ED-XRF analysis of vitex nigundo *Linn.*

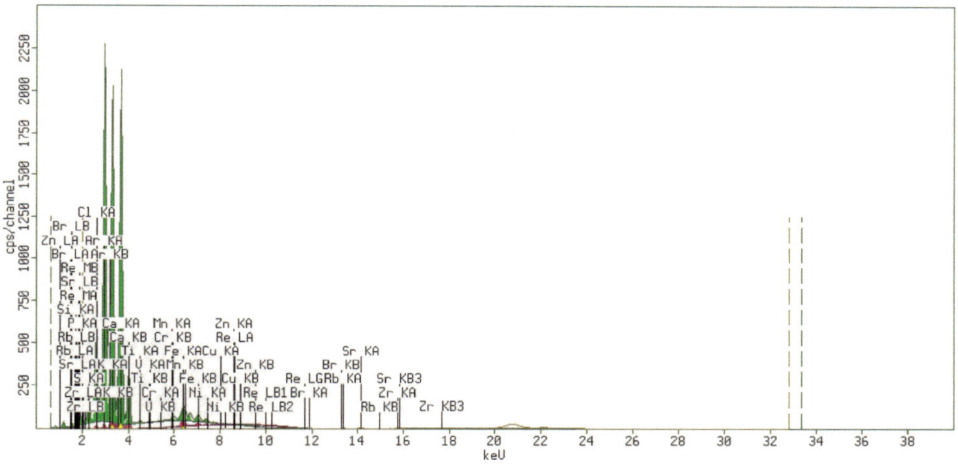

Figure 3.
ED-XRF analysis of Argemone Mexicana *Linn.*

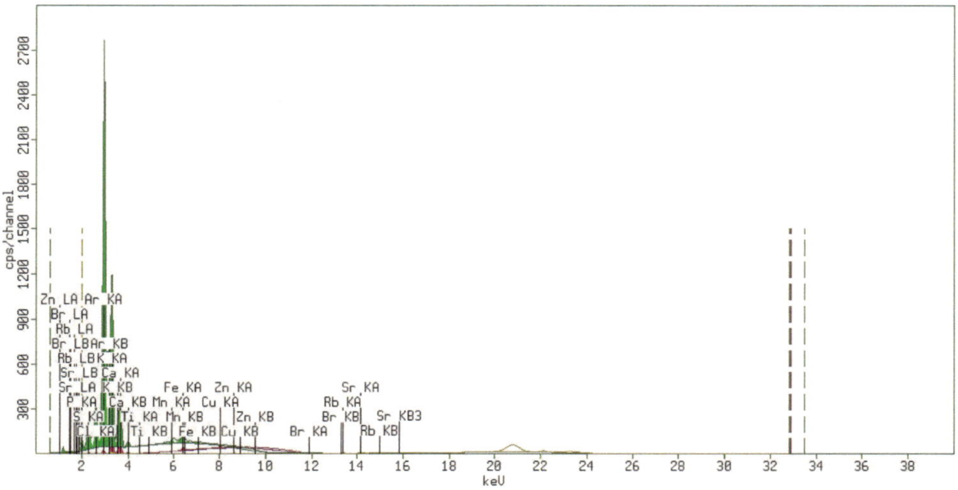

Figure 4.
ED-XRF analysis of T. foenum-graecum *Linn.*

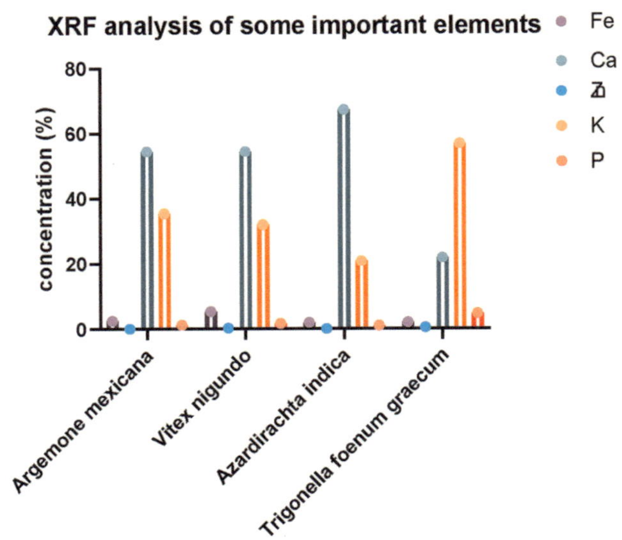

Figure 5.
XRF analysis of plant samples.

9. Results

Elemental analysis of *Vitex negundo* leaves by ED-XRF technique has been confirmed the presence of pharmaceutically active, major, minor, and trace elements. The results of elemental analysis were recorded in **Table 1**, which revealed presence of P (1.628%), K (31.975%), Ca (54.418%), Ti (0.842%), Mn (0.561%), Fe (5.387%), Ni (0.023%), Cu (0.054%), Zn (0.204%), Rb (0.019%) and Zr (0.008%) Si (0.224%), S (1.910%), Cl (2.611%), Sr. (0.087%). Toxic metals like Be, Ag, Sn, Ba, Pb, and Bi were found totally absent in *Vitexnegundo*leaves.

Elemental analysis of *T. foenum-graecum* seed by ED-XRF technique has been confirmed the presence of pharmaceutically active, major, minor, and trace elements. The results of elemental analysis were recorded in **Table 1**, which revealed presence of P (4.669%), K (56.797%), Ca (21.827%), Ti (0.176%), Mn (0.466%), Fe (2.022%), Cu (0.162%), Zn (0.411%), Rb (0.074%), Br (0.033%), Sr. (0.042%), S (5.184%), and Cl (8.138%). Toxic metals like Be, Ag, Sn, Ba, Pb, and Bi were found totally absent in *Trigonella foenum-graecum* seed.

Elemental analysis of *Argemone Mexicana* Linn leaves by ED-XRF technique has been confirmed the presence of pharmaceutically active, major, minor, and trace elements. The results of elemental analysis were recorded in **Table 1**, which revealed presence of P (1.195%), K (35.399%), Ca (54.450%), Ti (0.385%), Mn (0.225%), Fe (2.467%), Ni (0.010%), Cu (0.030%), Zn (0.049%), Rb (0.040%), Zr (0.003%) Br (0.022%), S (1.619%), Cl (3.971%), Re (0.004%), and Sr. (0.056%). Toxic metals like Be, Ag, Sn, Ba, Pb, and Bi were found totally absent in *Argemone Mexicana* Linn.

Elemental analysis of *Azardirachta indica* Linn leaves by ED-XRF technique has been confirmed the presence of pharmaceutically active, major, minor, and trace elements. The results of elemental analysis were recorded in **Table 1**, which revealed presence of P (0.966%), K (20.825%), Ca (67.265%), Ti (0.391%), Mn (0.371%), Fe (1.977%), V (0.107%), Cu (0.024%), Zn (0.047%), Rb (0.007%), Zr (0.001%), Br

(0.186%), S (1.733%), Re (0.000%), Sr. (0.154%), Si (0.213%), and Cl (5.733%). Toxic metals like Be, Ag, Sn, Ba, Pb, and Bi were found totally absent in *Azardirachta indica* Linn.

10. Discussion

Analysis of the present data revealed that Fe was observed with the adequate concentration in all the medicinal plants studied as compared to other trace elements recorded. The highest concentration of the Fe among the studied medicinal plants was found in *vitex nigundo* Linn.

Fe is the trace element plays an important role in the production of hemoglobin and oxygenation of red blood cells. It is also important for healthy immune system as well as energy production.

Fe plays an important role on immune system, the use of the medicinal plants in the treatment of skin diseases in the traditional system of medicine may be based on the amounts of Fe present in the plants.

Also, Mn is the important trace elements in immune system for regulation of immune responses of the body due to the breakdown of amino acids, production of energy, and utilization of foods.

Also, Mn is the component of the metalloenzyme manganese superoxide dismutase in the mitochondria and also the important constituent of the mitochondrial antioxidant defense system to give protection from the free radical, which are generated from the injured cells and are harmful to the skin.

Zn is also important element which is required for the metabolism of biochemical reaction in the body. It is found in tissue of plants and animals and plays an important role in maintaining healthy skin by controlling enzymes that are involved in the renewal of cells in our body. The highest concentration of the Zn among the studied medicinal plants was found in *T. foenum-graecum*, that is, 0.411%. Hence, the possible use of these medicinal plants for treating skin diseases in the traditional system of medicine can be understood.

Cu is very well known for the stimulation of immune system to fight against infection, involved in the repairing of injured tissues and promote healing. In addition, Cu is responsible for the formation of the connective tissues like cross linking of collagen and elastin. As Cu affects our immunity, so possess anti-infectant properties, so the presence of the maximum amount of Cu in all the plant samples studied support their role in curing skin diseases by the traditional practitioners in traditional system of medicine. Further, the role of V is limited and plays an important role in the treatment of diabetes, the main important function to provide protection against injury of tissues.

In the present study, Cu was found to be in varying concentrations in all the medicinal plants samples in the range of 0.024% to 0.162% with the highest concentration of Cu recorded again in the *T. foenum-graecum*.

Further, the role of V is limited and plays an important role in the treatment of diabetes, the main important function to provide protection against injury of tissues. Thus, the trace elements like Fe, Mn, Zn, Cu in addition to Co and V are responsible to defend the serious skin infections and diseases.

In this study, ED-XRF technique was used to trace the elemental composition of all the selected plants. It is evident that the elements present in the plant samples played a direct or indirect role in the control and treatment of the skin diseases and disorders.

The results of the current study suggest that the usage of medicinal plants in the traditional system of medicine for curing skin diseases since they are found to contain adequate amount of the Fe, Zn, Cu, Mn, and V.

11. Conclusion

The objective of the research work is to analyze trace elements present in selected medicinal plants using ED-XRF spectrometer and to estimate their elemental concentrations.

All four plants contain trace elements of different concentrations in medicinal plants selected for this study. It is believed that the various trace elements present in the plants play an important role in the management of skin diseases. The difference in the concentrations of these elements is mainly due to the differences in structure, as well as type of the soil, the cultivated field, age of the plant, climatic conditions, and irrigation facilities provided to the plants. The conventional treatment of dermal disease has many side effects, on the other hand, medicinal plant extracts are possesses similar therapeutic efficacy without any side effects. The present information will be helpful to prescribe the type of extract, dose, and mixture of these plants. The results justify that usage of these plants in traditional systems of medicine for the treatment of skin diseases contains the appropriate amount of Fe, Zn, Cu etc.

However, further research is needed to understand the relation between dermal diseases and trace elements. Finally, the study concluded that this information will be very beneficial for the researcher who would like to conduct research in the area of Herbal medicines. Also, it has been found that no excess quantities of toxic elements are present in selected medicinal plants and not harmful to health.

Acknowledgements

The authors are very much thankful to the authorities of Bits Pilani, Hyderabad for providing ED-XRF facilities in conducting this piece of research.

Author's contributions

Thonte. s.s analyzed and interpreted the data related to ED-XRF analysis. Yelmate A.A has given a major contribution for conducting the research and writing the manuscript. Both authors read and approved the final manuscript.

Funding

No funding was received.

Competing interests

No competing interest to declare here.

Consent for publication

Not applicable.

Availability of data and material

All required data and materials are available upon request.

Ethics approval consent for publication

Not applicable.

Plant Authentification

The plant parts were identified by Dr. C.S. Swami, department of botany, Dayanand science college, Latur. Deposition numbers for the herbarium of these samples were not given so it is not available.

Abbreviations

ED-XRF	Energy Dispersive X-ray Fluorescence

Author details

Archana A. Yelmate[1*], Sanjay S. Thonte[2] and Kranti L. Satpute[2]

1 Dayanand College of Pharmacy, Latur, Maharashtra, India

2 Channabasweshwar Pharmacy College, Latur, Maharashtra, India

*Address all correspondence to: archanayelmate1@gmail.com

References

[1] Sýkorová M, Jánošová V, Štroffeková O, Havránek E. Determination of some elements in plant samples by radionuclide X-ray fluorescence analysis. Acta Facultatis Pharmaceuticae Universitatis Comenianae. 2006;**53**:245-252

[2] Towett EK, Shepherd KD, B. Lee drake, plant elemental composition and portable X-ray fluorescence (Pxrf) spectroscopy: Quantification under different analytical parameters. X-Ray Spectrometry. 2015;**45**:117-124. DOI: 10.1002/xrs.2678

[3] Keizo I. Review PIXE and its applications to elemental analysis. Quantum Beam Science. 2019;**3**:12. DOI: 10.3390/qubs3020012

[4] Lokman H, Joynal A, Shirin A. For elemental analysis of domestic medicinal plants in Bangladesh. International Journal of Recent Advances in Physics. 2016;**3**:4

[5] Rajeshwari BM, Sharangouda JP, Rautary TR. Elemental analysis of some Indian medicinal plants by particle induced X-ray emission (PIXE) technique. Medicinal Plants. 2012;**4**(1):28-32

[6] Tiago T, José LF, Ana PN, Priscila LG, Ricardo AA, Paulo M. Simple procedure for nutrient analysis of coffee plant with energy dispersive X-ray fluorescence spectrometry (EDXRF). Scientia Agricola. 2013;**70**(4):263-267

[7] Jay PR, Kshetrimayum BS, Sanjiv K, Raj KM. Trace elements content in the selected medicinal plants traditionally used for curing skin diseases by the natives of Mizoram, India. Asian Pacific Journal of Tropical Medicine. 2014;7(1): S410-S414

[8] Khandelwal K. Practical Pharmacognosy. Pragati Books Pvt. Ltd; 2008. pp. 12.12-12.14

[9] Khandelwal K. Practical Pharmacognosy. Pragati Books Pvt. Ltd; 2008. pp. 18.15-18.18

[10] Khandelwal K. Practical Pharmacognosy. Pragati Books Pvt. Ltd; 2008. pp. 25.1-25.9

[11] Khandelwal K. Practical Pharmacognosy. Pragati Books Pvt. Ltd; 2008. pp. 23.8-23.11

[12] Khare CP. Indian Medicinal Plants: An Illustrated Dictionary. Springer Science & Business Media; 2008. pp. 295-297

[13] Khare CP. Indian Medicinal Plants: An Illustrated Dictionary. Springer Science & Business Media; 2008. pp. 84-85

[14] Duke JA. Handbook of Medicinal Herbs. CRC Press; 2002. pp. 461-464

[15] Duke JA. Handbook of Medicinal Herbs. CRC Press; 2002. pp. 178-185

[16] Duke JA. Handbook of Medicinal Herbs. CRC Press; 2002. p. 22

[17] Duke JA. Handbook of Medicinal Herbs. CRC Press; 2002. pp. 521-523

Chapter 13

Conservation and Sustainable Use of *Cryptolepis sanguinolenta*

Frank Opoku-Agyemang, Jessica Naa Offeibea Dodoo, Theophilus Elorm Hlomador, Kathleen Gilday and Jacqueline Naalamle Amissah

Abstract

Cryptolepis sanguinolenta (Cs) is a medicinal plant, indigenous to the West Africa sub-region and has been utilized in Ghana to treat malaria for generations. Besides being used as an antimalarial treatment in Ghana, Cs has been noted as being used in the US to treat Babesia, Lyme disease (*Borreliosis burgdorferi*), Bartonella, among others. The plant contains several indoloquinoline alkaloids, mainly concentrated in its root system, giving the plant its antimicrobial, antihyperglycemic, and anticancer properties. However, the destructive harvesting of the entire plant, along with its root system, is not sustainable over the long term and has already resulted in a substantial decrease in wild populations, threatening its long-term potential and survivability. This book chapter will discuss its uses, conservation strategies and cultivation protocols developed for Cs to ensure a reliable supply of plant material as well as its sustainable utilization.

Keywords: cultivation, malaria, medicinal plants, bioactive compounds

1. Introduction

Cryptolepis sanguinolenta (Lindl.) Schlecter is a scrambling thin twinning stemmed and flowering shrub belonging to the Apocynaceae family [1]. This all-important medicinal herb is classified into kingdom Plantae, phylum Magnoliophyta, class Equisetopsida, subclass Magnoliidae, order Gentianles, sub-family Periplocaceae, genus Cryptolepis and species sanguinolenta [2]. It is indigenous to West African countries like Ghana, Nigeria, Cameroon, Congo-Brazzaville, with reports of its existence in the Central African Republic, DR Congo, Uganda, Tanzania and Angola [3, 4]. It is mainly found in tropical rainforests, thickets, and mountainous ecologies usually near water, from sea level up to 850 m altitude [3, 5]. However, it does not grow well in areas with abundant shade, mushy and salty swamps of coastal regions.

In Ghana, it is commonly known as 'Nibima' in Twi, 'Kadze' in Ewe, 'Nurubima' among the Guans, 'Gangnamau' in Hausa, Ghanaian quinine and yellow dye root [4, 6]. *C. sanguinolenta* is mainly found growing in mountainous areas such as along the slopes of the Akwapim and Aburi mountains [5, 7]. It is also found in Ghana's

Ashanti Region, where it serves as the main vegetative cover for deserted farmlands around Lake Bosomtwe. The plant also thrives well in the woody savannah region and areas with a good supply of sunlight and water [4].

The cut stem contains an orange-colored sap that becomes red upon drying [8]. It has yellow flowers with tightly twisted petals. This open up to display a five star-shaped flower which develops into pods and matures at 9–10 months after planting (**Figure 1**).

In our eight years of working with *C. sanguinolenta,* insect pollinators have not been observed around its flowers, and this confirms our postulation that it is self-pollinated. Each plant produces an average of 90 boomerang-shaped pods which contains approximately 30 seeds. Its seeds are small (10–12 mm long), reddish-brown in color and oval in shape with a cluster of silky hairs fixed to one end of the seeds [4, 9]. The leaves are opposite, simple and petiolate with an uneven base. Its multi-root system, is found to contain high concentrations of the major alkaloid cryptolepine, and is the part of commercial value used in the preparation of herbal decoctions and tinctures for the treatment of several diseases including malaria.

The World Health Organization (WHO), reported about 241 million malaria cases worldwide with Africa having the highest incidence of about 228 million cases [10]. Sub-Saharan Africa alone, contributed to about 96% of global malaria deaths out of the 600,000 reported death cases [10]. In the quest to eradicate malaria, medicinal plants with potential anti-malaria properties such as *C. sanguinolenta*, a major medicinal plant with a long record of use in the treatment of malaria especially in Ghana [9, 11], should be given the needed scientific recognition. In developed countries such as the USA, this herb is appreciated for its anti-bacterial, anti-cancer, anti-diabetic, anti-fungal and anti-inflammatory properties and is been used to treat Babesia, Lyme disease (*Borreliosis burgdorferi*), and Bartonella [12]. Recently it was recognized as a potential treatment for tick-borne diseases in the USA and Europe.

The high demand for this all-important medicinal plant has resulted in its over-exploitation from the wild in non-sustainable ways [12]. It is therefore important to

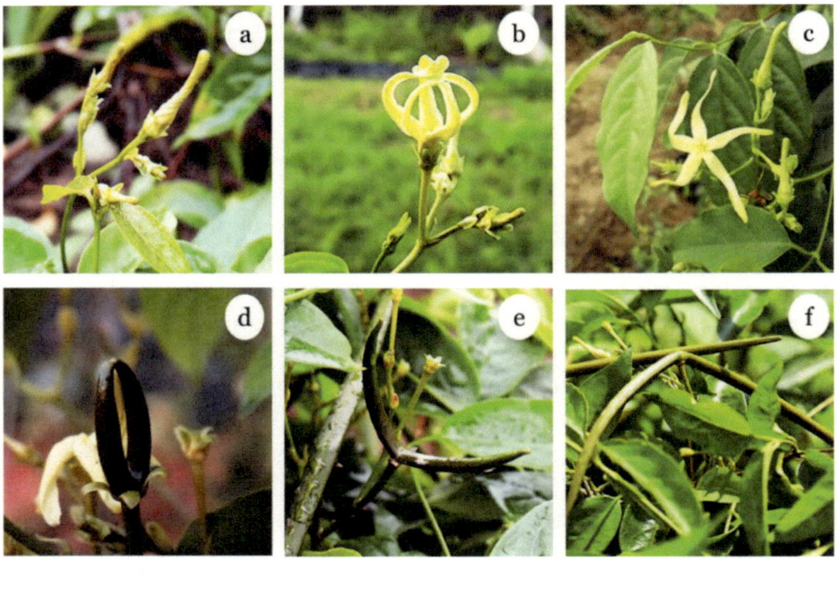

Figure 1.
Anthesis to pod formation stages of C. sanguinolenta *taken in the Sinna garden, Department of Crop Science, University of Ghana. Tightly twisted petals (a), unwound flower petals (b), completely opened five star-shaped flower (c), newly developed pods (d & e), fully formed pod (f).*

develop and adopt domestication and conservation strategies to ensure sustainable production and supply of *C. sanguinolenta* planting material. This chapter discusses active compounds, uses, conservation strategies and the prediction of suitable commercial production areas of *C. sanguinolenta* in Ghana.

2. Uses and active compounds in *C. sanguinolenta*

C. sanguinolenta, is recognized for its antimalarial [13], antimicrobial [14], anti-hyperglycemic [15, 16], and anti-amoebal properties. In the case of its use for the treatment of malaria, the bioactive indole alkaloid cryptolepine which is the major constituent of the root bark. It is reported to possess an anti-plasmodial property among other antiparasitic [3], anti-thrombotic [17], noradrenergic [18], vasodilator [17], hypoglycaemic [19, 20] properties. It also has anti-diabetic, anti-pyretic, anti-inflammatory, hypotensive, anti-thrombotic, and anti-plasmodial properties [2].

An aqueous extract of the roots yields a N-methyl derivative of quindoline and indoloquinoline alkaloids, mainly cryptolepine [21]. The roots also contain high concentration of indologuinoline and cryptolepine which has the most potent anti-plasmodial activity [22–24].

Cryptolepine was first isolated in 1931 by Delvaux and later from collected *C. sanguinolenta* accessions in Ghana [23] and Nigeria [25]. Several structurally related alkaloids found in the plant included, cryptoquindoline cryptoheptine, biscryptolepine, 11-hydroxycryptolepine, quindolinone, isocryptolepine (Cryptosanguinolentine), neocryptolepine, quindoline, and cryptospirolepine have also been isolated [21]. In prepared aqueous root extract used for the treatment of various ailments, only cryptolepine is isolated [3]. In the ethanolic root extract, the cryptolepine isomers called neocryptolepine, biscryptolepine and cryptoquindoline which are dimeric alkaloids have been isolated [26]. Research into the synthesis of the plant alkaloid cryptolepine and the development of its analogues as a way of understanding the mechanisms into its pharmacological effects have been carried out [27].

Among indigenous inhabitants where biomedicines are not readily available, herbal plants are usually the only source of remedy to treat various ailments [28]. The medicinal plant industry does not only play a major role in satisfying the health care needs of the populace but serves as a viable source of income to manufacturers and collectors of the raw herbal plant materials.

In African, *C. sanguinolenta* is widely use in the treatment of various ailments especially countries in the West African sub region. Traditional healers in Guinea Bissau use the root extract and the powdered leaf to treat fever, hepatitis and cicatrizant of wounds respectively. The boiled leaf is used as an infusion for the treatment of malaria [29]. In Uganda the prepared roots are used in the treatments of measles, hernia, snake bites and hypertension [3]. In Nigeria, the root is macerated to treat rheumatism and urogenital infection. In Ghana, the aqueous root extract is used to treat malaria, urinary, and upper respiratory tract infections [30]. It is also used for the treatment of colic, stomach complaints, amoebic dysentery, diabetes and diarrhea in other West African countries such as Senegal and DR Congo [31–33]. Due to its general use by traditional healers, it has been included in several herbal products sold on the market in Ghana, such as Class Herbaquine, Malaherb, Nibima, Phyto-Laria and Malacure. *C. sanguinolenta* is used in Central and West Africa for the treatment of infectious diseases such as amoebiasis and Covid-19 [34]. It is presently studied in clinical trials for the treatment of COVID-19 in Ghana [35, 36]. A recent study by Amissah et al. [12]

reported that cryptolepine extracts from plants aged between 9 and 12 months had the most antiplasmodial activity and drug selectivity index against *Plasmodium falciparum* Dd2. These cryptolepine extracts were identified for the effective management of cancer due to its cytotoxicity to Jurkat leukemia cell lines [12].

Besides its medicinal properties, the length of *C. sanguinolenta's* branches and twining nature enables its use as a rope to construct houses in Uganda [2]. In addition, the pulverized roots contain yellow pigment, which serves as a yellow dye in the leather, textiles, and fabric industry [3, 37].

2.1 Role of *C. sanguinolenta* as herbal medicine in the United States

An online survey was conducted in 2018 among 133 medicinal plant practitioners and clinics in collaboration with Woodland Essence LLC Ltd. (https://woodlandessence.com) to assess the use of *C. sanguinolenta* root extracts along with the quantities required in the United States of America. Medicinal plant practitioners were asked; 1) whether they knew the plant 2) whether they use the plant in their practice, clinic or personal protocol? 3) what conditions they use *C. sanguinolenta* to treat and 4) how much of the plant is used per month.

Findings from the survey revealed that majority of the respondents (131) representing 98.5%, were familiar with *C. sanguinolenta* whereas only 2 respondents representing 1.5% were not. It was revealed that 133 respondents (95.5%) used *C. sanguinolenta* in their practice, clinic or personal protocol whereas 6 respondents (4.5%) answering that they did not.

Regarding its uses, respondents mentioned Babesia (73.7%; 98 respondents), followed by Lyme disease (*Borreliosis burgdorferi*) (57.9%; 77 respondents), Bartonella (43.6%; 58 respondents), and as a systemic anti-bacterial (33.8%; 45 respondents) as the top four (4) conditions Cs is used to treat. Other conditions treated with *C. sanguinolenta* included anti-fungi infection (17.3%; 23 respondents), methicillin-resistant *Staphylococcus aureus* (MRSA) (14.3%; 19 respondents), urinary tract infections (11.3%; 15 respondents), external treatments (6.0%; 8 respondents), cancer (1.5%; 2 respondents), diabetes (1.5%; 2 respondents), and hepatitis (0.8%; 1 respondent) (**Figure 2**). Twenty-four (24) respondents representing 18.1% mentioned that *C. sanguinolenta* was used to treat conditions such as mold and deep lung infections, general antimicrobial, systemic anti-viral, prophylaxis with embedded deer tick, strep infections, gut bacterial outgrowth and recurring gastrointestinal (GI) tract

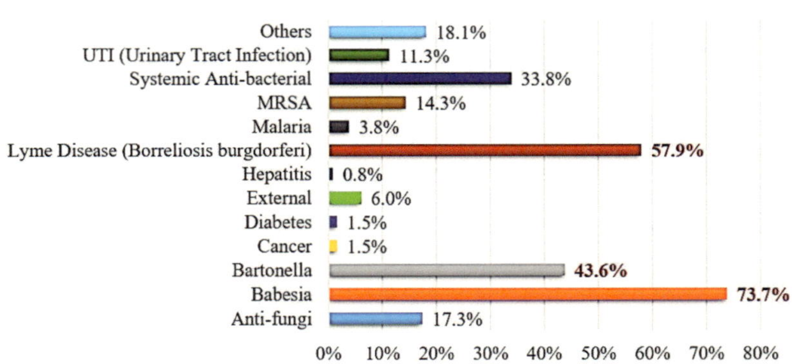

Figure 2.
Responses to the health conditions treated with C. sanguinolenta.

infections (**Figure 2**). According to the survey, medicinal plant practitioners and clinics testified to the efficiency of *C. sanguinolenta* in treating the medical conditions listed in (**Figure 2**).

"I suffered for over 8 months with recurrent Methicillin-resistant Staphylococcus aureus (MRSA) infections in the outer and middle ears. I tried over 6 different antibiotics (all resistant) and was getting ready to start IV antibiotics. My functional medicine practitioner had me take *C. sanguinolenta* in tincture form. Within a couple of weeks, I was cured! I have had a couple of flare up and the same protocol does the trick, and quick." (Respondent No. 12, personal communication).

"It is the only thing that has been effective in treating long-term staph infection." (Respondent No. 9, personal communication).

"It is literally saving my life from chronic GI tract bacterial infections, where no other medicine helps" (Respondent No. 11, personal communication).

Regarding dosage use, some respondents indicated using 40 drops twice a day for 14 days on and 14 days off (Respondent No. 25), 3/4 of a dropper of the CSA formula (Respondent No. 30) while another respondent (Respondent No. 41), reported its use in combination with other medicinal plants such as *Sida acuta* and *Alchornea cordifolia* as per Steven Buhner's protocols [38]. Respondent No. 51 indicated that patients usually take 1table spoon three times a day for approximately 4 months. In response to the duration of its use, respondent No. 50 reported a cycle of usage of 1–4 months on and 6 months to a year off.

Monthly quantities (ounces/milliliters) of *C. sanguinolenta* used by the respondents were indicated as follows; 1–4 ounces/ (54.9%; 73 respondents), followed by 4–40 ounces (34.6%, 46 respondents). Five percent (5.0%) and 2.3% of the respondents reported the use of larger quantities of between 40 and 162 and > 162 ounces respectively (**Figure 3**).

Findings from the survey point to the multipurpose use of *C. sanguinolenta* to treat ailments other than malaria including Babesia, Lyme disease (*Borreliosis burgdorferi*) and Bartonella among others. This confirms the importance of the herb on the US market, cementing the need for its conservation by encouraging its cultivation. *C. sanguinolenta* has since been tested with other botanical and natural products used by Lyme disease patients and found to be very active *in vitro* against stationary phase *Borrelia burgdorferi* [39] and *Babesia duncani* [40].

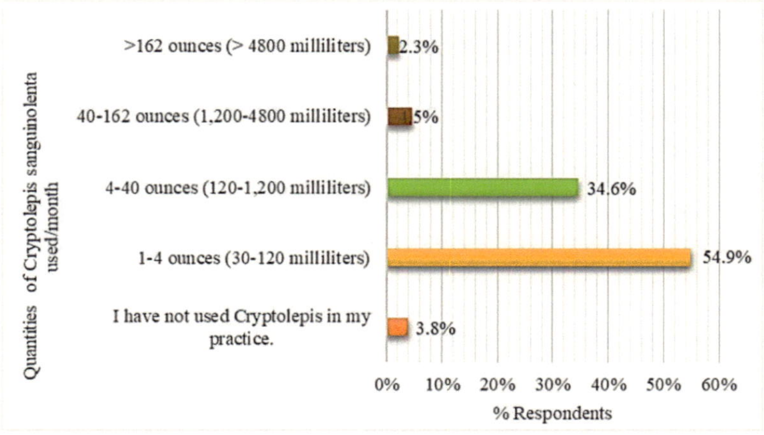

Figure 3.
Quantities of C. sanguinolenta *used per month as indicated by respondents.*

3. Conservation strategies

The local and international demand for *C. sanguinolenta* raises concerns about its continued availability especially since its root system is the part of economic importance. Conservation of plant species require the adoption of in-situ and ex-situ strategies complementing each other [41]. Ex-situ conservation strategies consist of using biotechnology-based methods such as tissue culture, cryopreservation and molecular diagnostics to maintain biological diversity outside a plant's natural habitat. On the other hand, in-situ conservation ensures that wild plant species are kept in their natural adaptive environment in order to ensure their maintenance and recovery in their natural habitats. The major concern with ex-situ conservation of medicinal plants is the risk of the plants losing the potency of their bioactive compounds. There is also the possibility of selecting their reproductive materials such as seeds for storage in seed banks for later use [41]. Seeds are referred to as the storehouse of plants genetic nature and a ready source of planting materials [42]. However, seeds of *C. sanguinolenta* have a low germinability which might be attributed to seed dormancy, storage conditions, inherent properties and or a thick seed coat (REF).

3.1 Seed storage environment and storage period effects on the germination ability of *C. sanguinolenta* seeds

The long-term conservation and domestication of *C. sanguinolenta* plant genetic resources require essential steps such as storage of seeds as *ex situ* germplasm. Storage of seeds under suitable environmental conditions is essential for the preservation of genetic integrity, maintaining seed viability, normal metabolism of seed and free from various environmental stresses [43, 44]. Some factors that may affect seed quality include temperature, insects and biotic stresses [45]. However, the most widely important factor which affects seed quality is the storage period [46]. According to [47], the viability of seeds is hugely influenced by the period of seed storage since the reduction in seed viability and increase storage period are directly proportional. Prolonged storage period can decrease seed germinability as result of the disintegration of the seed's metabolic system [48].

The present study was undertaken to test the effect of storage periods under different storage conditions on seed germination in *C. sanguinolenta*. To the best of our knowledge there is the first scientific report on the effect of storage periods and conditions on seed germination in *C. sanguinolenta*.

Freshly harvested *C. sanguinolenta* seeds from mature dried pods were used for the study. A 10 × 3 factorial experiments arranged in a Completely Randomized Design (CRD) with three (3) replications were used. Treatments consisted of two factors; Storage Conditions [Fridge (2–4°C), Room temperature (26° to 29°C), Freezer (−12° to −15°C)] and storage periods [0-week (freshly harvested seed), 2-week, 4-week, 6-week, 8-week, 10-week and 12-week] replicated three times. Germination measurements (germinability, synchronization, uniformity, mean germination rate, mean germination time, and co-efficient of variation) were calculated [49, 50].

The study identified storing freshly harvested *C. sanguinolenta* seeds (from mature dried pods) for 2 to 6 weeks as a suitable storage period for improving the germinability of seeds (**Table 1**). It has been observed severally that matured seeds of this plant when sown immediately after harvest yielded very low germination percentages. This observation corroborates the current study.

Seed Storage Age	G (%)	MT (Days)	MR	CV_1 (%)
Control	25.4	32	0.03	38.2
2WBS	62.7	20	0.05	32.0
4WBS	53.0	26	0.05	56.3
6WBS	50.8	25	0.04	30.5
8WBS	9.2	19	0.05	22.5
10WBS	25.8	16	0.07	35.6
12WBS	39.2	13	0.07	19.7
$P \leq 0.05$	**<0.001**	**<0.001**	**<0.001**	**<0.001**

G = germinability, MT = mean germination time, CV_1 = coefficient of variation of the germination time, MR = mean germination rate, WBS = Weeks Before Sowing.

Table 1.
Mean germination measurements of C. sanguinolenta *seeds under different storage periods.*

Seed Storage Conditions	G (%)	MT (Days)	MR	CV_1 (%)
Freezer (FZ)	41.8	21	0.05	32.2
Fridge (F)	33.8	22	0.05	32.7
Room Temperature (RT)	38.5	21	0.05	35.8
$P \leq 0.05$	**<0.001**	**0.766**	**0.732**	**0.325**

G = germinability, MT = mean germination time, CV_1 = coefficient of variation of the germination time, MR = mean germination rate.

Table 2.
Mean germination measurements of C. sanguinolenta *seeds under different storage conditions.*

Seed Storage Conditions	G (%)	MT (Days)	MR	CV_1 (%)
Control*FZ	25.7	32	0.03	38.2
2WBS * FZ	63.8	21	0.05	37.6
4WBS * FZ	73.3	24	0.06	45.8
6WBS * FZ	48.2	21	0.05	29.4
8WBS * FZ	12.5	21	0.05	18.2
10WBS * FZ	23.2	16	0.07	35.2
12WBS * FZ	46.0	14	0.07	21.0
Control * F	25.7	32	0.03	38.2
2WBS * F	55.0	20	0.05	29.5
4WBS * F	36.2	29	0.04	49.3
6WBS * F	47.2	24	0.04	31.0
8WBS * F	10.0	23	0.04	30.0
10WBS * F	28.9	14	0.07	34.6
12WBS * F	33.3	13	0.08	16.1
Control * RT	25.0	32	0.03	38.2
2WBS * RT	69.4	20	0.05	28.9

Seed Storage Conditions	G (%)	MT (Days)	MR	CV_1 (%)
4WBS * RT	49.5	24	0.05	73.8
6WBS * RT	57.1	29	0.04	31.0
8WBS * RT	5.0	15	0.07	19.4
10WBS * RT	25.4	16	0.07	37.1
12WBS * RT	38.2	13	0.07	22.0
$P \leq 0.05$	**<0.001**	0.480	**0.344**	**0.039**

G = germinability, MT = mean germination time, CV_1 = coefficient of variation of the germination time, MR = mean germination rate. WBS = Weeks Before Sowing, FZ = Freezer, F = Fridge, RT = Room Temperature, WBS = Weeks Before Sowing.

Table 3.
Mean germination measurements of C. sanguinolenta *seeds under different storage periods and storage conditions.*

Further evaluation indicated that seeds stored under freezer conditions prior to sowing produced higher germination percentage compared to those stored in the fridge and at room temperatures (**Table 2**).

Results from this study identified significant interaction between seed storage periods and storage conditions on germinability of *C. sanguinolenta* seeds where seeds stored for 4-weeks in the freezer prior to sowing recorded the highest germination (**Table 3**). Hence, freshly harvested *C. sanguinolenta* seeds are recommended to be stored at either room or freezer temperature conditions for a maximum of six weeks before sowing to achieve a higher germination percentage.

3.2 Priming effects on seed germination and seedling establishment of *C. sanguinolenta*

Seed priming is the process of hydrating seeds in water or synthetic compounds to kick start metabolic processes of germination and for the physiological conditioning of plants [51, 52]. Seed priming techniques include osmo-priming, bio priming, halo

Treatment	G	MT	CV_1	MR
0.1% KNO_3	34.67	19	40.50	0.05
−0.2 PEG 8000	17.33	27	34.84	0.04
−0.5 PEG 8000	20.00	26	25.08	0.04
H_2O_2	4.07	18	0.10	0.06
70% E + 50% B	29.33	22	35.68	0.05
1% KNO_3	33.33	23	31.29	0.04
0.5 KNO_3	29.33	20	34.07	0.05
dH_2O	26.67	26	38.30	0.04
Control	41.33	20	34.36	0.05
$P \leq 0.05$	**0.009**	**0.333**	**0.008**	**0.235**

G = germinability, MT = mean germination time, CV_1 = coefficient of variation of the germination time, MR = mean germination rate,

Table 4.
Mean seed germination measurements of Cryptolepis sanguinolenta *per priming treatment.*

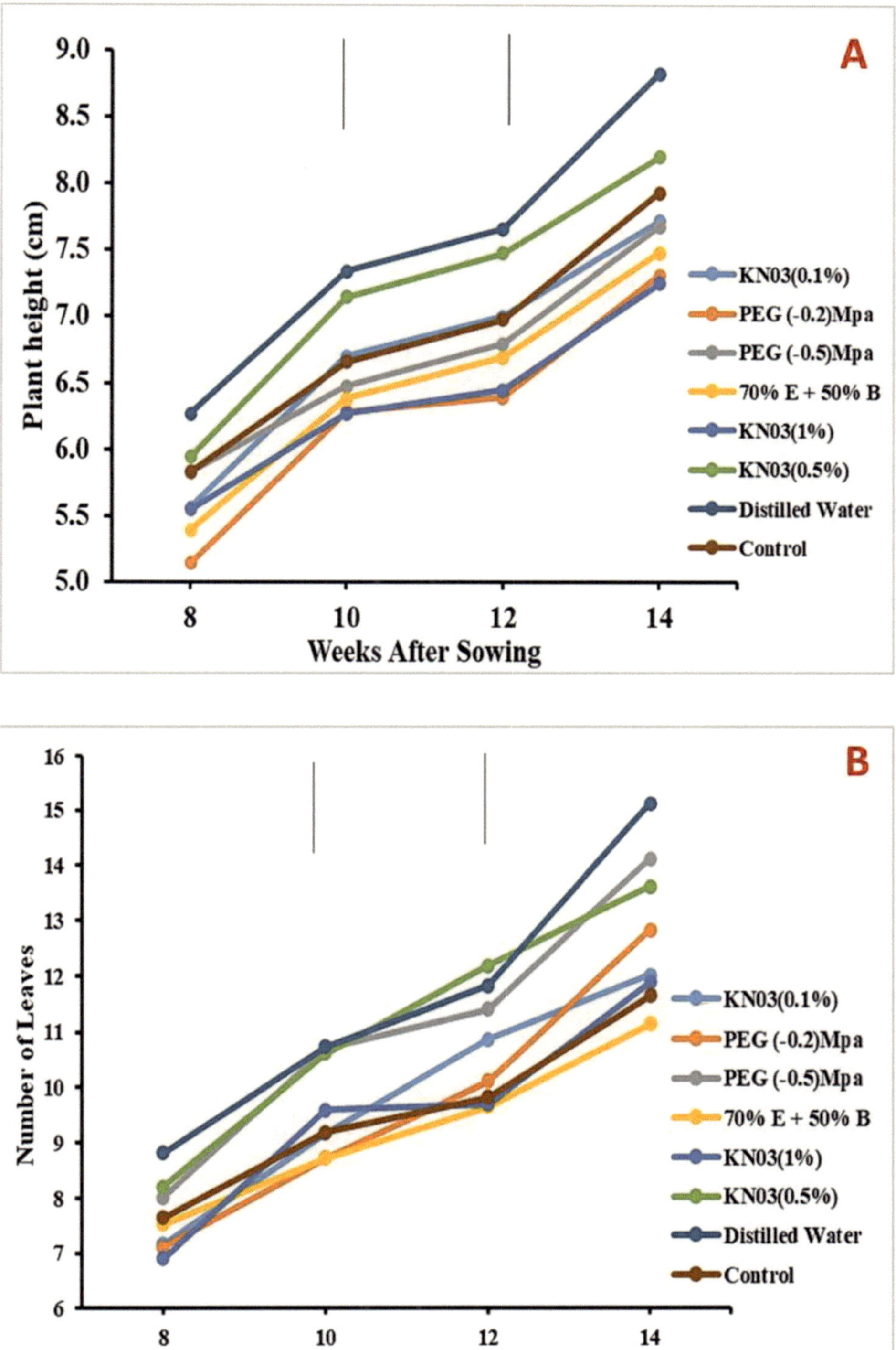

Figure 4.
Mean plant height (a) and mean number of leaves (B) of Cryptolepis sanguinolenta *seedlings at 8,10,12 and 14 weeks after sowing. The bars illustrated on the graph are LSD bars. KNO3 (potassium nitrate), PEG (polyethylene glycol 8000), 70% E + 50% B (70% ethanol +50% bleach).*

priming, hydro and matric priming [53]. Some factors influence the priming process and time, seedling vigor, plant development, and germination rate which include; plant species, priming duration, temperature, priming media, oxygen supply, aeration, light and storage conditions [54]. Seed priming provides faster and uniform germination [55] (Dawood, 2018), controls seed dormancy [56], increases percentage germination [57], increases water use efficiency in plants [58], reduces seed borne disease incidence [59], and increases crop yield [60].

Seed priming has been shown to offer the above-mentioned advantages in different crops such as wheat [61], sweet corn [62], mung bean [63], barley [64], lentil [65], and cucumber [66]. Hence, priming of *C. sanguinolenta* seeds could be a promising and effective technique in promoting germination and seedling establishment. A study on the effect of priming on germinability of seeds, growth and development of *C. sanguinolenta* seedlings was carried out.

A Completely Randomized Design with nine treatments (dH_20, 0.5% KNO_3, 0.1% KNO_3, 1% KNO_3, 70% Ethanol +50% Bleach, −0.2PEG 8000, −0.5PEG 8000, 3% Hydrogen Peroxide, Control), replicated three times was used. Germination measurements (germinability, synchronization, uniformity, mean germination rate, mean germination time, and co-efficient of variation) were obtained on approximately 3 months old seeds [49, 50]. Seedling parameters (including; plant height, plant girth, number of leaves, and chlorophyll content) were measured. Data was analyzed using GenStat software 19th edition.

The study identified 0.1% KNO_3 as a promising priming agent for improving the germinability of *C. sanguinolenta* seeds, however this was not significantly different from the unprimed (control) seeds (**Table 4**). Seeds primed with hydrogen peroxide rather recorded the lowest germination percentage.

Further evaluation of *C. sanguinolenta* seedlings indicated that the different priming agents used significantly influenced the plant height and number of leaves of the seedlings.

Distilled water treated seeds had the highest seedling parameters except for chlorophyll content in the leaves (**Figure 4**). Hence, priming seeds with distilled water could be used to improve seedling parameters of *C. sanguinolenta*, Other priming agents such as KNO_3 could be used to improve the germinability of the seeds.

4. Cultivation of *C. sanguinolenta*: Developing cultivation protocols (cropping cycle) and predicting suitable areas in Ghana for cultivation

In Ghana, *C. sanguinolenta* is adaptable in geographical areas with optimum rainfall such as the Akwapim and Aburi mountains [7]. It also thrives well in areas with a good supply of sunlight and water [4]. Wild harvesting for the treatment of malaria for decades has hugely contributed to the rapid decline in *C. sanguinolenta* populations and supply of this medicinal plant. This prompted the development of cultivation protocols including a cropping cycle for the species [9] as a conservation strategy to ensure sustainable supply.

To predict suitable cultivation areas for *C. sanguinolenta* in Ghana, GPS coordinates collected over an 8-year period from locations of wild germplasm across the different natural habitats were used. Additional data sources included; daily rainfall data

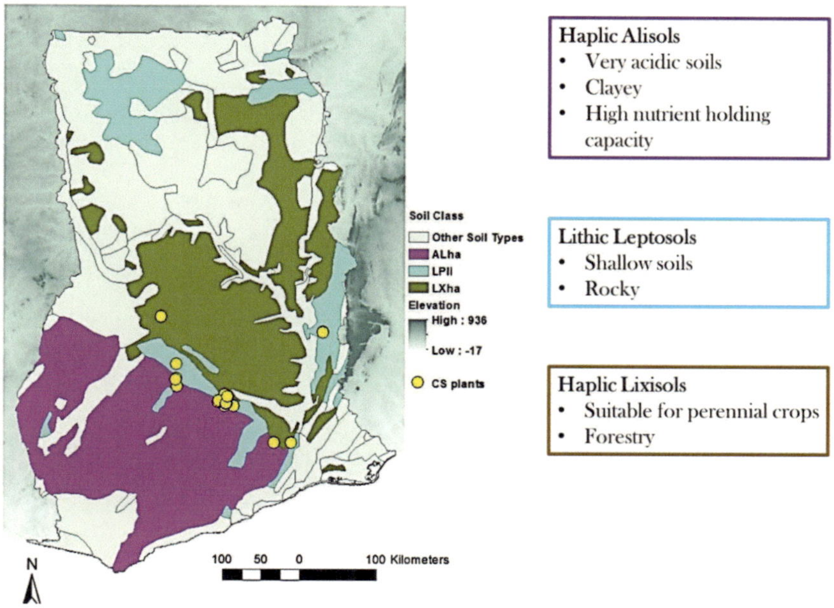

Figure 5.
Soil suitability map for C. sanguinolenta.

from 33 meteorological stations in Ghana, temperature data from climate-data.org and soil data from the EUROPEAN SOIL DATA CENTRE (ESDAC). Using the ArcGIS (version 10.6) Geo spatial software, the geographic data were analyzed by loading a layer of the map of Ghana open street map (OSM standard) and a digital elevation model (DEM). The GPS coordinates were superimposed on the map of Ghana. Based on 194 GPS records and 3 selected environmental variables (rainfall, temperature and soil classification), the suitable areas for the cultivation of *C. sanguinolenta* were predicted using spatial analyses in ArcGIS. The analysis identified Haplic Alisols (ALha), Lithic Leptosols (LPli) and Haplic Lixisols (LXha) as suitable soil classes for the cultivation of *C. sanguinolenta* (**Figure 5**).

These soil classes were found in the Ashanti, Bono, Eastern and Volta regions of the country. The suitable average temperature from collection areas which is optimum for the cultivation of *C. sanguinolenta* ranges between 27 and 31°C (**Figure 6**).

The analysis identified the mean annual rainfall 1100-1550 mm as a suitable rainfall amount for the optimum cultivation of *C. sanguinolenta* (**Figure 7**).

It was reported from the analysis that the predicted production areas suitable for the cultivation of *C. sanguinolenta* in Ghana had the following combined characteristics; clayey, acidic and shallow soils, temperature ranges of 27-31°C and mean annual rainfall of 1100–1550 mm.

Hence, fields for the domestication and cultivation of *C. sanguinolenta* can be established at these predicted suitable areas in the Ashanti, Bono, Eastern and Volta regions of Ghana for its production (**Figure 8**).

These predictable areas coupled with suitable conservation methods will ensure sustainable production of *C. sanguinolenta* thus ensuring its availability for long term use.

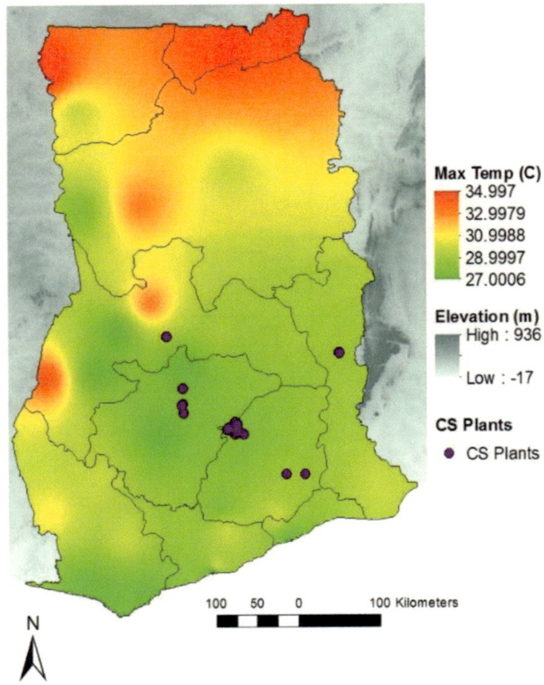

Figure 6.
Average maximum annual temperature for Ghana showing optimum temperature ranges suitable for the cultivation of C. sanguinolenta.

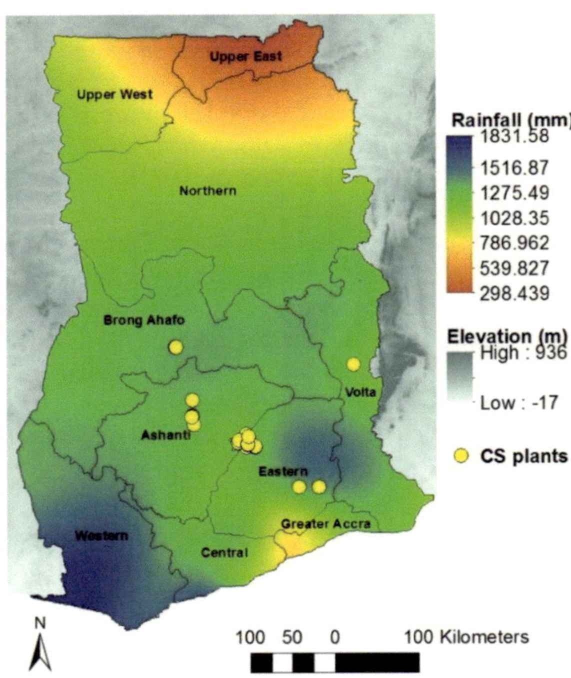

Figure 7.
Average annual rainfall distribution for Ghana showing optimum rainfall ranges suitable for the cultivation of C. sanguinolenta.

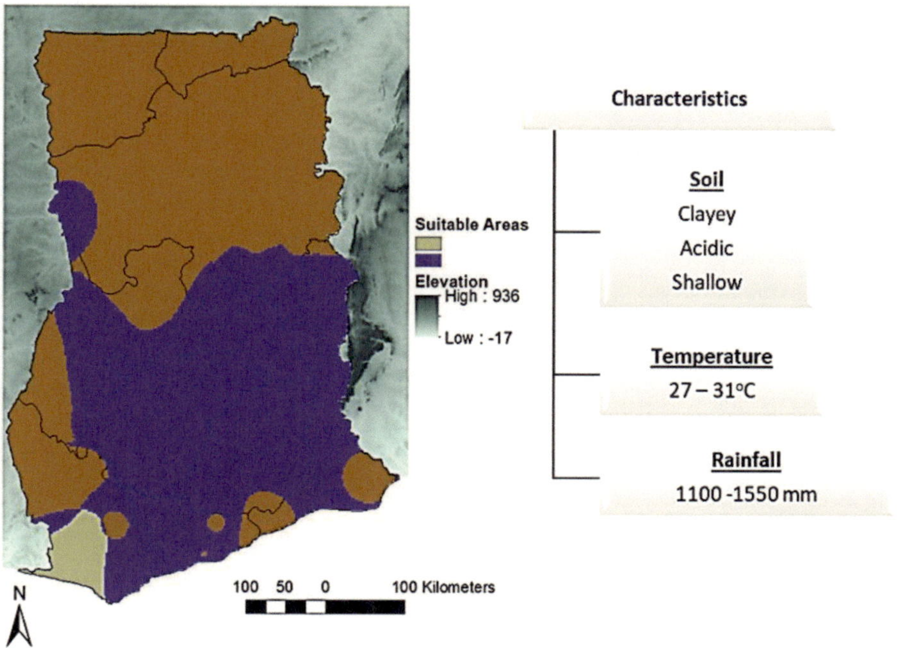

Figure 8.
Production areas for the cultivation of C. sanguinolenta *in Ghana.*

5. Conclusions

C. sanguinolenta was found to be used in the treatment of ailments other than malaria, pointing to its importance as a medicinal plant. To ensure sustainable supply of plant materials and prevent the plant from being extinct, conservation and domestication protocols developed are recommended for its sustainable large-scale cultivation. It is therefore imperative that proper management of high value medicinal plants through conservation receive the necessary attention to guarantee their long-term availability.

Small-scale farmers who also double as collectors of *C. sanguinolenta* from the wild can be encouraged to go into its cultivation as a way to supplement their income and improve their livelihoods. The predicted sites for cultivation of *C. sanguinolenta* opens the way for multi-location evaluation of the species to identify agro-ecological niches for cultivation. Although efforts have been made to investigate the properties, content and activity of bioactive compounds in medicinal plants, areas such as its conservation methods remain unexplored. In addition, further studies are needed to clarify the physiological and molecular mechanisms underpinning seed germination and dormancy in *C. sanguinolenta*.

Conflict of interest

The authors declare no conflict of interest.

Author details

Frank Opoku-Agyemang[1], Jessica Naa Offeibea Dodoo[1], Theophilus Elorm Hlomador[1], Kathleen Gilday[2] and Jacqueline Naalamle Amissah[1]*

1 Department of Crop Science, College of Basic and Applied Sciences, University of Ghana, Accra, Ghana

2 Woodland Essence, USA

*Address all correspondence to: jnamissah@ug.edu.gh

References

[1] McGuffin M, Kartesz JT, Leung AY, Tucker AO. Herbs of Commerce. 2nd. American Herbal Products Association. Silver Spring. 2000. 442p

[2] Osafo N, Mensah KB, Yeboah OK. Phytochemical and pharmacological review of Cryptolepis sanguinolenta (Lindl.) Schlechter. Advances in Pharmacological Sciences. 2017;**2017**:1-13

[3] Jansen PCM, Schmelzer GH. *Cryptolepis sanguinolenta* (Lindl.) Schltr. In: Schmelzer GH, Gurib-Fakim A, editors. Prota 11(2): Medicinal plants/ Plantes médicinales 2. [CD-Rom]. PROTA, Wageningen, Netherlands. PRO. 2010;**11**

[4] Ameyaw Y. Morpho-histological characters for the identification of Cryptolepis sanguinolenta (Lindl.) Schtr. International Journal of Science and Nature. 2012;**3**:331-339

[5] Addy M. Cryptolepis: An African traditional medicine that provides hope for malaria victims. HerbalGram. 2003;**60**:54-59

[6] Ansah C, Otsyina H, Duwiejua M, Woode E, Aboagye F, Aning K. Toxicological assessment of Cryptolepis sanguinolenta for possible use in veterinary medicine. Journal of Veterinary Medicine and Animal Health. 2009;**1**:011-016

[7] Barku V, Opoku-Boahen Y, Dzotsi E. Isolation and pharmacological activities of alkaloids from *Cryptolepis sanguinolenta* (Lindl) schlt. Journal of Biochemistry and Bioinformatics; 2012:**2**(3):58-61

[8] Paulo A, Houghton P. Chemotaxonomic analysis of the genus Cryptolepis. Biochemical Systematics and Ecology. 2003;**31**:155-166

[9] Amissah J, Osei-Safo D, Asare C, Missah-Assihene B, Danquah E, Addae-Mensah I. Influence of age and staking on the growth and cryptolepine concentration in cultivated roots of Cryptolepis sanguinolenta (Lindl.) Schlt. Journal of Medicinal Plants Research. 2016;**10**:113-121

[10] WHO. World Malaria Report. 2021. 322 p. Available from: https://www.who.int/publications/i/item/9789240040496

[11] Abebe D, Garedew B. Ethnobotanical survey of plants traditionally used for malaria prevention and treatment in indigenous villages of Tepi town south West Ethiopia. Journal of Pharmacognosy and Phytotherapy. 2019;**11**:9-16

[12] Amissah JN, Alorvor FE, Okorley BA, Asare CM, Osei-Safo D, Appiah-Opong R, et al. Mineral fertilization influences the growth, Cryptolepine yield, and bioefficacy of Cryptolepis sanguinolenta (Lindl.) Schlt. Plants. 2022;**11**:122

[13] Amoa Onguéné P, Ntie-Kang F, Lifongo LL, Ndom JC, Sippl W, Mbaze LM. The potential of anti-malarial compounds derived from African medicinal plants. Part I: A pharmacological evaluation of alkaloids and terpenoids. Malaria Journal. 2013;**12**:1-26

[14] Sawer I, Berry M, Ford J. The killing effect of cryptolepine on *Staphylococcus aureus*. Letters in Applied Microbiology. 2005;**40**:24-29

[15] Luo J, Fort D, Carlson T, Noamesi B, nii-Amon-Kotei D, King S, et al. *Cryptolepis sanguinolenta*: An ethnobotanical approach to drug

discovery and the isolation of a potentially useful new antihyperglycaemic agent. Diabetic Medicine. 1998;**15**:367-374

[16] Bierer DE, Dubenko LG, Zhang P, Lu Q, Imbach PA, Garofalo AW, et al. Antihyperglycemic activities of cryptolepine analogues: An ethnobotanical lead structure isolated from Cryptolepis sanguinolenta. Journal of Medicinal Chemistry. 1998;**41**:2754-2764

[17] Oyekan A, Okapor J. Effects of cryptolepine alone and in combination with dipyridamole on a mouse model of arterial thrombosis. Journal of Ethnopharmacology. 1989;**27**:141-148

[18] Noamesi B, Bamgbose S. The alpha-adrenoceptor blocking properties of cryptolepine on the rat isolated vas deferens. Planta Medica. 1980;**39**:51-56

[19] Herzenberg LA, Tung J, Moore WA, Herzenberg LA, Parks DR. Interpreting flow cytometry data: A guide for the perplexed. Nature Immunology. 2006;**7**:681-685

[20] Fort DM, Litvak J, Chen JL, Lu Q, Phuan P-W, Cooper R, et al. Isolation and unambiguous synthesis of cryptolepinone: An oxidation artifact of cryptolepine. Journal of Natural Products. 1998;**61**:1528-1530

[21] Ansah C, Gooderham NJ. The popular herbal antimalarial, extract of Cryptolepis sanguinolenta, is potently cytotoxic. Toxicological Sciences. 2002;**70**:245-251

[22] Cimanga K, De Bruyne T, Pieters L, Vlietinck AJ, Turger CA. In vitro and in vivo antiplasmodial activity of cryptolepine and related alkaloids from *Cryptolepis sanguinolenta*. Journal of Natural Products. 1997;**60**:688-691

[23] Dwuma-Badu D, Ayim JS, Fiagbe NI, Knapp JE, Schiff PL Jr, Slatkin DJ. Constituents of west African medicinal plants XX: Quindoline from *Cryptolepis sanguinolenta*. Journal of Pharmaceutical Sciences. 1978;**67**:433-434

[24] Tackie AN, Sharaf MH, Schiff PL Jr, Boye GL, Crouch RC, Martin GE. Assignment of the proton and carbon NMR spectra of the indoloquinoline alkaloid cryptolepine. Journal of Heterocyclic Chemistry. 1991;**28**:1429-1435

[25] Gellert E, Raymond-Hamet C, Schlitter E. The uses of the plant *Cryptolepsis sanguinolenta* in folklore medicine. Helvetica Chimica Acta. 1951;**34**:642-643

[26] Cimanga K, De Bruyne T, Pieters L, Totte J, Tona L, Kambu K, et al. Antibacterial and antifungal activities of neocryptolepine, biscryptolepine and cryptoquindoline, alkaloids isolated from Cryptolepis sanguinolenta. Phytomedicine. 1998;**5**:209-214

[27] Shnyder SD, Wright CW. Recent advances in the chemistry and pharmacology of Cryptolepine. Progress in the Chemistry of Organic Natural Products. 2021;**115**:177-203

[28] Cunningham A. African Medicinal Plants. Paris, France: United Nations Educational, Scientific and Cultural Organization; 1993

[29] Paulo A, Gomes ET, Steele J, Warhurst DC, Houghton PJ. Antiplasmodial activity of Cryptolepis sanguinolenta alkaloids from leaves and roots. Planta Medica. 2000;**66**:30-34

[30] Tempesta MS. The clinical efficacy of *Cryptolepis sanguinolenta* in the treatment of malaria. Ghana Medical Journal. 2010;**44**:1

[31] Paulo A, Pimentel M, Viegas S, Pires I, Duarte A, Cabrita J, et al. Cryptolepis sanguinolenta activity

against diarrhoeal bacteria. Journal of Ethnopharmacology. 1994;**44**:73-77

[32] Tona L, Kambu K, Ngimbi N, Cimanga K, Vlietinck A. Antiamoebic and phytochemical screening of some Congolese medicinal plants. Journal of Ethnopharmacology. 1998;**61**:57-65

[33] Ajayi A, Akhigbe R, Adewumi O, Okeleji L, Mujaidu K, Olaleye S. Effect of ethanolic extract of Cryptolepis sanguinolenta stem on in vivo and in vitro glucose absorption and transport: Mechanism of its antidiabetic activity. Indian Journal of Endocrinology and Metabolism. 2012;**16**:S91

[34] Adeleye OA, Femi-Oyewo MN, Bamiro OA, Bakre LG, Alabi A, Ashidi JS, et al. Ethnomedicinal herbs in African traditional medicine with potential activity for the prevention, treatment, and management of coronavirus disease 2019. Future Journal of Pharmaceutical Sciences. 2021;7:1-14

[35] Borquaye LS, Gasu EN, Ampomah GB, Kyei LK, Amarh MA, Mensah CN, et al. Alkaloids from Cryptolepis sanguinolenta as potential inhibitors of SARS-CoV-2 viral proteins: An in silico study. BioMed Research International. 2020;**2020**:1-14

[36] FDA. Food and Drugs Authority Approves First Herbal Medicine For Clinical Trial On Covid-19 Treatment. 2021. Available from: https://fdaghana.gov.gh/press.php?page=18

[37] Jansen PCM, Cardon D. Plant Resources of Tropical Africa 3. Dyes and tannins. PROTA Foundation, Wageningen, Netherlands/Backhuys Publishers, Leiden, Netherlands/CTA, Wageningen, Netherlands. 2005. pp. 216

[38] Buhner SH. Natural Treatments for Lyme Coinfections. Healing Arts Press, Rochester, Vermont: Anaplasma, Babesia, and Ehrlichia. Simon and Schuster; 2015

[39] Feng J, Leone J, Schweig S, Zhang Y. Evaluation of natural and botanical medicines for activity against growing and non-growing forms of *B. burgdorferi*. Frontiers in Medicine. 2020;**7**:6

[40] Zhang Y, Alvarez-Manzo H, Leone J, Schweig S, Zhang Y. Botanical medicines *Cryptolepis sanguinolenta*, *Artemisia annua*, *Scutellaria baicalensis*, *Polygonum cuspidatum*, and *Alchornea cordifolia* demonstrate inhibitory activity against *Babesia duncani*. Frontiers in Cellular and Infection Microbiology. 2021;**22**:1-15

[41] Chen S-L, Yu H, Luo H-M, Wu Q, Li C-F, Steinmetz A. Conservation and sustainable use of medicinal plants: Problems, progress, and prospects. Chinese Medicine. 2016;**11**:1-10

[42] Rajjou L, Debeaujon I. Seed longevity: Survival and maintenance of high germination ability of dry seeds. Comptes Rendus Biologies. 2008;**331**:796-805

[43] Lee YP, Baek K-H, Lee H-S, Kwak S-S, Bang J-W, Kwon S-Y. Tobacco seeds simultaneously over-expressing Cu/Zn-superoxide dismutase and ascorbate peroxidase display enhanced seed longevity and germination rates under stress conditions. Journal of Experimental Botany. 2010;**61**:2499-2506

[44] Long RL, Gorecki MJ, Renton M, Scott JK, Colville L, Goggin DE, et al. The ecophysiology of seed persistence: A mechanistic view of the journey to germination or demise. Biological Reviews. 2015;**90**:31-59

[45] Sultana N, Ali Y, Jahan S, Yasmin S. Effect of storage duration and storage devices on seed quality of Boro Rice variety BRRI dhan47. Journal of Plant Pathology & Microbiology. 2016;**392**:1-6

[46] Gebeyehu B. Review on: Effect of seed storage period and storage

environment on seed quality. International Journal of Applied Agricultural Sciences. 2020;**6**:3-9

[47] Bukvić G, Gantner R, Grljušić S, Popović B, Agić D, Stanisavljević A. Effects of storage period and temperature upon seed and seedling traits of perennial ryegrass (Lolium perenne L.). Poljoprivreda. 18 Dec 2015;**21**(2):3-9

[48] Zagorchev L, Seal CE, Kranner I, Odjakova M. A central role for thiols in plant tolerance to abiotic stress. International Journal of Molecular Sciences. 2013;**14**:7405-7432

[49] Ranal MA, Santana, D.G.d. How and why to measure the germination process? Brazilian Journal of Botany. 2006;**29**:1-11

[50] Ranal MA, Santana DGD, Ferreira WR, Mendes-Rodrigues C. Calculating germination measurements and organizing spreadsheets. Brazilian Journal of Botany. 2009;**32**:849-855

[51] Cumagun CJR. Advances in formulation of Trichoderma for biocontrol. In: Biotechnology and Biology of Trichoderma. MA, USA: Elsevier; 2014. pp. 527-531

[52] Li H, Li X, Liu S, Zhu X, Song F, Liu F. Induction of cross tolerance by cold priming and acclimation in plants: Physiological, biochemical and molecular mechanisms. In: Priming-Mediated Stress and Cross-Stress Tolerance in Crop Plants. London, United Kingdom: Elsevier; 2020. pp. 183-201

[53] Farooq M, Usman M, Nadeem F, Rehman H, Wahid A, Basra SM, et al. Seed priming in field crops: Potential benefits, adoption and challenges. Crop and Pasture Science. 2019;**70**:731-771

[54] Waqas M, Korres NE, Khan MD, Nizami A-S, Deeba F, Ali I, et al. Advances in the concept and methods of seed priming. In: Priming and Pretreatment of Seeds and Seedlings. Singapore: Springer Nature; 2019. pp. 11-41

[55] Dawood MG. Stimulating plant tolerance against abiotic stress through seed priming. In: Advances in Seed Priming. Singapore: Springer Nature; 2018. pp. 147-183

[56] Varier A, Vari AK, Dadlani M. The subcellular basis of seed priming. Current Science. 2010;**99**(4):450-456

[57] Shim K-B, Cho S-K, Hwang J-D, Pae S-B, Lee M-H, Ha T-J, et al. Effect of seed priming treatment on the germination of sesame. Korean Journal of Crop Science. 2009;**54**:416-421

[58] Dutta P. Seed priming: New vistas and contemporary perspectives. In: Advances in Seed Priming. Singapore: Springer Nature; 2018. pp. 3-22

[59] Rhaman MS, Rauf F, Tania SS, Khatun M. Seed priming methods: Application in field crops and future perspectives. Asian Journal of Research Crop Science. 2020;**5**:8-19

[60] Bagheri MZ. The effect of maize priming on germination characteristics, catalase and peroxidase enzyme activity, and total protein content under salt stress. International Journal of Bioscience. 2014;**4**:104-112

[61] Jafar M, Farooq M, Cheema M, Afzal I, Basra S, Wahid M, et al. Improving the performance of wheat by seed priming under saline conditions. Journal of Agronomy and Crop Science. 2012;**198**:38-45

[62] El-Hamed K, Elwan M, Shaban W. Enhanced sweet corn propagation: Studies on transplanting feasibility and seed priming. Vegetable Crops Research Bulletin. 2011;**75**:31

[63] Haider MU, Hussain M, Farooq M, Nawaz A. Optimizing zinc seed priming for improving the growth, yield and grain biofortification of mungbean (Vigna radiata (L.) wilczek). Journal of Plant Nutrition. 2020;**43**:1438-1446

[64] Wehner G, Kopahnke D, Richter K, Kecke S, Schikora A, Ordon F. Priming is a suitable strategy to enhance resistance towards leaf rust in barley. Phytobiomes Journal. 2019;**3**:46-51

[65] Biabani A, Azarnia M, Eisvand HR, Alamdari EG, Gholizadeh L. Effects of seed priming with gibberellic and salicylic acids and mycorrhizal inoculation on yield and yield components of lentil (Lens culinaris L.). InVIII International Scientific Agriculture Symposium, Agrosym 2017, Jahorina, Bosnia and Herzegovina, October 2017. Book of Proceedings. Faculty of Agriculture, University of East Sarajevo. 2017. pp. 294-300

[66] Anwar A, Xianchang Y, Yansu L. Seed priming as a promising technique to improve growth, chlorophyll, photosynthesis and nutrient contents in cucumber seedlings. Notulae Botanicae Horti Agrobotanici Cluj-Napoca. 2020;**48**:116-127